Is it hot in here?
Or is it me?

Is it hot in here?
Or is it me?
The Complete Guide to Menopause

Pat Wingert and
Barbara Kantrowitz

Foreword by Bernadine Healy, M.D.
FORMER DIRECTOR, NATIONAL INSTITUTES OF HEALTH

WORKMAN PUBLISHING · NEW YORK

To the women in our lives: our mothers, our sisters, our friends,
our daughters and those we love as daughters.
We wish you health and happiness.

Library of Congress Cataloging-in-Publication Data is available.

ISBN-10: 0-7611-3808-0; ISBN-13: 978-0-7611-3808-2 (paperback)
ISBN-10: 0-7611-4370-X; ISBN-13: 978-0-7611-4370-3 (hardcover)

Workman books are available at special discounts when purchased in bulk for
premiums and sales promotions as well as for fund-raising or educational use.
Special editions or book excerpts can also be created to specification.
For details, contact the Special Sales Director at the address below.

Cover design: Janet Parker / Interior design: Paul Hanson and Janet Vicario
Medical illustrations by Taina Litwak / Cartoons by Victoria Roberts /
Exercise illustrations by Munira Al-Khalili

WORKMAN PUBLISHING COMPANY, INC.
225 Varick Street
New York, NY 10014-4381
www.workman.com

Printed in the United States of Amercia
First printing November 2006
10 9 8 7 6 5 4 3 2 1

Foreword

Midlife women today don't fit yesterday's stereotype: ladies a tad frumpy, a lot depressed, mightily struggling with the mysteries of menopause as they waited to follow their ovaries into oblivion. We no longer buy into that silliness. The 40- or 50-something woman of today—smart, informed, involved, generally looking good and feeling healthy—is hardly defined by her menopausal status. But that does not diminish the fact that menopause is an important health consideration for every woman. Unique to the female of the species, the loss of ovarian function heightens the awareness of aging and age-related health vulnerabilities that mount in the second half of life.

The good news is that information is literally pouring out of the halls of medicine, putting old myths and taboos to bed and enabling women to deal practically with the biological and psychological issues surrounding this transition—or "change," as it was once called. And this information is *good*, based on high-quality research. This, too, is a change from just a few years ago. In the past, women's health research languished. Indeed, since the

male was the normative standard for health, studies unique to women were largely left undone.

The last decade of the 20th century saw an explosion in research on women. The Women's Health Initiative (WHI), which I began as a labor of love back in 1991 during my tenure as director of the National Institutes of Health, is a large, audacious, and in-depth study of women in the menopausal years. By design it looks holistically at the health of women and at the full range of threats that rear up during this time in a woman's life. The magnitude of this study, which blankets the country with its 40 clinical research centers and taps into an army of over 150,000 committed participants, is but one affirmation that women's health is no passing fancy, no "niche market," as a pharmaceutical executive once noted.

The myths and mystiques of menopause have crumbled under the weight of focused research, confounding conventional wisdom and shaking up some medical practitioners. But the message that has come through loud and clear in this vibrant era of women's health is not just the obvious—what works for men doesn't always work for women—but, more importantly, what's right for one woman is not always right for all women. Take hormone therapy. Not long ago, women were told it was good for every woman and for the rest of her life. Surprising findings from the WHI randomized clinical trials put a damper on *that* notion. Hormone therapy is a plus for some women and a hazard for others. And figuring out which is which for any given woman becomes more complex but more real as we learn a little more every day about how hormones interact with our brains, our breasts, our bones, and our hearts. Doctors have learned that they must individually tailor each woman's treatment plan, taking into consideration her age and health, her motivation and quality of life, and her own experiences and personal choices.

Research is also making it clear that how we live our lives, what foods we eat, how much we exercise, and how vigilant we are about our checkups and screens can make all the difference in our health. Both doctors and patients are beginning to realize that the future of women's health will be predictive, preventive, and personalized. This new approach to medicine will require each of us to be more actively engaged in making the health decisions that affect our lives. Working in partnership with our doctors and other caregivers, each of us needs to figure out just what is to be our own personal path.

But paths need objective guides and reliable roadmaps. And that is the mission of Pat Wingert and Barbara Kantrowitz. As they point out, menopause is not just the end of fertility and the child-bearing years that are so often seen as women's prime. It is the time for a woman to take charge of her health and make the changes that will carry her through her *second* prime time. I'm confident that Pat and Barbara's book will get you headed in the right direction.

—BERNADINE HEALY, M.D.

Contents

Chapter 4 ✤ Sleep / 71

Why insomnia often strikes now • The role of estrogen • Snoring: a sign of trouble? • Common sleep disorders • How to finally get the rest you need • Setting the mood for sleep • Why a glass of wine before bed won't do the trick • Foods that can keep you up and ones that make you sleepy • Is it depression? • Sex before bed (or not) • Why you're beating a path to the bathroom • Keeping a sleep diary • Physical problems that rob you of sleep • Hot and cold couples • The role of exercise • Sleeping pills and natural remedies

Chapter 5 ✤ Sex / 93

The rise and fall of libido • How to improve your sex life • Body changes that can make sex more painful • Getting expert help • Sex toys and where to buy them • Hormone therapy and libido • Why orgasm can be elusive • New thinking on women and sexual dysfunction • What you need to know about testosterone • Could Viagra be the answer? • Better-than-ever orgasms • The thrill is gone, and that's fine with me • How to fix lubrication problems • The connection between allergies and vaginal dryness • Vaginal estrogen cream and your partner • Alternative treatments • Yeast infections and how to fight them • Starting to date again • Why contraception and safe sex still matter • The right way to Kegel • Bleeding during sex • The depression-sex connection • Hysterectomy and sex drive • Chemo and libido • Sex after radiation • What's in the medicine chest? • What if it's his problem, not yours? • What you need to know about sexually transmitted diseases

Chapter 6 ✤ Bleeding / 135

Irregular bleeding and how you know when you need to go to the doctor • What does heavy bleeding really mean? • Causes of irregular bleeding • Could it be cancer? • Fibroids and how to treat them • What you can expect at the doctor's office • How to talk to your doctor about bleeding problems • What you should know about the newest procedures and medications • Should you worry about anemia? • Is the pill the answer? • Nonhormonal treatments that may work • Sex and bleeding • The pros and cons of hysterectomies • Should you try and keep your ovaries? • Why your uterus may be falling and what to do about it • Postmenopausal bleeding: a primer

Chapter 7 ✤ Aches and Pains / 161

A top-to-bottom compendium • Menstrual migraines and morning headaches: What they mean and new treatments for both • Burning mouth syndrome • What your gums reveal about your hormone levels • Thyroid problems: too much and too little • Can low thyroid make you fat? • To treat or not to treat: the debate over thyroid therapy • Torn rotator cuff • Frozen shoulder • Breast tenderness • Morning stiffness • Joints 101 • Beating arthritis • Talking to your doctor about incontinence • Foot problems and buying shoes that fit

Why We Wrote This Book

*I*s it hot in here, or is it me? This is the book we wanted to read the first time we asked ourselves that question. We went to our local bookstores looking for a guide to this confusing new phase of our lives, but everything we scanned seemed to be either about one woman's experience or a testament to one expert's opinion. We wanted a balanced, scientific, and comprehensive view, the menopausal equivalent of *What to Expect When You're Expecting*. But we wanted to know what to expect when you're *no longer* expecting. In other words, what happens next?

When we couldn't find the book we wanted, we decided to write it ourselves. We've been reporting and writing together at *Newsweek* magazine for 20 years. Although Barbara works in the magazine's New York office and Pat is in the Washington bureau, distance has never been a barrier. From the first story we worked on together to this book, we have been a team. Barbara's children are a little older than Pat's, but we often had similar questions and concerns as we struggled to combine work and home. For a long time, we covered parenting, children's health, and education—often generating story ideas directly from our own experiences as our children went from preschool to grad school. As we got older (yes, we admit that we have), we found ourselves increasingly concerned about our quality of life in the decades ahead. What could we do to stay healthy, happy, and active during and after menopause?

Like many of you, we were confused by the different messages we're getting about everything from hormones to hot flashes to low libido. So we decided to do what we've done in the past—to pore over the latest research, interview the best minds in the field, and attend conferences that brought all the experts together. We also spent a lot of time talking to "real people"—friends, friends of friends, neighbors, colleagues, members of our book clubs, church sodality groups, even the occasional unlucky soul who sat next to us on airplanes.

What we learned is that women are worried about too many sleepless nights, not enough sex, and those disturbing wrinkles that seem to multiply with every laugh and frown. But most of all, women are searching for a new way to look at this phase of life. It's not our mothers' menopause—but what will it mean for us?

Here's another thing we've discovered: There's no quicker way to end a cocktail party conversation with a man than mentioning that you're writing about menopause. Society at large just isn't all that comfortable with this topic. Talking about menopause is an admission that you're no longer 25 or even 35, but guess what? Keeping silent doesn't make you any younger.

If women talk to other women about what they're experiencing—if they break that taboo of silence—they'll find out that each woman experiences menopause in her own way. Some of us never miss a beat; others are felled by so many symptoms (hot flashes, mood swings, heavy bleeding) that they have a hard time functioning. Our reactions to the transition depend on where we are in the other parts of our lives. Maybe you've never had children and feel some regret now that it's no longer an option. Others of us are still raising young children. And still others relish the freedom that can only come when the kids are (finally) out of the house. But we all look in the mirror and wonder at the stranger staring back at us. In our reporting, we tried to represent all of you and provide guidance no matter what your path.

When we first started researching this book, one of the earliest studies we looked at made the point that women who know what to expect from menopause have an easier time of it. We were reminded of this at a recent party, when a friend in her late 40s told us about an experience she'd had not long ago. She had stopped at a convenience store en route to a soccer game to pick up a sports drink for her 13-year-old son. As she was about to pay, she felt a sensation of intense heat throughout her body and became nauseated and dizzy. The alarmed cashier asked if she needed help. Our friend shook her head and made her way outside. But when she and her son got back in the car, she panicked and told him to call 911 on her cell phone. She was sure she was having a heart attack. Within minutes, she heard sirens coming closer. It was only then, as the heat dissipated and she began to sweat, that our friend realized what had happened. She'd had her first hot flash! The emergency medical technicians, all in their early 20s, looked bewildered as she explained her mistake. But one thing was clear: The only thing she was dying of was embarrassment.

If only she'd had our book.

This is for her and for all the rest of us, too.

—PAT WINGERT AND
BARBARA KANTROWITZ

PART I
THE BASICS

CHAPTER 1

What's Happening?

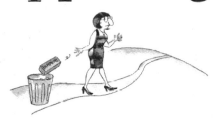

Your last period was shorter than usual. Or maybe it was longer. Somehow, the flow seemed a little different. It could be nothing— or it could be the first sign that you've entered perimenopause, the years before your last menstrual period. A few lucky women have regular periods to the end and then, almost overnight, no more tampons. But for most of us the transition takes four to six years. The journey may be marked by subtle changes that only the most attuned woman would notice, or it can be a bumpy ride. If it's the latter, you may struggle with a variety of symptoms: irregular bleeding, hot flashes, sleep problems, moodiness. You may wonder if you'll ever feel like your old self again. Understanding what's going on with your body is the first step toward being back in control.

WHAT YOU NEED TO KNOW

Remember when you were 13 and your girlfriends shared their complaints of menstrual aches and pains with you? Around that time, you probably realized that not everyone's periods were the same. After the initial shock of menstruating passed, some of your girlfriends hardly noticed a thing. Some got on a regular schedule pretty quickly, while others were so erratic they never knew when their "friend" would surprise

What Can Happen

❖ Disruptions in your regular menstrual cycles become more erratic over time. You officially reach menopause when you go 12 consecutive months without a period.

❖ Early signs that you're moving toward menopause (including small changes in your cycle or flow) may begin 10 to 15 years before menopause. The average age of menopause onset is 51.4 years.

❖ You might wake up one day and realize you missed your period, and never get another one. This would be normal. So would erratic periods for 11 years.

❖ Fluctuations in estrogen levels on the way to menopause cause symptoms such as hot flashes, breast tenderness, and decreased vaginal lubrication. Some women may also struggle with bleeding issues and fibroids.

❖ Menopause induced by surgery or chemotherapy may cause more difficulty with symptoms because of the sudden steep drop in estrogen levels.

❖ While most women reach natural menopause between ages 40 and 58, it occurs earlier about 1 percent of the time. The average age of premature menopause is 27 to 30 years.

---

them. Others were constantly popping aspirin for cramps, while a few of your pals were really troubled by premenstrual syndrome and were difficult to live with for about a week each month. Lots of other girls fell somewhere in between. In some respects, menopause is back to the future, because it often includes many of the same experiences in as wide a variation as menstruation. Just look at the chart on the facing page, and you'll see how little difference there is between the cycles of early menstruation and those of the menopause transition.

Natural menopause starts without your intervention; that's why it's sometimes described as "spontaneous." You might detect the first subtle hints of what's coming (slight changes in men-

strual duration and flow) 10 or more years before your periods stop. As you get closer to the end of your reproductive years, the timing may become more unpredictable and the level of flow may be unusually heavy or almost nothing at all. Some women experience problems like hot flashes (overwhelming waves of heat), night sweats, sleeplessness, less lubrication when sexually aroused, and moodiness as their hormone levels become increasingly erratic. All of these experiences are considered normal. You won't know for sure that you've reached menopause until you go a full year without a period. This can happen at any age from 40 to 58, although the average age is 51.4 years. A few women don't reach menopause until they're in their 60s.

Induced menopause, which can occur at any time after puberty, describes what happens to a woman whose periods have stopped because of some outside intervention such as chemotherapy, pelvic radiation, or the removal of both ovaries (sometimes as part of a hysterectomy). With chemotherapy and radiation, the perimenopausal transition can last for months. Sometimes fertility ends immediately. The most common type of induced menopause is surgical menopause, which occurs when both ovaries are removed. As a result, your body's main source of natural estrogen disappears immediately. This abrupt drop in hormones increases the likelihood that you'll experience menopausal symptoms such as hot flashes and verbal memory problems.

Premature (or early) menopause refers to any type of menopause (natural or induced) that occurs before age 40. While rare, premature menopause puts women at greater risk for bone loss.

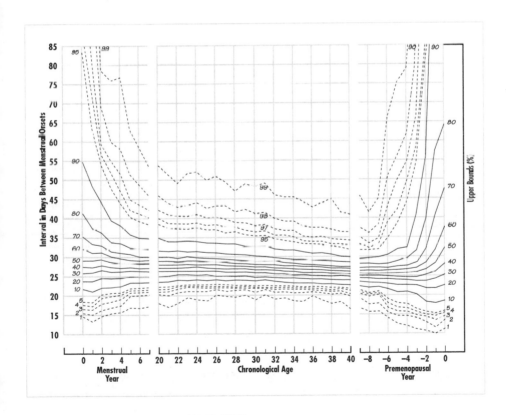

THE BEGINNING AND THE END

When the intervals between menstrual cycles are plotted out, as they were in this chart from the TREMIN Research Program on Women's Health, it's clear that early and late menstruation look amazingly alike.

When to See the Doctor

If you experience any of these symptoms, check with your physician:

❖ VERY HEAVY BLEEDING WITH CLOTS, OR PERIODS THAT LAST A WEEK OR MORE

❖ FREQUENT SPOTTING BETWEEN PERIODS

❖ BLEEDING WITH PAIN OR FEVER

❖ BLOOD IN YOUR URINE OR PAIN WHEN URINATING

❖ ABRUPT CESSATION OF PERIODS

❖ SYMPTOMS LIKE HOT FLASHES, NIGHT SWEATS, AND ERRATIC BLEEDING THAT ARE INTERFERING WITH YOUR ABILITY TO FUNCTION

❖ A MISSED PERIOD THAT COULD INDICATE PREGNANCY

❖ ANY BLEEDING THAT OCCURS AFTER ONE YEAR OF NO MENSTRUAL PERIODS

TIMING IS EVERYTHING

Q *I was surprised to learn that natural menopause typically occurs between the ages of 40 and 58. That seems like a really wide time span. What determines whether it happens early or late?*

A How many follicles (egg sacs) you were born with and the rate at which they deteriorate play a role. So does your lifestyle. Heavy smokers, long-time smokers, and current smokers reach menopause approximately a year and a half earlier than average. The same is true for women who have been treated for depression, epilepsy, or childhood cancer (specifically with pelvic radiation and certain anticancer drugs called alkylating agents) or who have been exposed to certain viruses or toxic chemicals. According to a few studies, heavier women and women with higher childhood cognitive test scores may reach menopause later than the average age. Women who have used supplemental estrogen (in oral contraceptives, for example) in the previous five years also tend to reach menopause later. The length of your menstrual cycles may give you a hint of what's coming. Women between the ages of 20 and 25 whose cycles are completed in 26 days or less tend to have an earlier menopause than those whose cycles last 33 days or more. If you've been pregnant more than once, you may have a slightly later menopause. If you've never been pregnant, you may have an earlier menopause. Here are some things that don't appear to affect the timing of your last period: the age when you started menstruating, race, marital status, and socioeconomic status.

THE STAGES OF MENOPAUSE

For a long time, doctors talked vaguely about different stages of menopause. Then, in 2001, a panel of experts from the National Institutes of Health, the North American Menopause Society, and the American Society for Reproductive Medicine convened the Stages of Reproductive Aging Workshop (STRAW) to develop a more formal description of female progression from puberty all the way to postmenopause.

While the STRAW model seems to imply a predictable transition from the reproductive years through perimenopause to postmenopause, women's real-life experiences actually vary tremendously. Soon after these stages were announced, the TREMIN Research Program on Women's Health (the oldest ongoing study of menstruation in the country, now based at Penn State) examined the menstruation diaries of 100 of their participants to test the assumptions put forward by STRAW. After reviewing up to 12 years' worth of records for each woman, the researchers found that the women followed 23 different patterns as they approached menopause. While most did follow the basic linear progression outlined by STRAW, many women flip-flopped between stages, stalled in one stage for a long time, or skipped a stage. Some skipped several stages. Others continued to have regular periods until one day when they stopped for good. A few postmenopausal women even crossed back over into perimenopause. So if your progression through perimenopause doesn't look like the STRAW model below, you're far from alone.

Final Menstrual Period

Stages:	−5	−4	−3	−2	−1	0	+1	+2
Terminolgy:	Reproductive			Menopause Transition			Postmenopause*	
	Early	Peak	Late	Early	Late**		Early**	Late**
				Perimenopause				
Duration of stage:	Variable			Variable			(a) 1 yr. (b) 4 yrs.	Until demise
Menstrual cycles:	Variable to regular	Regular		Variable cycle length (>7 days different from normal)	≥ 2 skipped cycles and an interval of amenorrhea (≥ 60 days)	Amen. x 12 mos.	None	
Endocrine***:	Normal FSH	↑FSH		↑FSH			↑FSH	

* Postmenopause is the time of life when you can no longer get pregnant. During stage +1 (less than five years since the last menstrual period), your ovaries' estrogen production may continue to decline until you reach a permanent low level. While the STRAW model delineates only two stages of postmenopause, researchers believe that more distinct segments may someday be identified.

** A stage when hot flashes and night sweats are most likely to occur.

*** This category refers to the level of follicle-stimulating hormone (FSH) found in your blood. FSH prompts egg sacs in your ovaries to begin maturing. As you progress through the transition, FSH levels spike and stay high as your ovaries fail to respond the way they did when you were younger.

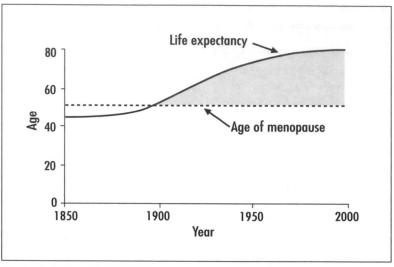

WE'RE LIVING LONGER
Thanks to modern medicine, better nutrition, and smarter lifestyle choices, women can expect to live a third of their lives past menopause.

ENDING EARLY

Q *Are premature menopause and premature ovarian failure the same thing?*

A Premature ovarian failure refers to the cessation of periods over several months or years, well before the typical age of menopause. It may be temporary if it's caused by drastic weight loss, an eating disorder, excessive exercise, or stress; once the aggravating cause is eliminated or reduced, menstrual periods may resume. It can be a permanent condition if it's related to genetic abnormalities or certain autoimmune diseases. In the latter case, it's synonymous with premature menopause.

AGE AND MENOPAUSE

Q *I know that the average age of puberty is lower in girls today. Does menopause come earlier, too?*

A Even though women are living longer than ever, the average age of menopause hasn't budged. As far as scientists can tell, it has always occurred around age 51. It's likely, however, that you'll live more of your life after menopause than your great-grandmother did.

NATURAL MENOPAUSE

Natural menopause is not a disease or a hormone deficiency disorder, although historically it has been treated

GORILLAS DO IT

We have something in common with female elephants, gorillas, lions, and certain whales, and we're not talking about that discouraging number on the scale this morning! We all go through menopause. The big question is why. In other words, what's the evolutionary function of menopause? The so-called "granny hypothesis" holds that older females who can no longer have their own babies become available to help care for the grandchildren, but this doesn't explain why granny baboons, for example, take part in raising their grandchildren even when they're still capable of producing offspring. And what about males? Why doesn't it happen to them? One theory is that females, as the primary caregivers, are genetically programmed to live long enough to raise their youngest. Males aren't as involved in child-rearing, so they can keep on reproducing until the end and count on females to finish the task of raising and launching future generations.

as both. These days, many women want to "de-medicalize" this life transition and embrace it as normal. It's probably safe to say that most get through it with little difficulty and have no need for any medication. You could well be part of that group.

But there's a reason that menopause has a bad rep and is a regular butt of jokes. A significant minority of women have a rough time. A few have a *very* rough time. Doctors think these women may be extra sensitive to hormonal changes or may have more rambunctious hormones. It's not always easy to figure out what to blame on menopause and what to blame on midlife, when you're more likely to have high blood pressure, obesity, diabetes, and thyroid problems. Some symptoms appear to be related to fluctuating estrogen: hot flashes, night sweats, heavy bleeding, vaginal dryness, decreasing bone density, breast tenderness, and headaches. Others appear to be indirectly related: sleeplessness, moodiness, and urinary tract and vaginal infections, as well as verbal memory and reading problems. Some are related to a drop in estrogen or an imbalance of estrogen and androgens: dry eyes, a low libido, abdominal weight gain, hair loss (or too much in the wrong places), wrinkles, and hearing loss. Health habits (such as sun exposure and smoking) affect the pace of many of these changes.

Before this list sends you screaming into the street, keep in mind that it's highly unlikely that any one woman will get hit with everything. You may experience a few of these problems over a period of months or years, or only intermittently. Some will be barely noticeable. Others

Is It True?

Fiction: Menopause is a fairly modern phenomenon. Before the 1900s, few women survived to age 50.

Fact: The average female life span in 1900 was 48.3 years, but that didn't mean that most women died in their late 40s. Half died before that age (usually in early childhood or while bearing children) and half died afterwards. A modern historian has calculated that women born in 1789 who managed to survive until age 20 were expected to live to age 56. Indeed, historical references to menopause date back to ancient Greece. So, while it's a fact that only starting in the 20th century did most baby girls have a high likelihood of living long enough to reach menopause, it's hardly a new experience for women.

will qualify as annoying, and still others may interfere with your ability to function. But you can learn to deal with all of them until that time when things actually improve. For example, some women's sex lives get better during the transition. (Yes, you read that right.) And no matter what else happens, by the end of this process you won't have to worry about unplanned pregnancies or contraception for the first time in decades. You're going to be just as smart as you ever were—and no doubt wiser. And you can use the rest of these changes to motivate yourself to start

doing all the things that your doctor has been telling you to do for years but that you've been putting off until tomorrow. Tomorrow is here. If you play it smart, you could be looking and feeling better when you reach postmenopause than you do right now. (See Appendix I for recommended screenings.)

But we digress. What exactly is happening to your body as you set out on this menopause journey?

It all started while you were still in the womb. Your body was set up differently from a boy's because of genes and hormones. When you hit puberty, you began to ovulate, and except when you were on hormonal contraceptives or pregnant, you've probably been doing this every month.

Ovulation 101

Just before you get your period, your body's levels of two hormones—estrogen and progesterone—take a nosedive. When they near bottom, the hypothalamus and pituitary gland in your brain receive the signal that it's time to get cracking. The hypothalamus sends pulsating doses of gonadotropin-releasing hormone (GnRH) to the pituitary gland, causing it to release the follicle-stimulating hormone (FSH). This signal is enough to get about a dozen eggs to start maturing and producing estrogen, prompting the lining of your uterus (the endometrium) to start thickening in preparation for a possible pregnancy. Just before you've reached the middle of

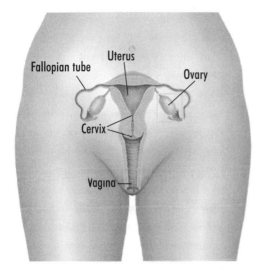

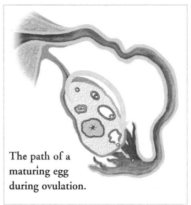

The path of a maturing egg during ovulation.

INTERNAL FEMALE REPRODUCTIVE ORGANS

your cycle, the uterine lining has tripled in size, one follicle has matured to the point that it's ready to release an egg, and your testosterone levels have risen, boosting your libido along with it. By now, so much estrogen is circulating that your body issues a jolt of luteinizing hormone that causes the follicle to release the egg, which moves through the adjacent fallopian tube and into the uterus. This process is called ovulation. The remains of the follicle, called the corpus luteum, secrete progesterone to further enrich the uterine lining. If the egg is not fertilized over the course of the next few days, the whole operation shuts down. Estrogen and progesterone start to nose-dive again, the corpus luteum shrivels up, the uterus starts to shed its lining, and menstruation takes place.

For most women, this cycle takes 27 or 28 days, but its length can vary widely. Usually, it's in the range of 21 to 38 days. But after monitoring women's menstrual cycles for 26 years, the TREMIN Research Program on Women's Health found that they can range in length from 11 days to more than 100 days. If you have cycles like those on the extremes, you should mention it to your doctor.

The Shift Begins

About 10 to 15 years before you reach menopause, your body starts giving you the first tiny hints that changes are coming. If you're self-aware, you might notice subtle differences in your periods. When you were in your early 20s, your cycle probably lasted about 32 days; by the time you reached your mid-30s, it had probably shortened to about 28 days. Even if it didn't happen exactly like this, your periods were coming more quickly. This would occur because your maturing follicles (specifically, the corpus luteum)

From the Past

We often use euphemisms to talk about subjects that make us uncomfortable, and menopause is no exception. Over the centuries, it has been called many things, including the cessation, the change of life, the time of life, Indian summer, hormone deficiency disease, and the climacteric. The word *menopause* comes from the Greek words for "month" and "cessation." It was apparently first used in 1816, when French physician C.P.L. DeGardanne referred to this phase of a woman's life as *le menespausie.* By 1821, he had shortened it to *ménopause,* and the word has been in common use since the mid-19th century.

were producing less progesterone during each cycle, shortening the period of time when the uterine lining thickened in preparation for a fertilized egg. As time goes on and perimenopause begins, the number and quality of follicles diminish to the point where not enough estrogen is produced to prompt ovulation and your periods become erratic. It's the mirror image of what happened when you started menstruating. As you approach the end of your reproductive years, these changes in duration and flow may become more obvious.

Other, quieter changes may also be under way. If you happen to have lab work done in the middle of a menstrual period, your doctor will notice that your FSH level is elevated. This happens because your ovaries are producing less estrogen and your brain tries to jump-start the process by sending more FSH into your bloodstream. The higher level of FSH prompts your ovaries to recruit more than the typical dozen follicles to produce estrogen for the next cycle. As a result, there may be times when your estrogen levels are unusually high and other times when they're unusually low. Both extremes can cause you to experience a variety of symptoms while you're still having regular menstrual cycles.

The perimenopause stage begins when your follicles' response to FSH becomes wimpy and erratic. This in turn makes your periods more irregular. During some of these cycles, your body will not release an egg. Other times, it may release more than one, which may explain why older moms have more twins.

Technically, you're in the early stage of perimenopause when the length of your cycle shifts by seven or more days from its normal track. As time goes on, you'll probably miss two or more cycles in a row. This signals that you're in the late stage of perimenopause. The length of time between

By the Numbers

◆ Average age of natural menopause in industrialized world: 51.4 years

◆ Typical age when menopause occurs: 40 to 58 years

◆ Average age when natural menopause transition begins: 47.5 years

◆ Possible length of transition: 1 to 12 years

◆ Typical length of transition: 5.8 years

◆ Average life expectancy of an American woman who survives to age 50: 82 years

◆ Total estimated number of postmenopausal women worldwide (2005): 477 million

◆ Total estimated number of postmenopausal women worldwide (2025): 1.1 billion

cycles can get longer and longer over several years.

Although there is tremendous variation in how women progress through the menopause transition, a typical pattern emerges. Before perimenopause, the average menstrual cycle lasts about 27 or 28 days. During the early part of the transition, the cycle may shrink to every 21 to 23 days. After a while, the intervals between periods begin to lengthen, and eventually menstruation stops altogether. But many women have a more unpredictable pattern. Some seem to speed through the stages; others dally for years. Some might get a couple of periods in a row and then experience a long hiatus before they get another one. It's fairly common to go six or nine months between periods toward the end. No one knows how to tell in advance what will happen to any one woman.

Out of Eggs?

Q *What makes the menopause transition begin? Is it because we're out of eggs?*

A No one knows exactly why menopause occurs when it does, but it could happen because of the significant reduction in the number of follicles in the ovaries. You were born with between one and two million of these follicles, but fewer than 500 of them will be used up as a result of ovulation. Many, many others will degenerate over time and die as part of a natural process called atresia, or cell death. (About 100,000 follicles are present at puberty; this number is reduced to

What to Tell Your Daughter

How you approach menopause will teach your daughter a lot about how she should view aging. Being open about it will show her that this change, like so many others in our lives, marks a natural beginning as well as a natural end.

somewhere between a few hundred and a few thousand at the approach of menopause.) It appears that the rate of atresia is steady until about age 37 and then accelerates. (However, there's a lot of variation from woman to woman.) It's possible that the follicles that remain in the ovaries after menopause will occasionally produce a little estrogen, but not enough to prompt ovulation.

For a long time, scientists assumed that women were born with all the follicles they would ever have. But recent studies at Harvard indicate that female mice produce new follicles during their reproductive years; this finding has generated speculation that the same thing might happen in humans. Scientists are also intrigued by indications that the material used to create these new follicles comes from bone marrow. This process may eventually explain the connection between stem cells, bone marrow, and human eggs.

SHOULD I SEE A DOCTOR?

Q *I'm 50 years old, and for the first time in my life I've gone three months without a period. I'm assuming this means I've moved on to the second stage of perimenopause. If I'm not having any problems (hot flashes, sleeplessness, etc.), do I need to see a doctor about this? Or can I wait for my next regular checkup with my ob-gyn to mention it?*

A If you've gone several months without a period and there's any chance that you might be pregnant, you should call your doctor immediately. If there's no chance of pregnancy and you're having no problems, you can wait until your next regular visit.

WHY 12 MONTHS?

Q *Why is menopause declared after 12 months without a period? What's so special about a year?*

A Frankly, nothing. It's just the time frame that a panel of experts agreed upon. They could have picked 10 months or 14 months or 24 months,

---

UPS AND DOWNS OF PERIMENOPAUSE

High estrogen levels are associated with:

◆ Breast tenderness

◆ Headaches

◆ Increased vaginal lubrication

Low estrogen levels are associated with:

◆ Decreased vaginal lubrication

◆ Painful sexual intercourse

Fluctuating estrogen levels are associated with:

◆ Hot flashes

◆ Night sweats

but they compromised on 12 because the vast majority of women never get another period after they've gone a year without menstruating. But remember this: Twenty percent of women resume menstruation after going three months without a period.

EARLY TRANSITION

Q *I'm only 37, but I've noticed some indications that I'm in the early stage of perimenopause. Does this mean I'll reach menopause early?*

A Not necessarily. Some women have a long transition and reach menopause at a "normal" age.

PERIODS AFTER MENOPAUSE

Q *Is it possible that I could get another period after more than 12 months without one?*

A Yes. About 4 in every 100 women get another period more than 12 months after their last. One woman in the TREMIN study started having irregular periods after a break of two years without one, then continued for a year before she reached menopause for good. The researchers found that stress (a death in the family, a career disappointment, a health crisis) often triggers this type of delayed period. (Conversely, stress can cause younger women to miss a period.) Because unusual bleeding is one of the few warning signs of gyneco-

logical cancer, make sure you report it immediately to your clinician. But don't panic. It often means nothing at all.

THAT OLD FEELING

Q *It's been more than 12 months since I had a period, but occasionally I feel internal stirrings like the ones I used to get just before my period.*

A There's a lot about the internal workings of menopause that we still don't understand, but you're not the only one who has felt those telltale changes and wondered what was going on. Some women do have another period after more than 12 months, so clearly their bodies keep trying to make it happen even after menopause has been officially declared.

TESTING FOR MENOPAUSE

Q *Pregnancy tests can tell if you're pregnant. Can a menopause test tell you that you're not going to have any more periods?*

A Neither a single blood test at the doctor's nor one over-the-counter kit can definitively confirm that you've reached menopause. What you *can* learn is whether you have an elevated FSH level at the exact time of the test. But because FSH levels fluctuate considerably during the course of a month (and because your cycles become less predictable during perimenopause), no single test can give you the whole picture. You might just happen to test on a day when your FSH is high, and it could fall again the next day. As a result, clinicians look for more than an elevated FSH level to determine whether or not you've reached menopause.

WHAT ABOUT PROGESTERONE?

Q *Will my ovaries still produce progesterone after menopause?*

A Progesterone is produced by the remains of the follicle after ovulation. When you stop ovulating, your ovaries no longer produce progesterone. That's why you need to add a progestogen if you take estrogen and still have a uterus.

ON THE PILL

Q *If I'm taking oral contraceptives, how will I know when I've reached menopause—or even that perimenopause has begun?*

A Oral contraceptives are very good at regulating menstrual periods and suppressing menopausal symptoms, so you may not be able to tell if you've reached menopause when you're on the pill. However, women who are well into the transition may stop having periods or experience hot flashes during the placebo week of their pill regimen. Most doctors recommend that their patients stop taking the pill, at least as a trial, around age 51 to see whether

they've reached menopause. If you no longer need to be on the higher levels of hormones required for contraception, you shouldn't be taking them.

ESTROGEN AFTER MENOPAUSE?

Q *After menopause, will my ovaries keep producing estrogen?*

A As you move toward menopause, your estrogen levels are declining. The first year after your last menstrual period, the drop in estrogen produced by the ovaries is the most dramatic. After that, the ovaries will continue to make less and less, until they're making next to nothing—or nothing at all. How long this takes depends on the quality and number of the remaining follicles. However, your ovaries will continue to produce testosterone, which your body can convert to estrogen through an enzyme called aromatase. Most postmenopausal women have about 90 percent less estrogen in their bodies than do premenopausal women, but there is variation from woman to woman.

OTHER ESTROGEN SOURCES

Q *Is there any other natural source of estrogen in my body after menopause?*

A The adrenal glands produce a substance called androstenedione, which circulates in muscles and fat and is turned into estrogen through aromatase. Testosterone is also converted to estrogen in your brain and around your heart. So, after menopause, you still have some naturally produced estrogen in your body—just less than you used to.

TOO LOW ON ESTROGEN?

Q *It sounds like my body really needs estrogen. Doesn't menopause mean I'll be deficient in something I really need?*

A The loss of estrogen related to natural menopause is an expected occurrence. It is not a deficiency. Still, some women may need more than their body produces to control symptoms like hot flashes, night sweats, a dry vagina, or painful intercourse. There are also women who just don't feel like themselves without supplemental hormones.

INDUCED MENOPAUSE

If you undergo chemotherapy or radiation in your pelvic area or if your ovaries are surgically removed, you can enter menopause abruptly and the symptoms (hot flashes from loss of estrogen, low sexual desire from loss of androgens) may be much more severe than those associated with natural menopause. Your body just doesn't have time to adjust. For many women, particularly those facing a serious illness like cancer, this is a difficult transition that requires extra emotional and medical support.

SURGERY. If both ovaries are removed (in a surgical procedure called a bilateral oophorectomy), ovarian hormone levels will decline within days. Fertility ends immediately, although pregnancy is still possible with the use of donor eggs if the uterus is intact. After a hysterectomy (surgery to remove the uterus), the ovaries still function and continue to be a source of estrogen and testosterone. However, if the operation disturbs the blood supply to the ovaries, natural menopause may occur two or three years earlier than average. After a hysterectomy, you stop menstruating and you can no longer bear children. This does not mean that you've reached menopause, which doesn't happen until you stop ovulating. Since women typically know they've reached menopause after no periods for a year, this determination is trickier if you don't have a uterus. Hot flashes would be a signal that your ovaries are secreting less estrogen.

CHEMOTHERAPY. Systemic chemotherapy affects all your cells—both the cancerous ones and the healthy ones. The ovaries are especially sensitive to chemotherapy, although its effect depends on the strength and length of the treatment. Loss of function can be gradual. Women under 30 may experience only temporary ovarian failure and are more likely to recover and start menstruating again. Women over 40 have a higher risk of permanent ovarian damage. In any case, if you're getting chemo, you're struggling with a serious illness as well as the potential loss of fertility—a double whammy. Most cancer hospitals offer patient support groups. You might also seek professional counseling to get through this difficult period. It's a major life trauma.

PELVIC RADIATION. This kind of radiation just targets tumors. High-energy waves or particles (such as X-rays, gamma rays, and alpha and beta particles) hit malignant cells to prevent them from growing and spreading.

Only radiation aimed at the pelvic area can affect the ovaries. As you might expect, high doses (used in treating cervical cancer, for example) have a more damaging effect on the ovaries than lower doses (which might be used to treat Hodgkin's disease). With lower doses, some ovarian function may even be recovered. During some radiation procedures, the ovaries can be shielded to prevent damage. Ask your doctor.

SOLO EFFORT

Q *I have a large cyst on one ovary, and my doctor thinks it will have to be removed. Will I go into menopause? I'm only 41.*

A As long as you have one ovary, you'll still produce estrogen. Your remaining ovary will work that much harder to stabilize your hormone levels. You shouldn't notice any major changes.

REVERSING MENOPAUSE?

Q *Because of my family history, I'm at very high risk for breast cancer and am thinking about having my ovaries removed as a precautionary measure. I've heard that you can reverse menopause by having an ovary frozen and implanting the tissue elsewhere in your body. Could this be true?*

A A procedure called ovarian cryopreservation and transplantation is being developed, but it has been used in only a few cases and is still considered highly experimental. In this procedure, an ovary is surgically removed and checked for cancer cells. If healthy, the ovary is sliced up, mixed with an antifreeze solution, and frozen very slowly. Later (in one case of a breast cancer survivor, six years later), the pieces are implanted elsewhere in the body— under the skin of the lower abdomen or inner arm, for example. About three months after surgery, the tissue may begin functioning and menopause is reversed. Eggs may be retrieved for *in vitro* fertilization. One baby has been produced through this method, but very little is known about long-term safety to the mother.

Other techniques, such as embryo or egg freezing, are more commonly available. Before you decide to have your ovaries removed, it would be wise to meet with a fertility specialist who will review your medical history and discuss the options available to you.

PREMATURE MENOPAUSE

Spontaneous menopause (12 months without a period) before age 40 is called premature or early menopause. Unlike amenorrhea (a temporary disruption of menstrual periods that can be related to stress, weight loss, or over-exercising), premature menopause is a permanent condition. About 1 percent of American women enter menopause early; as a result, these women are at greater risk for health problems such as osteoporosis or heart disease when they're older. Premature menopause can also be emotionally traumatic if a woman hasn't yet had all the children she wants. Grief is a natural reaction to finding out at age 27 or 30 (the average age of premature menopause) that you may never give birth to a child that's genetically yours. You may feel that your body has failed you, or you may blame yourself for bringing it on by some past unhealthy behavior. In fact, the causes of premature menopause are not clear; it could be genetics or an autoimmune disease.

Women who reach menopause early generally have the same symptoms as women whose fertility ends in their late 40s or 50s: hot flashes and night sweats, irregular periods, dry vagina. Some women, however, exhibit no symptoms and continue to have what appear to be normal periods. These women are diagnosed by testing levels of the follicle-stimulating hormone (FSH). Consistently elevated levels indicate that the brain is trying extra hard to get the ovaries to work properly. Sometimes doctors will also do an ultrasound of the ovaries to determine if the supply of follicles is depleted. Hormone therapy helps to alleviate bothersome symptoms and can provide some protection against bone loss and perhaps heart disease. In this case, your doctor would probably prescribe it to you until you reach the age

SOME POSSIBLE CAUSES OF PREMATURE MENOPAUSE

In about two-thirds of cases, women never learn why their ovaries stopped functioning prematurely; however, some diseases and conditions are associated with early menopause. These include:

- Thyroid disease
- Hypoparathyroidism
- Rheumatoid arthritis
- Diabetes
- Pernicious anemia
- Adrenal insufficiency
- Vitiligo
- Lupus
- Fragile X syndrome
- Androgen insufficiency syndrome

of natural menopause, around 51. You'll likely get a higher dose than the hormones given to older menopausal women because the goal is to replace the estrogen that normally would be in your system. Usually, you'll get a patch to deliver estrogen and a pill to provide a progestin. The patch provides a continuous flow of estrogen into the bloodstream, which is closer to the way the body delivers estrogen.

Premature menopause can put a woman at risk for other diseases. In a recent study, 27 percent of women with ovarian failure had low thyroid function, compared with 2 percent in the overall population. Taking thyroid hormone in a pill treats this problem.

FAMILY FACTORS

Q *I'm having hot flashes, my periods are becoming irregular, and my doctor says my FSH levels are high. I'm only 36. Why is this happening so early?*

A It could be genetic. About 10 to 20 percent of women who enter menopause early have a relative who stopped menstruating before 40. A genetic mutation may also cause some women to produce fewer eggs. You could have been born with fewer follicles or with follicles that don't live as long as other women's. Or you might have an abnormal or missing X chromosome, which determines gender. Females need two X chromosomes to make an adequate number of follicles; if part or all of one X chromosome is missing, your body may not have made enough to start with or you may run through them too quickly. This scenario accounts for about 2 to 3 percent of these cases. In other cases, the immune system attacks the follicles. This explains about 5 percent of ovarian failures; as yet, researchers don't know why this happens.

TESTS AND TECHNOLOGIES

Q *My sister, who's older, stopped menstruating early. How can I find out if this will happen to me?*

A Since there's a history of premature menopause in your family, especially on the part of someone as close as a sister, you should consult with a fertility specialist as soon as possible. An ultrasound of your ovaries will show how many follicles remain. Your hormone levels can also be checked to see if you show any early signs of change; regular monitoring can identify even slightly elevated levels of hormones, which may signal that your system is progressing unusually fast through your reproductive years. New technologies, including freezing eggs and freezing ovarian tissue, might prove effective in enabling you to conceive later than you otherwise could. Once sure signs of menopause have appeared, however, it's probably too late to intervene.

ANY HELP?

Q *Is there any treatment that works? I haven't had children yet, and now I may never be able to.*

A As of this writing, there's no proven treatment to restore normal ovarian function. In randomized clinical trials, researchers have looked at the effectiveness of a wide range of therapies. None of these brought back fertility.

However, between 5 and 10 percent of women with premature ovarian failure do become pregnant without any treatment. Researchers have no explanation for this. It could be as simple as luck—a rare healthy egg is fertilized.

Another option is the procedure in which a fertility specialist combines a donor egg and a sperm cell in a laboratory and implants the embryo in your uterus. This isn't always successful, however. For success and failure rates of different reproductive technologies, check out the website of the Centers for Disease Control and Prevention: www.cdc.gov/ART/index.htm.

BETTER SAFE THAN SORRY

Q *If I can still get pregnant with ovarian failure, does that mean I need to stay on the pill? The chances seem so slim.*

A Slim, yes, but not impossible, so you do need to use contraception. Birth-control pills may be a good choice if you have no risk factors such as high blood pressure, a history of smoking, or blood clots. However, for some women with ovarian failure, oral contraceptives are not as effective in preventing pregnancy. Barrier methods—a diaphragm or condoms—might be a better choice. You need to consider your medical history in choosing the best contraception. Talk to your doctor about it.

THE PILL

Q *I didn't know my ovaries had failed until I went off the pill. Could oral contraceptives have caused this problem?*

A Researchers haven't found any connection between the use of oral contraceptives and ovarian failure.

PREGNANCY AND PERIMENOPAUSE

A re you done having children? Did you ever want any? Are you still hoping to get pregnant someday? The answers to these questions are among the most powerful determinants of how you feel about approaching menopause. As more women wait longer to start a family, this has only become truer.

For the woman who is all done or who never wanted to get pregnant, menopause may be a relief. No more contraception! But for the woman who waited—for whatever reason—the realities of biological limits can come as something of a shock. If we can prevent unwanted pregnancies through the easy availability of oral contraception, surely we should be able to schedule pregnancies as well. But we are not in control of our fertility—a reality that may be especially difficult to deal with if your body's timetable is set earlier than others.

Although more moms of toddlers have a little gray in their hair these days, doctors still consider a woman over 35 to be of "advanced maternal age." You may be in great shape and look like 25, but your ovaries aren't fooled. After age 35, the rate at which your eggs naturally deteriorate and die is likely to increase significantly. If you get pregnant during this time, you face a higher chance of miscarriage. By age 45, more than half of all pregnancies end in miscarriage. The chances of complications for either the pregnancy (cesarean delivery, premature labor, fetal mortality) or the fetus (chromosomal abnormalities) increase with age. (See Appendix I.) Research has also indicated that consistently elevated follicle-stimulating hormone levels are a sign that the quantity or quality of your eggs isn't what it used to be. (Of course, one test indicating a high level is not enough to prove anything.)

That said, midlife women are having many more babies than ever before. Fertility research has given many women the chance that nature itself would deny them. Twenty years ago, it was unusual for a woman in her 40s to carry a baby to term; now it's much more common.

Still, it's hard to predict how easy or difficult it will be for an individual woman to get pregnant later in life or how much professional help she'll need.

AGE BARRIER

Q *Is it all about age? If you're close to 50, is it no longer possible to carry a baby to term?*

A Advanced age does tend to predict a harder time getting pregnant and completing a pregnancy, but there's a lot of individual variation. Occasionally, chronological age doesn't track with ovarian age. Consider the fact that "normal" menopause can occur anytime between 40 and 58. Research indicates that some women are born with more follicles than average. The rate of follicle deterioration increases with age, but the rate for some women is steeper than for others. This means that some women have more eggs in better shape for a longer period of time. There have always been women who assumed they were no longer fertile but suddenly found themselves pregnant with an unplanned "bonus baby."

While fertility specialists can determine whether you still have lots of eggs and what's happening with your hormones right now, they have a limited ability to predict the future. If getting pregnant is something you're serious about, you need to see a good fertility specialist as soon as possible and have yourself evaluated.

ERRATIC PERIODS

Q *I got married late, and my husband and I are trying hard to have a baby right away. Unfortunately, my periods are already becoming erratic. How does this affect my fertility?*

A As long as you're getting a period, there's a chance that you can become pregnant. However, as you get closer to menopause, you may have more cycles that include menstrual bleeding but not ovulation; in other words, no egg is released for possible fertilization because your estrogen levels never get high enough. On the other hand, perimenopause is all about fluctuating hormone levels. Sometimes, estrogen levels are very high.

Another thing to think about: There's a greater-than-normal chance that more than one egg will be released during a menstrual cycle and that pregnancy could result in a multiple birth.

So far, science doesn't have all the answers about the relationship between erratic periods and fertility and whether some perimenopausal women have a better chance than others of taking a pregnancy to term. However, a fertility specialist can help you gauge your own chances of a successful pregnancy by inspecting your ovaries with ultrasound and literally counting the follicles inside. Monitoring your hormone levels can also determine how far down the track you are. The general rule is that you can get pregnant until 12 months have gone by without a period—in other words, until you have officially reached menopause.

Risk of Miscarriage

It is more difficult to get pregnant as you get older. There's also a greater chance that the pregnancy will end in miscarriage.

MATERNAL AGE	PERCENTAGE OF PREGNANCIES ENDING IN MISCARRIAGE
15 to 19	10%
20 to 24	10
25 to 29	10
30 to 34	12
35 to 39	18
40 to 44	34
45 and above	53

WORRIED ABOUT MISCARRIAGE

Q *If I'm trying to get pregnant in my late 40s and my periods are erratic, does that mean I'm likely to miscarry?*

A We know that some women are able to get pregnant late in the game and carry a baby to term. We also know that the older you are, the more likely you are to miscarry. When you get pregnant in your 40s, there's also a greater chance of complications for you and the baby. But scientists just don't know how the regularity of periods affects any one woman's ability to sustain a pregnancy to term.

Q *If it's possible to get a period after more than 12 consecutive months without one, is it possible to get pregnant after that?*

A It is theoretically possible for a woman to get pregnant after more than 12 months without a period, but the chances are remote. As we mentioned earlier, about 4 in 100 women get a period after 12 months without one. Follicles remain in the ovaries after menopause, and occasionally they will produce a little estrogen, though presumably not enough to result in ovulation.

WELCOME TO THE REST OF YOUR LIFE

A s you can tell from this chapter, your body is going through major changes. Some can be liberating (no more periods!) and others leave you feeling wistful (no more periods!). If you're like most of us, you're probably experiencing some mix of these emotions. No matter how young you look or feel, you're bound to be anxious about what lies ahead.

Menopause is definitely a turning point you can't ignore, but it's also a great opportunity to begin again and get yourself in the best shape of your life. You'll see lots of evidence throughout the rest of this book that the changes you make now will have a huge influence on how you age. Pay more attention to eating right and exercising daily. Schedule regular doctors' checkups and screenings. Reexamine your social, emotional, and intellectual worlds. Do your friends and family get to see enough of you? Are there activities or interests you've always wanted to explore? This is the time.

You're not 25 anymore—and that's a good thing. You've been around long enough to know what you want and how to get it. You're no longer cowed by authority figures; in fact, you're one yourself. Back in the 1970s and '80s, when many of us came of age, we were all in such a hurry to get somewhere—although a lot of us weren't exactly sure where that "somewhere" was. Now we've arrived. So take a good look around your new neighborhood. And don't forget to enjoy yourself.

CHAPTER 2

The Hormone Question

On the morning of July 9, 2002, an announcement from the National Institutes of Health (NIH) struck menopausal women and their doctors like a bombshell. The NIH was abruptly halting a major study of combined hormone therapy because early results showed that women taking estrogen and a progestin were at higher risk for breast cancer, stroke, blood clots, and heart attack. This news shocked millions of American women taking hormone therapy. Until then, doctors had routinely prescribed hormones to protect their midlife patients against heart disease, to keep their brains healthy and their bones strong—and even to smooth out pesky wrinkles. As a result, doctors were bombarded with calls from frightened and often angry women: Should I throw out my pills? Am I going to die of a heart attack? How could you do this to me?

Many women did quit hormone therapy after learning about the study, called the Women's Health Initiative (WHI). Some, still struggling with symptoms like hot flashes and vaginal dryness, ultimately went back on estrogen. In the years since then, the number of women using hormone therapy has dropped dramatically, but the controversy continues. Some doctors believe that scientists will someday prove that estrogen is indeed the elixir of youth. Others contend that women should make every effort to ride out symptoms like hot flashes without medication

What Can Happen?

For a generally healthy woman in her early 50s, the overall risks of hormone therapy are low; your particular medical history determines your own vulnerability. The Food and Drug Administration requires manufacturers of products used in hormone therapy to state on their package labels that estrogen should not be taken by:

❖ Women who are pregnant

❖ Women with a past or current history of breast cancer or one of the other estrogen-sensitive cancers (such as endometrial cancer) and women with liver disease

Oral estrogen should not be used by:

❖ Women with very high triglyceride levels that put them at risk for coronary heart disease

❖ Women who have had blood clots in their lungs or legs

Many women who try hormone therapy stop within a year because of side effects such as nausea, headaches, and breast tenderness. If you experience any of these but want to stay on hormones to deal with menopausal symptoms, talk to your doctor about lowering the dose or using other products (e.g., patches instead of pills).

---

because so little is known about the long-term consequences of hormone therapy.

Before you work up too much of a sweat about taking hormones, we want to point out that this isn't the most important health choice most women will make during these years. Menopause is a time to rethink a lot of issues, including your heart health, the strength of your bones, your diet, and the amount of exercise and sleep you get—even the quality of your most intimate relationships. All of these things can have a much more significant effect on your future well-being than whether or not you use menopausal hormone therapy.

With that caveat, you do need to understand the often contentious debate over taking estrogen. Menopause is a natural process, not a disease. You may choose hormone therapy because you and your doctor believe it will improve your quality of life. That's not the same thing as curing an illness. In this chapter, we explain what scientists currently know about the pros and cons of taking estrogen in all its forms and combinations so you can work with your doctor to decide what's right for you.

ALL ABOUT ESTROGEN

As a hormone, estrogen functions as a chemical messenger in your body, telling cells what to do. As a sex hormone, it performs the important task of regulating the parts of your body that make you female.

Before menopause, most of your estrogen is produced in your ovaries (see Chapter 1 for more details). Much like flipping a switch, this connection sets off a series of responses. During puberty, estrogen tells your breasts to grow; later on, it helps to maintain pregnancy by regulating the levels of another sex hormone, progesterone, and by kick-starting the development of the fetal brain, liver, and other organs and tissues.

Estrogen travels through your bloodstream looking for special receptors present in your breasts and uterus, as well as your brain, heart, liver, and bones. Researchers used to think there was only one kind of estrogen receptor. Then, a few years ago, they found another one, which they called estrogen receptor beta to distinguish it from the original estrogen receptor alpha. Alphas are more prevalent in the reproductive system and the liver. Betas are more commonly found in bone, the lungs, and the urogenital tract, as well as in blood vessels. Both alpha and beta receptors are abundant in the ovaries and the brain. As we learn more about estrogen receptors, the hope is to one day defeat estrogen-related cancers.

During the menopause transition, the ovaries gradually stop making estrogen. This is a natural process, not a sign of illness. Levels can go up and down for years before the final cutoff. Fluctuating hormone levels and the eventual loss of estrogen are behind troubling menopausal symptoms such as hot flashes and vaginal dryness.

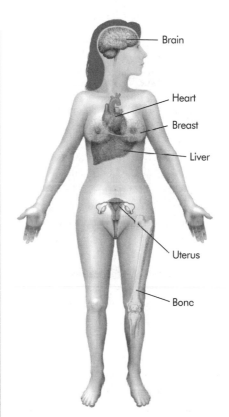

Brain

Heart

Breast

Liver

Uterus

Bone

MAIN TARGETS OF ESTROGEN

The risk for certain other medical conditions increases when estrogen is lost at menopause. Bones are likely to become more fragile, which can lead to osteoporosis. (By age 60, 25 percent of Caucasian and Asian women develop spinal compression fractures.) After menopause, the risk of cardiovascular disease begins to climb. Many researchers think this happens because estrogen has been providing some heart protection by keeping blood vessels elastic and clear of cholesterol.

Although their production of estrogen winds down at menopause, the ovaries

When to See the Doctor

*I*f hot flashes and night sweats are seriously disrupting your life and making it difficult for you to function, talk to your doctor about how your medical history affects the potential risks and benefits of hormone therapy for you. If you're troubled by vaginal dryness, ask your doctor if you're a candidate for new therapies that target this problem. You should also ask about other remedies, especially lifestyle changes that can minimize hot flashes.

continue to produce testosterone, which is converted to estrogen in liver and fat tissue. Other parts of the body also produce hormones in the testosterone family, which are converted in the same way. Women with a lot of fatty tissue, especially in their buttocks, abdomen, and thighs, produce more of these hormones and thus have more estrogen than thinner women do. This may be why heavier women are at higher risk for breast cancer and other estrogen-sensitive cancers.

All in all, estrogen activity is a very delicate mechanism that scientists are only beginning to understand.

Hormone Therapy Basics

Are you considering taking estrogen to relieve menopausal symptoms like hot flashes, those sudden waves of heat that leave you red-faced and dripping with sweat, or vaginal dryness that's making sex uncomfortable, or just because you're longing to feel a little more like your old self? If you're entering menopause prematurely because of illness or surgical removal of your ovaries, your doctor may recommend that you take estrogen until you reach the age of natural menopause. For some women, hormone therapy may also be recommended to slow bone loss (if there are problems with other drugs for osteoporosis) or to improve mood and thinking.

You and your doctor will have lots of choices. Hormone therapy varies according to the type and dose of estrogen, the dosing regimen, and the method of delivery. Which one you pick depends on your medical history, your preferences, and the problem you're trying to fix. Prescription estrogen comes in pills, creams, gels, patches, and vaginal rings. Most of these circulate estrogen throughout your body and would be prescribed if you're looking for relief from hot flashes. There are also products that send estrogen locally to your vaginal area; you would use these if vaginal dryness is the only issue. (See Appendix I.)

If you still have your uterus, you will also take the hormone progesterone or a progestin (a synthetic form of progesterone) to make sure there's no uncontrolled growth of the tissue in your uterine lining, called the endometrium. Uncontrolled growth could put you at risk for endometrial cancer. Progesterone causes the endometrium to shed every month. It's a little like getting your period, except that you're not ovulating. Women who've had a hysterectomy (an operation that removes the uterus) need only estrogen.

In general, hormone therapy is for women who are on the verge of menopause or who are postmenopausal. Women who are perimenopausal and need supplemental hormones often get oral contraceptives, which help to control their hot flashes while regulating their periods, controlling bleeding, and protecting against a possible pregnancy.

Hormone therapy increases the risk of stroke, blood clots, and, in some cases, breast cancer. Like almost all medications, prescription hormones have potential side effects, including bloating, breast tenderness, breakthrough bleeding, nausea, and headaches. Hormone patches can also cause skin irritation in some women.

SYSTEMIC THERAPY. You can get systemic estrogen in pills, patches, creams, and gels. There's also a vaginal ring that delivers estrogen to your whole body; it's more potent than the ring used to treat vaginal dryness alone. All women are at increased risk for blood clots when they're on hormone therapy, but obese women are at the greatest risk and would more likely get non-pill forms of estrogen (gel, patches, or vaginal estrogen) because estrogen delivered in these forms doesn't pass through the liver and is therefore less likely to raise the level of clotting factors

---

THE "P" WORD

Menopausal women took estrogen alone until 1975, when research discovered a link between estrogen therapy and a rise in endometrial cancer. That's when scientists added a form of the hormone progesterone to trigger sloughing of the uterine lining, which normally occurs at the end of the menstrual cycle. Like estrogen, progesterone comes in different forms:

Natural progesterone. Produced by the ovaries after ovulation and by the placenta during pregnancy, progesterone prepares the uterus for implantation of a fertilized egg and helps to maintain pregnancy.

Synthetic progesterone. This is chemically identical to the progesterone produced by your body, but it's created in a laboratory. Progesterone crystals are micronized (ground very small) to facilitate absorption.

Progestins. These synthetics mimic most or all activity of progesterone but do not have the same chemical structure.

Progestogens. This category includes both naturally occurring and synthetic progesterone, as well as the synthetic progestins.

---

in the blood. You might also rely on the preferences of your doctor. Many clinicians now consider non-pill forms of estrogen their first choice for all patients because of the reduced clotting risk. Progesterone and progestins also come in different forms: tablets, a gel, and a device placed in the uterus. Both progesterone and progestins are referred to as progestogens.

LOCAL THERAPY. You can get relief from vaginal dryness with an estrogen tablet that you place in your vagina or with estrogen creams or a ring inserted in your vagina that delivers estrogen in measured doses. Although there is some evidence of endometrial thickening with local therapies, doctors are divided on whether and how often you need to take a progestogen with these drugs. Some will give you a progestogen once or twice a year; a few might suggest periodic ultrasound monitoring of the endometrium or biopsies. Make sure you understand your doctor's point of view on this.

COMBINATION THERAPY. Women who still have a uterus usually take estrogen in combination with a progestogen. There are two forms of combination therapy: cyclic or sequential (estrogen taken every day; progesterone or a progestin taken only 10 to 14 days in each cycle) and continuous (estrogen and a progestin taken daily without a break). Prempro, the drug used in the WHI trial, is prescribed for continuous combined hormone therapy. Cyclic therapy is gaining favor among doctors who think it most closely mimics natural menstruation. You and your doctor will decide which therapy regimen is best for you.

ESTROGEN ALONE. Women who have had a hysterectomy take only estrogen. If you've also had your ovaries surgically removed before the age of natural menopause, your doctor might recommend estrogen to replace the missing hormone until you're around 51. This may offer some short-term protection against heart disease and osteoporosis. Women who lose their ovaries but still have a uterus need estrogen and a progestogen.

ORAL CONTRACEPTIVES. Perimenopausal women can use low-dose oral contraceptives to ease symptoms like hot flashes and irregular bleeding. For younger women, this is often the preferred approach. Before menopause, fluctuating hormone levels cause problems. The pill regulates your cycle and prevents unwanted pregnancy. In any case, you need to use some form of contraception until you've gone a year without a menstrual period.

WHERE DO I BEGIN?

Q *What's the most important thing to know before I make a decision about hormone therapy?*

A You should understand the background of the Women's Health Initiative (WHI) if you want to make the most informed choice about hormone therapy. Because WHI partici-

From the Past

In the early 20th century, when doctors first discovered hormones and began to understand how they worked, many people believed that these chemicals had enormous potential as an elixir of youth. Pharmaceutical companies rushed to produce them, hoping to make gold out of that promise. In the 1960s, hormones got a big boost from a book called *Feminine Forever*, by a New York gynecologist named Robert Wilson. The author, a fervent estrogen evangelist, describes how a distraught husband demanded treatment for his menopausal wife. "She's driving me nuts," the man told Wilson. "She won't fix meals. She lets me get no sleep. She makes up lies about me. She hits the bottle all day." Wilson gave the woman what he describes as "intensive twice-a-week estrogen injections" after the husband pulled a gun out of his pocket and said, "If you don't cure her, I'll kill her." (Wilson claims he later discovered that the husband was a prominent member of the Brooklyn underworld, so apparently this threat was real.) After three weeks, the woman's disposition "improved noticeably" and she was busy taking care of her husband, who, it turned out, was dying of tuberculosis. "I received an invitation to his elaborate funeral," Wilson says. "His widow felt genuine grief at his death." Estrogen apparently had a more cosmic benefit as well. The widow later told Wilson that during the last weeks of her husband's life, she had been able to instill in him a sense of repentance and of "religious hope for the salvation of his otherwise-lost soul." A miracle drug indeed.

pants took only two specific estrogen products—Premarin and Prempro—no one really knows if the results would be the same for less potent pills or patches (although doctors assume they would be). It's also important to understand that the women in the WHI study were generally older and farther from their last menstrual period than the average woman who goes on hormone therapy. Because age and time since menopause increase a woman's risk of heart problems, the WHI's usefulness to newly menopausal women is limited. Finally, the WHI was looking at hormone therapy's effectiveness as long-term prevention against chronic disease, not as a short-term treatment for hot flashes and vaginal dryness—the two most common menopausal symptoms.

CONFLICTING RESULTS

Q *A lot of other studies have tried to assess the relative benefits and risks of hormone therapy. How do their results compare with the WHI data? I'm afraid I find the whole subject very confusing.*

What You Need to Know About Medical Research

Scientists know much more about how our bodies work than they did even a decade ago, but it's important to realize that each study brings them only a little closer to a full picture. The more studies that are done on a certain topic, the more scientists feel they're on the right track. You could compare this scenario to the process of getting to know a friend. The first time you meet, you learn certain things about her. Maybe you don't even like her. Then you work together on a project, visit her house, have your first fight, or go on vacation together. With each encounter, you learn a little more. Were your first impressions wrong? No, they were right—based on the limited knowledge you had back then. But as you understand more about this person, your sense of who she really is becomes deeper and more nuanced.

The same is true of medical knowledge. Some scientific experiences are more meaningful than others.

Observational studies. Closely monitoring the behavior of large groups over time, researchers examine, test, and question each participant. These studies often give scientists a clue that a particular result may be connected to a certain behavior. In the 1980s and '90s, observational studies alerted researchers to the fact that women who were using menopausal hormone therapy had fewer heart attacks than did women who did not take hormones.

Though important, observational studies have a major limitation: people choose their own behaviors or experiences. There's no way to know what would have happened to them if they had chosen something else. For example, would the healthy women on hormone therapy have been just as healthy without it? Maybe they had fewer heart attacks because they had access to better medical care or because they watched their weight and exercised regularly.

A It's not surprising that you're confused. Lots of doctors are, too. After ads touted its potential to keep women young forever, estrogen rode a wave of popularity until about 1975. That's when researchers linked it to a surprising increase in endometrial cancer. Sales plummeted until doctors started giving their patients a progestin along with estrogen. The progestin triggers sloughing of the endometrium, the uterine lining, and decreases the risk of endometrial cancer. That estrogen-progestin mix is the basic combination used today for women who still have a uterus.

Over the next couple of decades, endorsements by celebrities helped popularize the idea of hormone therapy as a way to keep women healthy and vigorous. Medical science appeared to support that view. Before the WHI, more than 30 epidemiological studies followed women over a period of years and found that those who used estrogen or a combination of estrogen and a progestogen had a lower risk of heart disease than did those who

Randomized controlled trials. In these clinical studies, designed to determine cause and effect, subjects are randomly assigned to different experiences. The best of these studies reduce the likelihood that the results are due to something else, including chance.

Placebo-controlled studies. Participants in these studies are divided into two distinct groups: subjects who receive a specific medical intervention and those who are given a placebo. In a *single-blind study*, the participants don't know which group they belong to. (Interestingly, those taking the placebo often report feeling better; this is called the placebo effect.)

In a *double-blind study*, the people analyzing the data don't know which group is which, so there's no chance of bias as they look at the results.

As you no doubt have figured out by now, the best studies are *randomized placebo-controlled double-blind studies*.

Study results are measured by statistics; formulas determine whether the results are "statistically significant," or likely to be true. Studies that include larger groups of people are generally more reliable. When results are replicated by independent studies, researchers are even more confident that they understand a particular phenomenon.

Still, you can end up with conflicting information. Some test results address only a narrow slice of a bigger question. Or the researchers may reconsider their theories and start mapping out new projects that will get them closer to a resolution—part of the two-steps-forward, one-step-back process that characterizes scientific progress.

All the studies mentioned in this book reflect the current state of knowledge about menopause. We've tried to signal when evidence is based on a lot of studies or only a few, or is simply a theory. You can use this information in working with your doctor to make the best decisions.

did not use hormone therapy. These studies also found that women on estrogen appeared to have stronger bones and less chance of developing dementia. Although no clinical trial (a cause-and-effect study) had shown that hormone therapy was safe, annual prescriptions tripled in the 1990s. The WHI, started in 1991, was an attempt to get better information about estrogen as a preventive medicine for aging women—not as a treatment for menopausal symptoms. In 2002, when the estrogen-progestin part of the study

was halted, 14 million American women were on hormone therapy. After the WHI, that number dropped to 6 million and has stayed low ever since.

You should also understand that medical research is constantly evolving. Since 2002, researchers have continued to follow the women in the WHI trial and have published new studies that provide more nuanced information about the results; more are on the way. However, in science, the only certainty is that there will always be unresolved questions.

A BRIEF HISTORY OF HORMONE THERAPY

Researchers have been analyzing the risks and benefits of hormone therapy for more than three decades. Here's a rundown of the most significant studies:

Nurses' Health Study. In this 1972 observational study, scientists followed 59,337 nurses aged 33 to 55. After 16 years, the investigators found that the risk of coronary heart disease was lower in women who chose to use estrogen and a progestogen than in women who did not use hormones. But they also reported that the hormone users were less likely to be smokers or to have a family history of heart attacks or diabetes. Moreover, they were slightly younger and leaner and more likely to take multivitamins. All of these factors could help explain why they had fewer heart attacks, except that they also ate more saturated fat and had higher cholesterol levels, which could have put them at greater risk for heart disease.

Postmenopausal Estrogen/Progesterone Interventions (PEPI) trial. This three-year study of 875 healthy women aged 45 to 64 at the start was launched in 1987 by the National Institutes of Health and seemed to show a heart-protective benefit for estrogen. The women were given either estrogen alone or estrogen and a progestin, depending on whether or not they'd had a hysterectomy. A third group of women received a placebo. All the women who took hormones showed a significant rise in their levels of HDL cholesterol (the good kind) compared with the women in the placebo group. The women who received estrogen alone increased their HDL levels by more than twice as much as the women who received estrogen and a

progestin. Women with the biggest increases in HDL levels cut their heart disease risk by 25 percent. All groups reduced their levels of LDL cholesterol (the bad kind), although the reduction in the placebo group was relatively insignificant.

Heart and Estrogen/Progestin Replacement Study (HERS). The results of this study, released in 1998, cast doubt on estrogen's heart-protective role. The study followed 2,763 postmenopausal women whose average age was 67 and who had suffered heart attacks or chest pain caused by blocked arteries or had undergone heart surgery. In other words, they were very different from the PEPI subjects, who were healthy at the start of that trial. The goal of HERS was to test whether estrogen and a progestin would prevent a second heart attack or other coronary event. It found no such effect after four years. In fact, hormone therapy seemed to increase the risk of blood clots in the legs and lungs during the first year. A follow-up to the HERS study tracked the same women for about three more years and found no long-term decrease in heart disease among hormone users.

Women's Health Initiative (WHI). This study, launched in 1991, was designed to test whether hormone therapy's perceived benefits (protecting women from heart disease, bone loss, dementia) outweighed the increased risks of breast cancer, endometrial or uterine cancer, and blood clots. Two clinical trials, an observational study, and a community prevention study involving more than 161,000 average postmenopausal women made it one of the largest women's health studies ever conducted in the United States. In the estrogen-alone arm, 10,739 women who had had hysterectomies were given either a placebo or estrogen in the form of Premarin. In the estrogen-progestin arm, 16,608 women who still had a uterus took either a placebo or the combination pill Prempro. Premarin and Prempro were chosen because they were commonly prescribed at the time and also because in earlier studies they appeared to improve women's health. Participants ranged in age from 50 to 79 at the start of the study; the average age was about 63. (See Appendix I.)

The estrogen-progestin arm of the study was stopped three years early, in 2002, because researchers found that *as a group* the women taking estrogen and a progestin were at higher risk for blood clots, heart attack, and stroke, as well as breast cancer. The risk of heart attack for these women was greatest in the first year and continued high for several years afterwards; the risk of blood clots was greatest in the first two years—four times higher than that of placebo users. The risk of breast cancer increased in the fifth year. In the benefits column, combination therapy reduced the chance of fractures and appeared to cut the risk of colon cancer. The estrogen-alone arm was halted in 2004 because the results showed that estrogen increased the risk of stroke and did not cut the risk of coronary heart disease for the *average* woman in the study. Its effect on breast cancer depends on the woman's overall health history, but there is evidence that it can reduce vulnerability in women not already at high risk.

An ancillary study called the WHI Memory Study found that women 65 and older who were taking combination therapy had twice the risk of dementia as women on placebo and were not protected against mild cognitive impairment, a less severe loss of memory and reasoning. Estrogen alone somewhat increased the rate of dementia and mild cognitive impairment.

Overall Results of the Women's Health Initiative		
	TYPE OF TREATMENT	
RISK	ESTROGEN PLUS PROGESTIN	ESTROGEN ALONE
Heart attack	Increased risk	No effect
Stroke	Increased risk	Increased risk
Blood clots	Increased risk	Increased risk
Breast cancer	Increased risk	Varies, but can reduce risk in some women
Colon cancer	Reduced risk	No effect
Bone health	Fewer fractures	Fewer fractures

WHAT'S IN A NAME?

Q *I've seen it called hormone therapy, hormone replacement therapy, and menopausal or postmenopausal hormone therapy. Why do they keep changing its name?*

A At the start of the WHI, it was generally known as "hormone replacement therapy." But afterwards the FDA did a little replacing of its own and now uses the term "hormone therapy" to refer to this class of medications. Some doctors and scientists would like to call it "menopausal hormone therapy" or "postmenopausal therapy" to differentiate taking estrogen from other uses of hormones.

THE AGE FACTOR

Q *How important is your age if you're about to start hormone therapy?*

A The WHI showed that age is one of the critical factors to consider as you and your doctor decide what to do. Only a third of the women in the study were under 60, and only 16 percent were within five years of their last menstrual period—the time when women are most likely to take estrogen to relieve menopausal symptoms. The data look significantly different for women in their 50s, 60s, and 70s. Initiating hormone therapy is clearly a problem for women in their 70s and somewhat worrisome for those in their

60s, but the data for women in their 50s are less threatening—especially if they stay with the therapy for only a year or two. (See Appendix I for a comprehensive breakdown of WHI results by age group.)

ANOTHER TURNAROUND?

Q *Since scientists are still studying the pros and cons of hormone therapy, does this mean that someday they might find that estrogen does protect women against heart disease?*

A Many doctors still believe that estrogen protects against heart disease before menopause. It may be many years before we have all the answers about what happens when you start on estrogen around the time of menopause and continue to take it for an extended period of time. Scientists suspect that giving women estrogen early may help reduce the risk of heart disease for a while—although they don't

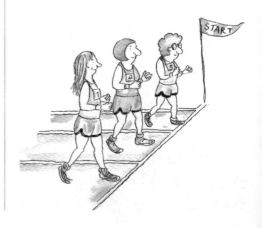

UNDERSTANDING RISK

Risk means one thing to scientists and quite another to the general public. Scientists look at risk from many angles to more fully understand the significance of the results of their studies. In their terms, *relative risk* estimates the difference in risk between two groups because of the presence or absence of a specific factor such as a medication. *Absolute risk* measures individuals' chances of developing health problems over a specific time period.

Many media reports about the Women's Health Initiative emphasized the relative risks, usually expressed in percentages. For example, in the estrogen-progestin arm of the study, there was a 29 percent increase in coronary heart disease risk for women aged 50 to 59. But that actually means only 5 more cases for every 10,000 women. You can see how expressing something in terms of relative risk makes a big difference in how you perceive it. While it's helpful for people making public policy decisions to hear about relative risks, it may not be useful to an individual woman whose choice depends on her overall health history, age, and time since menopause. When you're making a decision about a certain treatment or medication, absolute risk is often more useful in estimating your chances of a problem. And for healthy women under 60, the absolute risk for breast cancer, stroke, heart attack, and blood clots could be less than 3 in 1,000. Remember, however, that the risk is cumulative. This means if it's 1 in 1,000 the first year, it's 2 in 1,000 the second year, and 1 in 100 the 10th year. This is why most women should stop taking hormones as soon as possible. You can find links to the WHI studies and other information on hormone research at the WHI website: www.nhlbi.nih.gov/whi.

know for how long. Eventually, aging affects vascular health and a woman's arteries begin to lose elasticity. The extent and timing of atherosclerosis, or hardening of the arteries, depends on lifestyle and genetics. Doctors think that for each woman there is a point where estrogen becomes a negative rather than a positive. Right now, no one can predict where that point will be for most women and certainly not for an individual woman. But it is now clear that starting hormone therapy many years past menopause can be dangerous. Studies currently under way on younger women may help scientists understand when hormones might help fight heart disease and when it's clearly too late to start taking them. Until we have those answers, doctors are not recommending hormone therapy for prevention. It should be considered only for short-term relief of menopausal symptoms.

OTHER RISK FACTORS

Q *Other than my age, what else should I think about if I want to use hormone therapy?*

A If you're struggling with hot flashes and vaginal dryness, you should check out nondrug measures first. (See Chapters 3 and 5 for more details.) Exercising more and losing weight if necessary have proven helpful for many women and improve overall health at the same time. But if these and other measures don't work, you and your doctor need to evaluate your personal risk, taking into account your age, the time since your last menstrual period, and your overall health. If you have a personal or family history of heart disease, estrogen-related cancer, or blood clots, your doctor needs to know about it. Smoking also raises your risk of cardiovascular disease, and a recent study indicates that it may increase your chances of getting breast cancer if you take estrogen. Diabetics are already at risk for heart disease; if you're diabetic, your doctor may not want you to take estrogen. The interplay of all these factors determines your personal risk.

WHAT'S THE DIFFERENCE?

Q *Is the estrogen that's used in hormone therapy the same as the estrogen my body produces? Where does it come from?*

A It depends on the product. The most commonly prescribed form of estrogen comes from the urine of pregnant horses; that's why it's called Premarin (for pregnant mare urine). Why pregnant horses? Well, because they're large animals that pee a lot and it's relatively easy to "harvest" their estrogen-rich urine. Years ago, scientists tried to get urine from pregnant women, but that was impractical for a number of reasons, including the smell, taste, concentration of estrogen, and difficulty of collection. Apparently, pregnant women just aren't as predictable and easy to manage as pregnant horses.

A variety of estrogens are used in hormone therapy. Some are created in the lab, but don't be turned off by that; many safe and effective products are synthetic, and some natural estrogens are more potent and may be potentially less safe. *Estradiol,* the primary estrogen produced by your ovaries, is available in gels, creams, tablets, and patches; derivatives of *estrone,* the most abundant estrogen in your body after menopause, are less potent than estradiol but more easily absorbed in pills. Estrone and estradiol are the primary components of hormone therapy. Estrone derivatives are found in products labeled conjugated equine estrogen (from pregnant horses) and esterified estrogens (from plant-based material). *Estriol,* made in the liver from estradiol and estrone, is produced in large amounts during pregnancy. And finally, there's a group of weak, estrogen-like substances called *phytoestrogens* that are found in soy and hundreds of other plants; their effect on the human body is uncertain.

WHY NOT MORE FOR ALL?

Q *If all women are low on estrogen after menopause, why don't we all need hormone therapy?*

A You're not "low" on estrogen; you just have less than you used to. If you're going through natural menopause in your late 40s or early 50s, your loss of estrogen is part of the normal aging process and you don't have to replace it in order to be healthy. All you really need to do is eat right, exercise frequently, and schedule regular doctor visits. Most women get through these years without too much trouble, but some require treatment for symptoms like hot flashes or vaginal dryness and this is where hormone therapy comes in. Estrogen reduces hot flashes and alleviates vaginal dryness by up to 90 percent. But it's not the only treatment for these problems. Many women find relief from hot flashes simply by keeping the bedroom cool at night or wearing layered clothing. Other medications, like certain antidepressants, can also help. (See Chapter 3.) The average woman has hot flashes for only a few years, usually just before and after the final menstrual period. Unless your hot flashes are significantly interfering with your daily functioning (an estimated 10 to 15 percent of women), you'll probably be fine without medication. Lubricants and vaginal moisturizers can ease a dry vagina (more on this in Chapter 5), but these may not be enough for some women. If you do decide to try hormone therapy, current recommendations are to start on the lowest possible dose for the shortest possible time consistent with the goals of treatment. You and your doctor will have to decide what that recommendation means for you.

HOW BAD IS BAD ENOUGH?

Q *Right now, I only have two or three hot flashes a week, and I'm okay with that. How will I know when my symptoms become bad enough to warrant thinking about hormone therapy?*

A Believe us, you'll know. If your hot flashes are so frequent and severe that they're interfering with your ability to function normally, you need to talk to your doctor about your options. Chances are, you'll never reach that point; the majority of women find other ways to handle the discomfort of hot flashes. In any case, it's very much an individual decision. Some women find four or five hot flashes a day too many; others brush off twice that number. Some women's hot flashes are simply annoying; others are so severe that they become debilitating. For women dealing with a lot of stress, handling hot flashes can be harder than it is for women whose lives are more relaxed.

If you're feeling overwhelmed, talk to your doctor about nonpharmaceutical solutions as well as medication. Together, you can decide what's best

Thinking About Hormone Therapy?

These guidelines are not hard and fast, but they do give you a general idea of what's being recommended for most healthy nonsmoking women. The current recommendation for anyone using hormones is to take the lowest effective dose for the shortest time needed to meet treatment goals.

(Key: OC = oral contraceptives; E = estrogen alone; E&P = combination of estrogen and a progestogen)

Age	What's Going On	General Advice	Type of Therapy
Under 40	Premature menopause; intact uterus	Recommended	E&P
Under 50	Significant perimenopausal symptoms such as hot flashes that are not responding to other therapies; uterus intact	Recommended	OC
Under 50	Irregular and/or heavy perimenopausal bleeding; uterus intact	Recommended	OC
Under 50	Natural menopause with uterus intact; significant symptoms	Recommended	E&P
Under 50	Hysterectomy including removal of ovaries	Probably recommended*	E
Early 50s	Natural menopause with significant symptoms that don't respond adequately to nondrug interventions; uterus intact	Worth considering	E&P
Early 50s	Natural menopause with few symptoms that don't respond adequately to nondrug interventions; uterus intact	May be considered**	E&P
Early 50s	Natural menopause with no symptoms	Not recommended	
Early 50s	Hysterectomy with removal of ovaries; significant symptoms	Probably recommended*	E
Early 50s	Menopause reached years after hysterectomy; ovaries retained; significant symptoms not responding to nondrug interventions	Worth considering	E
Mid to late 50s	Natural menopause with significant symptoms that don't respond to nondrug interventions	May be considered, depending on time since menopause and duration of hormone therapy	E&P
All ages	Estrogen-related cancer	Not recommended	
All ages	Significant vaginal dryness; no uterus	Local (vaginal) hormones may be recommended	E
All ages	Significant vaginal dryness; uterus intact	Local (vaginal) hormones***	

*Depends on reason for hysterectomy/oophorectomy.

**Too hard to generalize; lots of variation here, depending on desires of patient and philosophy of doctor.

***Some doctors will recommend combination therapy; some, estrogen alone with endometrial monitoring.

for you, based on your medical history. The important thing to remember is that you don't have to suffer silently; there is help.

OTHER USES?

Q *The WHI showed that hormone therapy helped with osteoporosis and may offer some protection against colorectal cancer. Are these good reasons to use it?*

A Most medical organizations say no. There are other preventive measures against both diseases that don't carry the risks of hormone therapy. Also, the bone health benefits disappear when you stop using it. That's important because women are at greatest risk of fractures in their 70s and 80s. Hormone therapy begun in your 50s and used for only a year or two wouldn't have any effect on your fracture risk two decades or more after you stop. As far as its effect on colorectal cancer is concerned, much more research has to be done in this area.

BREAST CANCER

Q *I have terrible night sweats, but my mother and my aunt had breast cancer and I'm worried about hormone therapy. It is an option for me?*

A If there's breast cancer in your family history, you need to tell your doctor about it when discussing hormone therapy. Your chances of getting the disease depend on a number of

factors, including your own medical history and the age at which your mother and aunt developed cancer. Hormone therapy makes breast tissue more dense and mammograms harder to read— something you need to know if you're worried about cancer. To ease your menopausal symptoms, your best bet at this point would probably be some lifestyle changes and certain antidepressants, which have been shown to be effective in breast cancer patients. (For more information, see Chapter 3.)

In the WHI study, women who took estrogen and a progestin had a higher chance of getting breast cancer after five years, while the women who took estrogen alone generally showed no higher risk of the disease (although women at high risk increased their risk by taking hormones). This led some scientists to wonder if there was a connection between progestogens and breast cancer risk. If there is, it's still unclear.

WEIGHT GAIN

Q *I've already put on several more pounds than I need. Will estrogen make me gain more?*

A You've discovered one of the downsides of the menopause years—it's easier to gain weight and much harder to lose it. Your metabolism is slowing down as you age, and you're probably getting less exercise than you used to. Hormone therapy won't affect that either way; there's no evidence that

What to Tell Your Daughter

The continuing debate over the benefits of hormone therapy reminds us that scientific research is always a work in progress. When today's headlines trumpet a new medical advance, keep in mind that a contradictory discovery may come along someday. That's why we all need to be educated consumers of medical care and an active partner in decision-making with our doctors. Encourage your daughter to ask questions.

you'll either gain or lose weight when you take it. The only solution for excess pounds (at any age) is a healthier diet and more physical activity.

SKIN DEEP

Q *Does hormone therapy help you look younger?*

A There's no strong evidence of this, although some small studies indicate that hormone therapy may improve the collagen content of your skin. If you're concerned about avoiding wrinkles, you have to start young. Use sunscreen, don't smoke, and avoid big changes in weight. Most of the rest is up to your genes. If you've been careful before, keep it up. If not, start now. (For more suggestions on how to protect aging skin and improve what you've got, see Chapter 15.)

PROGESTERONE CREAM

Q *I have a friend who uses natural progesterone cream from a health food store, and she says it stops her hot flashes. Is this possible?*

A Progesterone cream from a health food store may be made from wild yams or soybeans. It is not the same as the synthetic progesterone used in hormone therapy or the natural progesterone produced by your body. There's some evidence that it may help with hot flashes, but its content is not carefully regulated, so you really don't know how much you're getting and what level might be dangerous. In addition, progesterone cream should not be used to counteract the effects of estrogen in hormone therapy since it doesn't protect against endometrial cancer. Any natural products or supplements should be taken only with a doctor's okay.

THE RIGHT DOSE

Q *I understand that the current advice on hormone therapy is to take the smallest effective dose. How does my doctor know what that is?*

A The women in the WHI study took 0.625 milligram of Prempro or Premarin because that was the standard dose at the time. One of the benefits of the study was that it inspired drug companies to offer a variety of lower-dose versions of hormone therapy. Many women find that these lower doses are just as effective. But this is where it gets a little tricky. No one knows how much an individual woman should take to alleviate her symptoms. It's really a matter of trying one dose and seeing whether it works. If it doesn't, you and your doctor can decide whether you want to try a different dose. This process can be time-consuming, since it takes up to about eight weeks to tell whether the hormone therapy is working.

IS LESS SAFER?

Q *So, are lower doses the safest way to go?*

A No one knows. The assumption is yes, but no studies have been done to confirm this. As more women take the lower doses, scientists will be able to make a better estimate of the risks. For now, however, it's just an educated guess.

TIME FRAME

Q *I'm told that if I decide to use hormones, I should take them for the shortest possible time. That's so vague. How will I know when I don't need them anymore?*

A That's another mystery. You have to stop for a while and see if your symptoms continue. If they do, you can choose to begin hormone therapy again. Some doctors say you should go off every six months; others say annually. If your doctor doesn't give you some sense of how long you'll be on hormones, ask about it.

SYMPTOM TIMING

Q *How long do menopausal symptoms like hot flashes last in most women?*

A In general, hot flashes peak just before the last menstrual period. By a year or two after menopause, most women report feeling much better. But, as we keep saying, there's a great deal of individual variability among women—and not just in symptoms. One woman might barely notice a severe flash, while another could be bothered by relatively small ones. And there's no way to tell how long hot flashes will last in any one woman. You could decide to try hormone therapy for a year and find that your hot flashes have stopped when you get off—or you could find that they've returned and may even have gotten worse. That's one of the things that make this decision difficult. No one can predict what your individual experience will be. However, based on the averages, you should be done with hot flashes a year or two after your last menstrual period.

RISKY YEAR

Q *What if I choose to stay on hormone therapy for only a year just to get me over the hump? Is a shorter time safer?*

A It might not be. The women in the estrogen-progestin arm of the WHI had a slightly higher risk of blood clots and stroke in the first year of therapy. So, for an individual woman, the first year could actually be the most dangerous. Remember, those were overall numbers. For the youngest women in the study, the risks were lower than for the oldest women. Many researchers think the blood clot and stroke risks were the result of preexisting but undiagnosed vascular problems. The theory is that the estrogen aggravated the condition, causing plaque that had accumulated in arteries to rupture and form blood clots. This seems less likely to happen in younger, healthier women who start taking hormones around the time of menopause, when their arteries should still be relatively healthy. It's important to talk to your doctor about your medical history, especially any history of cardiovascular disease.

WAITING IT OUT

Q *Wouldn't my symptoms stop even if I took nothing?*

A That would be the case for many women, though there's no way of knowing in advance if you're one of them. Some women have hot flashes for just a short time; a very few suffer for decades after menopause. A good rule of thumb is to try wearing layered clothing and keeping the bedroom cooler (along with other lifestyle changes) for at least six months and see if the hot flashes subside. If they don't, talk to your doctor about alternatives.

STILL IN TRANSITION

Q *I'm 49 and having periods every couple of months. I'm also having hot flashes. What's the best remedy?*

A You should first try nondrug measures: get more exercise, stop smoking, learn stress-reduction techniques (for more on this, see Chapter 3). If none of these works and hot flashes are really interfering with your normal functioning, your doctor may suggest medication. As long as you're ovulating and could get pregnant, you still need to worry about contraception. A low-dose birth-control pill would solve both problems for now. Generally, doctors do not prescribe menopausal hormone therapy for women in your situation because the estrogen wouldn't be potent enough to inhibit ovulation and you could still get pregnant.

Many women in their 40s and 50s may be reluctant to take birth-control pills because they remember that, many years ago, the pills were considered dangerous if you took them after age 35. That's no longer the case. Today's lower-dose pills are considered safe for midlife women who need contraception, as long as they don't smoke and are not at risk for blood clots. And birth-control pills can have some health benefits as well. Research has shown that they may reduce the risk of ovarian cancer, endometrial cancer, and pelvic inflammatory disease.

HORMONAL CONTRACEPTION

Q *Since menopausal hormone therapy is less potent than the pill and you should take the lowest possible dose, why can't I start hormone therapy before menopause and use another form of contraception such as a diaphragm or IUD, at least until I'm 51 or so?*

A Menopausal hormone therapy and the pill ease symptoms in two different ways. Before menopause, you get hot flashes and irregular bleeding because your hormone levels are fluctuating. After menopause, you get hot flashes and vaginal dryness because your body hasn't adjusted to lower levels of estrogen. That's why oral contraceptives are a better choice for many women before their last menstrual period. When you're perimenopausal, the pill will regulate your hormone levels and cut down on symptoms. The less potent menopausal therapy doesn't regulate hormone levels. It also won't prevent pregnancy if you're still ovulating. Having a baby in your 40s or 50s can be dangerous to both your health and the baby's (see Chapter 1).

Low-dose birth-control pills or the patch can hide changes in your cycle that would signal the onset of menopause. The pills or patch might affect your level of follicle-stimulating hormone (FSH), which is tested to determine whether you're approaching menopause. Many doctors tell women to stop hormonal contraceptives around age 51, since that's the average age of menopause. The general recommendation is that you should be off by age 55. If you're still having significant symptoms, then you could consider menopausal hormone therapy.

MAKING THE SWITCH

Q *At what point is menopausal hormone therapy a better choice than oral contraceptives to get rid of hot flashes?*

A If you haven't had a period for three or four months and your FSH is consistently high, your doctor will probably want you to start hormone therapy if lifestyle changes haven't relieved your hot flashes. Again, the current recommendation is to take the lowest effective dose to help your symptoms. What that means for you is something you will work out with your doctor. In general, you would want to reassess at least annually and see whether you still need estrogen to help ease your hot flashes or other symptoms.

STICKY PROBLEMS

Q *I'm using a hormone patch that leaves icky black lines when I change it. I've tried scrubbing the marks off with a sponge and a loofah, but nothing works. Suggestions?*

A When you're getting ready to put the patch on, make sure your skin is clean and dry. Don't use lotion or talcum powder near that area (your upper arms or lower torso are the usual choices). Also, don't place the patch under your bra strap or waistband. If you still get those black lines, rub your skin with baby oil. That should fix it.

WHEN YOU'RE DONE

Q *What's the best way to stop hormone therapy? What if I still have hot flashes?*

A You'll just have to see how you react; there are no clinical guidelines for this. More than half the women in the WHI study had hot flashes after quitting hormone therapy. They were six times more likely to have these symptoms than the women in the placebo group. They were also twice as likely to report an increase in overall stiffness and pain, another very common symptom at menopause. This was puzzling, since none of the women had severe menopausal symptoms when they started. They were chosen precisely for that reason; women who had severe symptoms would have known whether they were taking estrogen or a placebo. In another study of women who stopped estrogen after WHI, more than 70 percent had some hot flashes. Most of these ended in a couple of months, but 25 percent of the women decided to resume hormone therapy.

Of course, these women stopped taking estrogen suddenly. That left doctors wondering whether a gradual tapering off might be better. There's some evidence to back up this approach, but in another large study of women who stopped hormone therapy after hearing about the WHI results, only a quarter developed troubling symptoms. In addition to hot flashes, some women have heavy bleeding for a few days after they quit hormone therapy.

So, when you go off estrogen, you're essentially performing a little experiment on yourself. If your hot flashes come back, give yourself a few weeks to see if the symptoms get better with time and lifestyle changes. If they don't, your doctor may suggest going back on a low dose of hormone therapy and then tapering off slowly. A very small group of women may want to stay on hormones indefinitely because they feel better on them. If that applies to you, you need to understand your risks (which are cumulative) and make sure you're carefully monitored by your doctor.

Here's a tip: To find out if you'll still have hot flashes without hormones, try your experiment during the colder months. High temperatures can trigger hot flashes, making it harder for you to tell whether the heat wave you're feeling is internal or external.

HAPPILY EVER AFTER?

Q *Could I stay on hormone therapy the rest of my life and not suffer any ill effects? An 80-year-old friend of my mother's says she's been taking estrogen for 20 years and still feels great.*

WHAT ARE BIOIDENTICALS?

To most doctors, *bioidentical* refers to a wide variety of FDA-approved drugs that are structurally identical to the hormones produced by a woman's ovaries. But in recent years, *bioidentical* has also come to refer to made-to-order hormone treatments created by compounding pharmacies based on saliva tests. Celebrity promoters and Internet sites are aggressively marketing these new types of bioidentical hormones as safer and more "natural" than the hormones made by drug companies. Some even promise that these new bioidenticals protect against heart disease, dementia, and breast and endometrial cancer—or argue that they're not drugs at all. It sounds too good to be true. And guess what? It is.

The truth is that all hormone treatments—whether made by Big Pharma or by a compounding pharmacy—are drugs. All of them alter the chemistry of your body, and that's the definition of a drug. Secondly, none of them are "natural." You may like the fact that some start out as wild yams or soybeans, but by the time they've been converted to hormone therapy, they're all synthetics. Saliva tests have also been shown to be an unreliable way to measure hormone levels. There's no good evidence that these drugs are safer or more protective against disease. The same risks that apply to other hormones should apply to these products. There is evidence, however, that drugs made by compounding pharmacies are less likely to contain uniform content or the right potency. As a result, the FDA and the American College of Obstetricians and Gynecologists, among others, discourage their use, and most doctors won't prescribe them.

So, rather than take a chance on faddish drugs that we know even less about, we suggest taking advantage of the positive change prompted by the WHI: a much wider variety of FDA-approved products to choose from. These include bioidenticals whose primary ingredient is 17-beta estradiol. Some products to consider are Estrace, EstroGel, and Estrasorb. Low-dose hormone therapy now comes in many dosages and forms, including pills, patches, gels, and vaginal rings. (For more information, see Appendix I.)

Women have become much savvier about claims by pharmaceutical companies. That same skepticism should apply to hormone products that are not FDA-regulated.

A It's possible, and indeed there are women like your mother's friend who have been on estrogen for decades and won't give it up. Quality of life is important, and if hot flashes significantly affect your ability to function, you may want to stay on estrogen longer. It's your decision—just be sure you're fully informed about the risks you're taking. If you choose to stay on hormone therapy, you'll have to be rigorous about scheduling regular checkups with your doctor to make sure you don't develop any health problems related to estrogen. And at every visit you should reevaluate your decision.

CASE STUDIES

Every woman has her own reason for choosing or rejecting hormone therapy. Here's how five hypothetical women might go about making the decision.

ANNA: Hot Flashes After a Hysterectomy
Age: 43

How she entered menopause:

Because of heavy bleeding caused by persistent fibroids, Anna had her uterus and ovaries removed. Within days, she began experiencing severe hot flashes and night sweats that interrupted her sleep. Her 67-year-old mother has been diagnosed with osteoporosis, and Anna's own slender build (she's 5'3" and 105 pounds) and lack of exercise put her at risk as well. She asks her doctor for help with hot flashes.

What she needs to know:

Anna's doctor explains that her loss of estrogen is occurring eight years earlier than that of the average woman in the industrialized world. Her most significant health concern from this early loss is the effect on her bones, particularly since she's already at risk for osteoporosis. Her doctor orders a bone mineral density (BMD) test; the results show that her bones are already somewhat more fragile than average. Taking estrogen will stem further bone loss while she's on hormone therapy. Some evidence also suggests that she may get additional protection from heart disease during this time.

Anna's hot flashes are especially severe because of the sudden loss of estrogen after the removal of her ovaries. Her body had no chance to adjust. Night sweats that frequently disrupt her sleep could make her vulnerable to mood problems. Taking estrogen will probably stop the hot flashes and night sweats or at least significantly reduce them. The doctor checks Anna's medical history and tells her she has no particular risk factors that would argue against hormone therapy.

Her decision:

Anna chooses to take low-dose estrogen. Because she no longer has her uterus, she doesn't have to take a progestogen to protect the uterine lining. Her doctor plans to keep her on estrogen until she's 51. At that point, they will decide whether she would benefit from other bone-building medications or she should stay on hormone therapy longer. When she does stop taking estrogen, she'll taper off gradually in an effort to avoid "rebound" hot flashes. Between now and then, she'll see her doctor annually to assess her overall health and decide whether estrogen therapy is still the best course for her. She will also get annual BMD tests. In the meantime, she's doing weight-bearing exercises at the gym to increase her bone strength while making sure she has adequate calcium and vitamin D in her diet.

BECKY: The Queen of Mean
Age: 52

How she entered menopause:

Shortly after her 50th birthday, Becky started getting hot flashes. Her periods had always been regular, but they began to get closer together and then farther apart. At this point, she hasn't had a period for seven months, but night sweats are ruining her sleep and making her cranky. To get through the day, she drinks four or five cups of coffee. She isn't exercising the way she used to, and she's gained a few pounds. She's also under a lot of pressure at work. And when her husband and teenage children call her the Queen of Mean, everyone but Becky thinks it's funny. Finally, she asks her doctor about hormone therapy.

What she needs to know:

Becky's doctor sympathizes, but says he doesn't want to start her on medication until she's made changes in her lifestyle that might ease the hot flashes. Her FSH level is high, which means she could be nearing the end of the menopausal transition. He tells Becky that most women have hot flashes for only two to three years around the time of their last menstrual period, so she might already be through the worst of it. Becky has never had breast cancer or blood clots, which could make hormone therapy risky, but her doctor says she should reduce her stress and find other ways to improve her sleep before she takes hormones.

Her decision:

Becky is skeptical, but she agrees to do something about her high level of stress and report back to her doctor in three months. She signs up for a morning yoga class at her local gym, and although it's hard for her to get up early, she finds that her stress level is noticeably lower after only a few weeks. She buys a fan for her side of the bed and keeps it on all night, which cools her off considerably without disturbing her husband. She also switches to a lighter blanket and cuts down on caffeine—especially her late afternoon latte. Before bed, she takes a leisurely bath just to relax. These changes, too, are surprisingly successful. Although she still wakes up occasionally, Becky is able to go back to sleep fairly quickly and feels much more rested in the morning. When she returns to her doctor three months later, they both decide she should forgo hormone therapy for now. It's an option they'll revisit if the night sweats return.

CHRISTINE: A Survivor
Age: 45

How she entered menopause:

When she was 42, Christine was diagnosed with breast cancer. The tumor was caught early, and she was treated with surgery and radiation; she hasn't had any recurrences. Now, three years later, Christine is getting some of the first signs of menopause: irregular periods and hot flashes. The hot flashes aren't bad at night, but she's been caught red-faced one too many times at work. Most of her colleagues are 35 or younger, so she's a little self-conscious about being in her late 40s. A big part of her job is making presentations to clients, and she's noticed that the more important the client, the more likely she is to have a hot flash during the meeting. She's already tried wearing layered clothing so she can take off her jacket when the flash begins, and she's cut back on caffeine and spicy foods. She's even tried carrying a bottle of cold water so she can take a swig when a hot flash starts. But nothing seems to help. Christine has regular doctor visits to make sure she's still free of breast cancer. She brings up the issue of her hot flashes at one of these visits.

What she needs to know:

The doctor tells Christine that hormone therapy is risky for women who've had an estrogen-sensitive cancer like hers. In fact, the FDA specifically states that such women should not take hormones. Some studies have shown that more estrogen might spark a recurrence, although others have found no effect. Hormone therapy pills, which send estrogen throughout the body, could also make her breasts denser, so her mammograms would be harder to read—not a good thing for a breast cancer survivor. The doctor tells Christine that for all these reasons, hormone therapy is not a good option for her.

Her decision:

Since lifestyle changes haven't worked, Christine's doctor recommends an antidepressant to relieve her hot flashes. Research has shown that some antidepressants can be very effective in this area. Of these, Effexor (venlafaxine) has produced the best results. In several placebo-controlled studies, this drug reduced hot flashes up to 61 percent in a month, compared with 27 percent for a placebo. Christine's doctor explains that there might be some side effects, such as dry mouth, decreased appetite, nausea, and a lower libido, although most patients tolerate Effexor without these problems. (Side effects generally disappear within weeks.) After her doctor explains all this to her, Christine decides that Effexor is worth a shot. Six weeks later, she returns to tell her doctor that she has had far fewer hot flashes and has been able to get through several important presentations without the slightest blush. She and her doctor decide she will stay on Effexor for the foreseeable future and periodically reevaluate whether she should continue on the drug.

DEIRDRE: Reluctant Lover
Age: 56

How she entered menopause:

Unlike many of her friends, Deirdre found that menopause was largely a nonevent in her life. By the time her periods starting becoming irregular, all three of her children were out of the house. With just Deirdre and her husband at home, housework seemed a breeze and she was able to focus more energy on her career with a satisfying outcome: a promotion to a job she loves. She had a few hot flashes, but nothing really distressing, and she felt relief when her periods stopped completely at age 51. Now, just as she's enjoying her freedom, a new problem is emerging. Although Deirdre and her husband have always had a satisfying sex life, she has become more and more reluctant to make love. Her vagina feels dry and itchy, and intercourse is painful—no matter how much foreplay. She's tried a vaginal moisturizer, but it isn't doing enough. Deirdre generally avoids medication, even aspirin for a headache, but her relationship with her husband is beginning to suffer. Although she finds it embarrassing to bring up the subject, she asks her doctor for help.

What she needs to know:

Sensing her discomfort, Deirdre's doctor reassures her that vaginal dryness is a common problem after menopause. Since Deirdre is a longtime patient, her doctor also understands that she wants to avoid medication and is reluctant to use hormone therapy. He explains that as Deirdre's estrogen levels dropped, the tissue lining of her vagina and the opening to her bladder became thinner, drier, and less

elastic. Many postmenopausal women experience burning, itching, and discomfort during intercourse. Vaginal lubricants and moisturizers work for a lot of women. Frequent sex helps, too, because any stimulation increases blood flow to the vaginal tissues. However, even with all that, some women find that sex is more pain than pleasure.

Her decision:

Since vaginal dryness is her only symptom, Deirdre doesn't need the more potent systemic estrogen therapy offered by pills or patches. Instead, her doctor suggests she try estrogen delivered directly to her vaginal area. This local therapy involves a much lower dose, which alleviates some of Deirdre's concerns about hormones. Her choices are an estrogen cream, a tablet, or a ring inserted in the upper part of her vagina. Because it seems simplest, Deirdre decides to try the ring, which slowly releases estrogen over a period of 90 days. After that time, she returns to her doctor and reports that sex is much less painful. The doctor suggests that she now use vaginal lubricants and moisturizers regularly (as well as continuing to enjoy frequent sex). If the problem returns, she can always try local therapy again to get back on track.

EMILY: Stuck in the Middle
Age: 47

How she entered menopause:

She's not quite there yet, but something is definitely happening. Her periods are becoming irregular (20 to 40 days apart), and her flow can be embarrassingly heavy. At one point, she had to wear extra-strength pads for 21 straight days just to keep everything under control. She's also beginning to have some hot flashes, which are making it difficult to get a good night's sleep. Emily is single, but there's a man in her life. She's not quite sure about him, however, and she's worried that even at 47 she might get pregnant. She feels stuck in the middle, as worried about pregnancy as she was in her 20s and yet concerned that menopause is just around the corner. She asks her doctor how to balance all these issues.

What she needs to know:

Because she's still ovulating, Emily needs contraception. She also wants help with menopausal symptoms. The solution her doctor suggests surprises her. The doctor tells her that because she's a non-smoker in good health with no history of blood clots, she should take a low-dose oral contraceptive. When she was in her late 20s, Emily took the pill, but she stopped after hearing that it was dangerous. Now she can't believe her doctor is telling her to take it! Her doctor explains that the very low-dose pills available these days are indeed safe for women her age and that they work really well at regulating fluctuating estrogen levels and controlling bleeding.

Her decision:

After talking to her doctor, Emily decides to go on the pill. Six weeks later, most of her perimenopausal symptoms have abated. She's also feeling more relaxed with her partner because she's not worried about an unwanted pregnancy. Emily and her doctor decide that as long as she's feeling okay, she'll stay on oral contraceptives until she's 51. Then she'll go off for a month to see whether she's reached menopause. Her doctor may also test her FSH level 10 days after she gets off the pill to see if it's elevated—another indication of her menopausal status. If she still needs relief from hot flashes, she and her doctor will decide whether menopausal hormone therapy would be a good idea for a few years.

PART II

WHAT
YOU'RE FEELING
NOW

CHAPTER 3

Hot Flashes

The first time it happened, you had just polished off a spicy dinner and you blamed it on the jalapeños. The next time, you woke up in the middle of the night, bewildered and drenched in sweat. A few days later, you were talking to a colleague at work when, without any warning, you felt that ominous warmth creeping up your torso. That's when you finally understood what was happening: hot flashes, the menopause symptom we dread the most because they're so . . . *public.*

Well, if it's any comfort, you're not sweating alone. More than three-quarters of North American women suffer from hot flashes during the menopause transition. This means, of course, that a lucky minority of women don't. Our question is: Who are these women and where are they hiding? Everyone we know has experienced the unwelcome sensation of sudden heat more than once and often in an embarrassing situation: in the middle of a conversation, during an introduction to someone new, or rushing to meet a deadline.

Most of us suffer silently and hope that this phase, too, will pass—like acne and the troubling penchant for shoulder pads that came over us in the 1980s. And for many women, that will indeed be the case. It's estimated that fewer than 20 percent of women have hot flashes so severe that they require treatment. Many women get relief by wearing lighter clothing, drinking lots of water,

What Can Happen

❖ A sudden sensation of heat in your torso and face, sometimes preceded by feelings of anxiety and a rapid heartbeat

❖ Sweating as the flash dissipates and your body tries to cool down

❖ Occasional chills as the flash comes to an end

❖ Increased sensitivity to relatively small increases in temperature

losing weight, and getting regular exercise. If you do need medication, hormone therapy is still an option for some women, even after all those scary headlines. If you can't take hormones for medical reasons, there are other drugs that can help. And when all else fails, you can always take a walk down the frozen food aisle!

RELIEF WITHOUT AN Rx

Small lifestyle changes can help a lot. Before you consider hormone therapy or other prescription medication, try these suggestions for a few months:

GET MOVING. Researchers still debate the effect of regular exercise on the frequency and severity of hot flashes, but many women say working out for an hour three or more times a week helps. Exercise does reduce stress, a common hot flash trigger. You might experience what seems like a hot flash while you're exercising, but the gym is one place where you won't stand out if you get all hot and sweaty!

DRESS IN LAYERS. At work, try a sleeveless top under your suit. If you need to take off the jacket, you'll get an extra dose of cooling air. Avoid turtlenecks. Also, make a point of slightly underdressing for the weather. And welcome winter. Chilly temperatures are your best friend.

A FASHION STATEMENT

Waking up drenched with sweat is no fun. It doesn't happen to all women, and it might happen to you only a few times. But if it's a persistent problem, you could try sleepwear and bedding made of high-tech fabrics designed to keep you cool and dry. The idea is to "wick away" moisture. The same material is used in a lot of active wear, so if you already own T-shirts or leggings made of this stuff, you could try sleeping in them for a few nights before you invest in more. Brand names include Hot Mama, Wicking J Sleepwear, DryDreams, CoolDryComfort, and HotCoolWear. These companies also make T-shirts and underwear that can help with hot flashes during the day. Some clothing lines are sold through the web; others can be found in department stores. Try Googling brand names for outlets near you.

TONING TRICEPS

Wearing a sleeveless top doesn't do any good if you're embarrassed to take off your jacket because of arm jiggle. This exercise from the National Institute on Aging strengthens the muscles in the backs of your upper arms. Stand or sit in a chair with your feet flat on the floor, spaced so that they're even with your shoulders. Hold a weight in your right hand and raise your right arm all the way up so that it's pointing to the ceiling, palm facing in. Support your right arm by holding it just below the elbow with your left hand. Slowly bend your right arm until the weight in your right hand rests between your shoulders. Take three seconds to straighten your right arm to point to the ceiling again. Hold this position for a second. Take three seconds to lower the weight back toward your shoulders by bending your elbow. Keep supporting your right arm with your left hand throughout the exercise. Pause, then repeat 8 to 15 times. Repeat the exercise with your left arm, then do one more set with each arm.

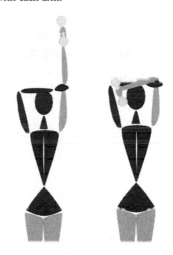

RELAX. Paced respiration, a form of deep breathing, works for a lot of women. You'll need some training to get it right, so check with your health-care provider. Yoga, meditation, and massages are also good ways to cut stress.

LOWER THE THERMOSTAT. Keep your house a little cooler than usual, especially at night. To get an extra boost of cold air, try aiming a fan at your side of the bed.

STOP SMOKING. Here's a good incentive to quit. Long-time smokers are more likely to have moderate to severe hot flashes. And the more you light up, the more you'll heat up. In one study, women who smoked more than a pack a day were more than 2.5 times more likely to report bad hot flashes than women who never smoked.

LOSE WEIGHT. Heavier women get more hot flashes and have a harder time cooling off, possibly because fat acts as insulation. In any case, if you're carrying around more pounds than you should, this is a good time to start eating wisely.

COOL DOWN YOUR DIET. Spicy food triggers hot flashes in many women. Too much caffeine can also bring on the sweats.

When to See the Doctor

*Hot flashes are normal occurrences during the menopause transition,
but they can also signal other medical problems.
Talk to your doctor if your hot flashes*

✤ ARE SO FREQUENT AND SEVERE THAT THEY INTERFERE WITH YOUR NORMAL
  FUNCTIONING.

✤ ARE ACCOMPANIED BY UNEXPLAINED LOSS OF WEIGHT.

✤ DON'T RESPOND TO LIFESTYLE CHANGES LIKE GETTING REGULAR EXERCISE.

DRINK WATER. At night, keep a glass of ice water by your bed; it might help cool you down if you wake up with a hot flash. You should also make a point of staying hydrated during the day.

WHAT'S GOING ON?

Q *I just had my first hot flash, and it was a freaky sensation. What exactly is going on in my body?*

A Hot flashes are completely normal and usually nothing to worry about. But knowing this doesn't help when you suddenly start sweating in the middle of a meeting or at some other equally inappropriate time. During a hot flash, you feel a sensation of warmth—even intense heat—spreading up from your torso to your face. Some women actually appear flushed; many experience rapid heartbeat. This can happen a few times a day or almost every hour. There's no rule. Generally, you'll cool down in a few minutes, although some women have individual hot flashes that last as long as half an hour. (See, it could be worse!) The average length is between 30 seconds and 5 minutes.

No one knows exactly what happens to your body during a hot flash, but it appears that changes in brain chemistry have something to do with it. One theory is that these changes may affect the hypothalamus, a region of the brain that controls all kinds of things: blood pressure, fluid and electrolyte balance, and body temperature. The hypothalamus gets input from all parts of your body as it goes about the job of keeping you running efficiently. When it senses a problem, it springs into action, adjusting heart rate and blood flow to the skin, among other things. It may be that during a hot flash fluctuating estrogen levels and hormones from your pituitary gland confuse the hypothalamus. Even before you feel the heat, the hypothalamus may be getting an incorrect message that your skin is too hot, so it tries to cool you off. Your heart pumps faster, the blood vessels in your skin dilate to circulate more blood (and get rid of the heat), and your sweat glands spring into overdrive. The "flushed" effect comes from the dilated blood vessels.

Newer studies suggest that another mechanism might be at work here. Dr. Robert R. Freedman and colleagues at Wayne State University in Detroit have used functional magnetic resonance imaging (fMRI) to observe the brain during a woman's hot flash. The area that showed the most activity was the insular cortex, which is responsible for understanding internal body events. Mysteriously, no activity was seen in the hypothalamus. Dr. Freedman's theory is that women who get hot flashes have a very narrow "thermo neutral zone"— the temperature(s) at which the body is neither sweating nor shivering. Women with frequent hot flashes have virtually no thermo-neutral zone; in women with no flashes, that zone is about 0.4 degrees Centigrade. Estrogen appears to widen the thermo-neutral zone, which would explain why hormone therapy reduces hot flashes. More research is under way, raising all our hopes that we may soon understand not only what causes hot flashes but also how to prevent them.

From the Past

"The blood surges to the head at the slightest provocation, making the eyes dim and the ears to ring and roar . . . swift waves of heat flash and throb from feet to crown, and one lives for a gasping minute in a furnace heated seven times hotter than an August noon."
—from *Eve's Daughter, or Common Sense for Maid, Wife and Mother,* by Marion Harland (1882)

Long before they were called "hot flashes," these symptoms were well known to women. Popular 19th-century treatments ran the gamut from useless to debilitating to toxic—opium, camphor, henbane, quinine, acetate of lead. If none of those worked, doctors ordered women to be bled. (One popular medical book of the era suggested draining 12 ounces.) But well into the 20th century, a lot of physicians thought hot flashes were more fantasy than fact. In his *Text-Book of Gynecology* (1901), Dr. C.A.L. Reed characterized them as a "subjective sensation and . . . not real."

WHEN WILL THEY STOP?

Q *Is there any way to tell how long my hot flashes will last?*

A Some women get a few hot flashes for a year or two around the time of the menopause transition. Others suffer for many years, and a very small percentage report occasional hot flashes for the rest of their lives. For women who are undergoing natural menopause, more severe hot flashes seem to indicate more years of fanning yourself. Still, there's no firm rule about this. Women who undergo surgical menopause also are more likely to have severe and long-lasting hot flashes; in one study, 90 percent of patients experienced continuing symptoms for more than eight years. But don't panic. Barring other complications, chances are that you will have passed the worst of it within a year or two of your last menstrual period.

DAY AND NIGHT

Q *What's the difference between hot flashes and night sweats?*

A Nothing, really, except timing. Hot flashes that occur at night are called night sweats. Doctors lump them both into the category of vasomotor symptoms. Sometimes night sweats are so bad that you have to change your nightclothes or even your bedding—and live with daytime grumpiness. In fact, many women think waking up drenched with sweat in the middle of the night is one of the worst symptoms of menopause. It's also one of the most unpredictable. In sleep studies of menopausal women, researchers have found that the majority sleep through many of their hot flashes. And the hot flashes that do wake us up aren't necessarily the longest in duration or the ones that raise our skin

temperature the most. No one knows why this is.

Night sweats can also be symptomatic of medical problems ranging from thyroid disease to some cancers. If you're waking up frequently, check with your doctor to make sure nothing else is going on.

FREQUENT FLASHER

Q *Some friends of mine say they hardly ever get a hot flash, but I think I have about 20 a day! What makes me so unlucky?*

A All women are not created equal when it comes to hot flashes. Frequency and duration can be the

---

FLASH FACTS

You say tomahto. You'll see them called hot flashes in some medical books and hot flushes in others. Both refer to the same pesky problem.

Why you're yawning. A National Sleep Foundation poll found that 44 percent of U.S. women going through menopause and 28 percent of postmenopausal women have hot flashes an average of three nights a week.

Hot spots. No one knows why, but hot flash rates vary widely around the world. In Hong Kong, only about 10 percent of women report getting hot flashes, compared with 62 percent in Australia, 68 percent in Canada, and 83 percent in the United Kingdom.

result of many factors, including your ethnic background, body weight, and even the amount of exercise you get. For reasons no one yet understands, African-American women have more hot flashes than Hispanic or Caucasian women do. Dutch women have more than women in North America. And Chinese factory workers in Hong Kong have far fewer than their Western counterparts. Frequency increases during perimenopause, when estrogen levels tend to fluctuate the most. You're also most likely to get them in the early evening, a few hours after the highest body temperature of the day. A history of premenstrual complaints, such as PMS, is also associated with hot flashes.

But not everything is preordained. Some lifestyle factors that can increase frequency include hot room temperatures, being overweight, current and past smoking, a lower level of physical activity, and lower socioeconomic status.

GOING BUGGY

Q *Just before a hot flash comes on, I get this creepy feeling—as if bugs are crawling all over me. Am I going crazy?*

A You're not crazy. That creepy feeling actually has a name (you'll love this): *formication*, which comes from the Latin word for "ant." You may also experience some other unsettling but not

harmful sensations, such as palpitations or a sudden increase in your heart rate. Some women also report a tingling in their feet or hands.

IS IT SOMETHING ELSE?

Q *I know hot flashes are normal during menopause, but could they also indicate some other medical condition?*

A Hot flashes can indeed be a sign of something else. That's true of many symptoms women get at midlife, so you should not neglect regular doctor visits during this period (or any other

Is It True?

Fiction: Men don't get hot flashes.

Fact: Men do get hot flashes if their testosterone levels drop suddenly. This kind of dramatic change happens, for example, when men with prostate cancer have their testes surgically removed or take medication that lowers their testosterone levels. And just as women can experience hot flashes for other reasons, so can men. Hyperthyroidism, some cancers, and even too much MSG can make a guy sweat. Any man who gets hot under the collar more than occasionally should talk to his doctor. A blood test can help decide if low testosterone or something else is the problem.

> ### HOT FLASH EMERGENCY KIT
>
> If you're worried about hot flashes at the office, here are some supplies to keep in your desk drawer:
>
> ◆ A package of moist towelettes so you can clean up in the restroom
>
> ◆ A clean bra and a T-shirt that's nice enough to go under a suit jacket
>
> ◆ A small bottle of cologne to make you feel better after you've changed
>
> ◆ A plastic bag for transporting soggy clothing

time, for that matter). Other causes of hot flashes include thyroid disease, epilepsy, infection, leukemia, and certain cancers. Some drugs, such as tamoxifen and raloxifene, also can cause hot flashes. In general, you should tell your doctor about any new symptom that continues for more than a week or two. You should also report changes in your body to your doctor if they interfere with your normal functioning. Don't be embarrassed to ask questions!

HOW HOT IS HOT?

Q *How hot do you really get in a hot flash? I feel like I'm burning up, but I know that there's a limit to how high my temperature gets.*

A Skin temperature can rise as much as seven degrees, although generally it's between one and four degrees. That's just the skin temperature; your internal body temperature (what you measure with a thermometer) doesn't change. After the initial flash, your skin temperature gradually returns to normal. That can take up to half an hour. It makes us grouchy just thinking about it.

A HOT AND COLD COUPLE

Q *I've controlled most of my night sweats by turning our bedroom into Antarctica. The air conditioner now runs on high 365 days a year (don't even ask about the electric bill). But while I'm finally getting enough sleep, my husband shivers all night and is threatening to decamp to the guest room.*

A Ah, the bedroom wars. During the menopause years, it's all a matter of degrees. No simple answer here, but you could try an electric blanket with dual temperature regulators. Another possibility is placing a fan near your side of the bed so your husband isn't disturbed by the breeze. You could also position the air-conditioner vents so they focus solely on you. Experiment a little. Maybe you don't have to keep the air conditioner on full blast; a few degrees cooler might be enough for you and won't make your husband feel as if he's in the deep freeze. Although a hot flash makes you feel like your body heat has skyrocketed in seconds, the actual change in temperature is small, sometimes only a few tenths of a degree. A slightly chilly room instead of a truly frigid one might be enough to let you both keep your cool.

IN THE OFFICE

Q *This is actually an etiquette question. Is it ever okay to explain why you're feeling uncomfortable if you have a hot flash at work? People don't mind saying they're getting over the flu or they were up all night with a sick kid. But I've never heard anyone say she's having a hot flash.*

A Your question reflects the fact that we live in a youth-obsessed society and hot flashes are a sign that you're getting older. It would be great if we could all acknowledge these things and just deal with them, but that's not where we are right now. So our answer is a mixed one. Generally, we would say you should dress in layers and just soldier on if you have a hot flash at the wrong moment. One surgeon we know says she does just that when she feels a hot flash in the middle of an operation. If she can keep going, you can, too! A possible exception might be when you're in a group of women you know well . . . and we mean *really* well, not just casual acquaintances. Then you could say something briefly. If it's a group of women close to your own age, try to make a joke out of it. Don't whine or complain—a good rule to follow for most tricky situations at work.

FROM SWEATING TO SHIVERS

Q *Maybe I'm just weird, but the worst part of a hot flash for me is afterwards, when I feel like I'm in Alaska. What causes that?*

A It's the contrast between your raised skin temperature during a hot flash and the return to normal, similar to what you experience when a fever suddenly breaks. You may find, for example, that if you have a hot flash at night, you first throw off the covers and then snuggle down into them in an effort to keep warm. The simplest way to deal with this is to wear lightweight pajamas and start off sleeping with the minimal bed covering or blanket. If you're cold later on, you can always add a throw blanket. During the day, dress in layers. You can take off a jacket or shawl if you feel hot without attracting too much attention and then put it back on when you've cooled down.

STRESSING OUT

Q *I can go for days without a flash, and then suddenly I'll start sweating when I'm talking to my boss. Is it just bad timing?*

A A lot of women find that stress brings on hot flashes, which is unfortunate since this is a time of life when stress is all around you—whether it's dealing with children, aging parents, or extra pressure in the office. Try relaxing with yoga sessions or meditation.

Regular physical activity can also help reduce overall tension. You might ask your clinician about paced respiration, a deep-breathing technique that has been found to decrease hot flashes in some women. You'll need some training to master it, but paced respiration basically involves breathing about a third slower than normal from deep in your abdomen, much like doing yoga breathing exercises.

TRACKING TRIGGERS

Q *I've noticed that I'm more likely to get hot flashes after I've had too much coffee or when I've had a spicy meal. Could these be the cause?*

A Although many women say there's no pattern to their hot flashes, others find they sweat in specific situations. These are called triggers. If you avoid your particular triggers, you could decrease the frequency of your hot flashes without medication. A good way to pinpoint triggers is to keep a hot flash diary (see below) for a few days and see if you can find any connection between what's going on in your life and the onset of the hot flash.

FEELING COOKED

Q *I understand that you're more likely to get hot flashes when you're stressed, but I get them even when I'm doing things I enjoy. Just the other day, I got one while making my specialty, banana bread. What happened?*

A We've seen absolutely no studies linking banana bread baking to hot flashes. However, it's possible that sticking your head into a hot oven might

---

Excerpt from a Hot Flash Diary

Day	Time	What I Was Doing
Monday	10:30 A.M.	Rushing to get to a meeting. I was late.
	3 P.M.	Just started drinking my mid-afternoon latte (second of the day).
	10:30 P.M.	Got into bed and was thinking about all I have to do tomorrow.
Tuesday	9 A.M.	Ran into Gina. Remembered I had forgotten to send her a thank-you note for the birthday present.
	1 P.M.	Ordered a sandwich at the deli and realized I had left my wallet back at the office.
	11 P.M.	Woke up after a nightmare.

have something to do with it. Many things can trigger a hot flash, and one of them is ambient heat—the temperature around you. So the reason you got a flash while cooking could well have been because that delicious bread baking in the oven pushed the thermometer up a few degrees too many. The best piece of advice we can give you is one you've probably heard before: If you can't stand the heat, get out of the kitchen.

SUDDEN CUTOFF

Q *Why are hot flashes so much more severe after induced menopause?*

A In natural menopause, your body gradually shuts down production of ovarian hormones. It's a process that usually takes years. But induced menopause—whether the result of surgery or radiation during cancer treatment—means that you're losing those hormones all at once and the shock to your body is greater.

WORK IT OUT

Q *Why does exercise help hot flashes? Doesn't it raise your body temperature? I certainly get all sweaty after a good workout.*

A The evidence about exercise and hot flashes is mixed. In observational studies, women who engaged in regular physical activity reported fewer

and less severe hot flashes than did sedentary women.

However, very strenuous exercise can actually trigger a hot flash in some women. So you're right to wonder about the effect of body temperature; there does seem to be a connection. But that's no excuse to avoid strenuous exercise. If you enjoy it and it keeps you fit, fine. Just be ready with a bottle of cold water in case you need to cool down in a hurry.

IS IT TIME FOR HORMONES?

The first line of defense against hot flashes should always be lifestyle changes. Quit smoking, lose weight, get regular exercise, wear layered clothing, and cut down on spicy foods and caffeine. If these or similar measures don't work and your hot flashes significantly interfere with your daily functioning, then you should talk to your doctor about drug therapy such as hormone treatment.

Although recent headlines have scared off many women, hormone therapy (estrogen together with a progestogen or estrogen alone) has been the prescription treatment of choice for hot flashes since the 1960s. By the '70s, doctors had concluded that their patients on hormone therapy appeared healthier and younger-looking than other women and started prescribing it not only for symptom relief but also as a preventive measure against heart disease and other ailments. Then came the Women's Health Initiative (WHI) and its findings that 1) combined therapy led to an increased risk of stroke, blood clots, and breast cancer, and 2) estrogen alone for women who'd had a hysterectomy offered no protection against heart disease and increased risk of stroke and blood clots. (See Chapter 2.) Many women threw out their pills; others kept taking them while worrying about the long-term effects. Before you reject this option, you should know that the WHI was designed to see if estrogen could prevent heart disease, as many doctors believed. That's why the average age of the women in the study was 63—a long way from menopause. It's not clear how the results apply to younger women who want to take estrogen for a few years to ease hot flashes.

So what's the bottom line? Now that doctors have had time to review the WHI data, many say they would still prescribe hormones for women who are suffering from moderate to severe hot flashes as long as the patient has no risk factors: basically, no history of breast or endometrial cancer, heart attack, blood clots, or stroke. If you're still perimenopausal, you might get a low-dose birth-control pill as long as you don't smoke and have no other risk factors. Women who are just about at menopause and still have a uterus get a combination of estrogen and progesterone (or a progestin) because of the risk of endometrial cancer if estrogen is taken alone. Women who've had a hysterectomy take only estrogen. (See Appendix I for a comparison of different approaches.)

Patients need to wait at least four weeks before they feel the full effect of hormone therapy. Current recommendations are to prescribe the smallest effective dose for the shortest amount of time consistent with treatment goals. When you stop hormone therapy, your vulnerability to hot flashes could be over. Unfortunately, that's not true for everyone, and some women go back on hormones because of recurring hot flashes.

At this point in the research, the decision is very much an individual one. There is no single right answer. You have to weigh the potential risks and benefits in consultation with your doctor. And you can stop at any time. In fact, you should always revisit your decision during your annual checkup.

MORE THAN PILLS

Q *What if I don't want to take pills? Are there any other forms of hormone therapy that help with hot flashes?*

A In the United States, most women choose to use the pill form of hormone therapy because they're used to taking medication orally, but women in other countries are more likely to take hormones in the form of a patch, a gel, a cream, an intrauterine device, or a shot. One of these, especially the patch, may be a smarter way to go. The advantage of the non-pill forms is that they aren't processed by your liver and go directly into your bloodstream or to the area of your body that needs help (like your vagina). Avoiding the stomach or liver also seems to decrease the risk of blood clots. Which form you choose may depend on your reason for using hormone therapy. Creams, gels, and patches applied to your arms, legs, or torso would be a good option for you since hot flashes are your top complaint. For women troubled by vaginal dryness or pain during intercourse, vaginal rings or vaginal tablets might work best. As with oral hormone therapy, risks and benefits must be evaluated on an individual basis.

WHAT ABOUT ANDROGENS?

Q *I know that estrogen isn't the only sex hormone swirling through my body. Do androgen levels change during menopause? And could that play any role in hot flashes?*

A Although we don't understand the exact mechanism of hot flashes, fluctuating levels of estrogen are the most likely culprit. Levels of androgens are lower as well, but the drop isn't dramatic. Testosterone and other androgens reach a peak when you're about 20; by about age 45, the level has fallen by 50 percent and continues to decline gradually for the rest of your life. An estrogen-androgen product called Estratest is marketed to women whose hot flashes aren't responding to standard hormone therapy, but there are no strong clinical data to confirm that the testosterone in it adds anything to the mix. (Estratest is often prescribed to treat lack of sexual desire during the menopause transition, but it is not FDA-approved for this purpose.) In addition to the risks of hormone therapy, too much androgen can induce male sexual characteristics such as deepening of the voice and facial hair. The North American Menopause Society does not recommend the combination of estrogen and androgen for women whose hot flashes aren't responding to hormone therapy.

WHAT ELSE IS OUT THERE?

Q *What if you don't want to try hormone therapy? Is there any other medication that helps?*

A The anticonvulsant Neurontin (gabapentin) can help with hot flashes and is recommended by the North American Menopause Society for women who cannot use other medications. Neurontin has been shown to be more effective than a placebo in reducing hot flashes in randomized controlled studies and seems to be a safer choice than hormone therapy for someone who has had breast cancer. Doctors at the Mayo Clinic who researched gabapentin as a treatment for hot flashes sometimes use it in combination with antidepressants. Catapres (clonidine) is an antihypertensive drug that reduces the frequency of hot flashes in some women. You can't take it if you have certain heart conditions, and it can cause arrhythmias in high dosages. It's also recommended by the North American Menopause Society. But again, you need to ask your doctor if they're appropriate for you.

ANTIDEPRESSANTS

Q *If antidepressants can help control hot flashes, should I try one even if I'm not feeling blue?*

A Antidepressants may be a good option for women who have had breast cancer or who can't take hormone therapy for some other reason. Women who have been on hormone therapy for at least a few months and are still suffering from hot flashes might also want to try them. Three drugs have been shown to help: Effexor (venlafaxine), Paxil (paroxetine), and Prozac (fluoxetine). Effexor can reduce hot flashes from 40 to 60 percent (depending on the dose) and works fairly quickly, within two weeks. Paxil seems to be similarly effective. Prozac was shown to work better than a placebo in one study but does not appear to work as well as Effexor or Paxil. All of these drugs have possible side effects, including sleepiness, sexual dysfunction, and dizziness, and may interact with other medications.

HOT FLASHES FROM TAMOXIFEN

Q *I'm taking tamoxifen for breast cancer and have started having hot flashes. What can I do to make them less bothersome?*

A Hot flashes are the most common side effect of tamoxifen, probably because it blocks the effects of estrogen in many parts of your body. And those declining estrogen levels produce all the symptoms of menopause, including hot flashes.

The best recommendation is to try the lifestyle routine before you consider other steps. Exercise regularly, lower the room temperature, wear light clothing. If these don't work, talk to your doctor about medication. This is tricky because the most effective treatment, hormone therapy, is not recommended for breast cancer patients since estrogen could stimulate growth of cancer cells. You can try antidepressants such as Effexor, Prozac, and Paxil, but ongoing research indicates that some antidepressants, Prozac in particular, may reduce tamoxifen's effectiveness. Another option for you may be clonidine, a drug used in the treatment of high blood pressure. It's been shown to be effective in studies, but the side effects can be rather unpleasant: insomnia, dry mouth, and constipation.

So there's no easy answer here. You may just have to wait it out. Hot flashes from tamoxifen usually subside in three to six months.

Q *I'm 46 years old, and I've been getting hot flashes for the past few months. The hot part doesn't really bother me, but the redness does. My face is a mess. It almost looks like I have acne. What's happening to me?*

A Falling estrogen levels and hot flashes can trigger a skin disorder called acne rosacea even if you've never had it before. This is particularly true if you're fair-skinned. No one knows what causes rosacea, but the symptoms are hard to hide: pimples and facial redness that is often accompanied by stinging or burning. In the early stages, it looks like a bad sunburn; more advanced cases can be disfiguring. Rosacea, which usually starts in your 30s or 40s, can also affect your eyes, neck, and back. There's no surefire cure, but for women your age doctors might prescribe hormone therapy or an antidepressant to cut down on the flushing. A topical cream or antibiotic can also be used for more severe cases of rosacea. Your doctor will help you decide which treatment approach to take.

WHAT ELSE CAN YOU DO?

A ctivities that promote relaxation— such as yoga, massage, meditation, or even a nice long bath—can help to reduce the frequency and severity of hot flashes. This is especially true if you notice that stress and tension are triggers for you. Although there are no controlled clinical trials that prove this, we think they're certainly worth a try. At the very least, they'll provide a few moments of peace.

Other alternatives include soy products, black cohosh, ginseng, evening primrose oil, and vitamin E. Read on to learn the pros and cons of each.

SOY. Many women swear that soy products help to decrease the frequency and intensity of hot flashes, but the science on this is unclear. We should have more answers in a few years, when we get results from a major soy study funded by the National Institute on Aging. In the meantime, it probably won't hurt to add soy milk or tofu to your diet. Using soy supplements is more problematical. Soy contains plant chemicals called isoflavones, which may help fight cancer. But isoflavones mimic estrogen and scientists worry that women at risk for breast cancer might consume too much and trigger growth of malignant cells. If you're considering soy supplements, the recommended dosage is 40 to 80 milligrams a day, but talk to your doctor about your medical history before you run out to the health food store.

BLACK COHOSH. A traditional treatment for the ills of menopause, black cohosh has been prescribed in Germany for more than 40 years to ease hot flashes, depression, and sleep problems. However, just because it has been used for a long time doesn't mean it's safe. (We thought hormone therapy was perfectly safe until the WHI results.) There's a lot we don't know about black cohosh, including how it works—or even if it works at all. At this point, there are no convincing data to support using it. Most of the studies have been relatively short—just a few months. Also, not all black cohosh products are the same. One study found that 3 of 11 supplements contained no black cohosh at all. The North American Menopause Society specifically warns women with breast cancer to stay away from black cohosh because of contradictory evidence about its safety for them. Recent studies have indicated that black cohosh may cause liver damage in some women. In fact, the agency that regulates health care products in the United Kingdom has determined that all products carrying black cohosh should carry a warning.

HERBS AND OILS. Get together with a group of women and you'll probably hear someone sing the praises of products like ginseng, evening primrose oil, dong quai, licorice, and Chinese herb mixtures. Because there's no clinical evidence of their safety, the North American Menopause Society doesn't recommend any of them, and even giving them a try without your doctor's okay can be risky. In large enough doses, they can interfere with your prescription medications and may bring on debilitating side effects such as cardiac arrhythmias (licorice), uterine bleeding (ginseng), and diarrhea (evening primrose oil). These products are unregulated, which means you don't know what you're taking. Why do your friends say they work? It could be the placebo effect. In studies of hot flash drugs, participants taking a placebo frequently report an impressive decline in symptoms close to that produced by the medication being tested. In other words, just thinking you're getting help often does the trick.

VITAMIN E. In 2004, Johns Hopkins researchers, investigating the theory that vitamin E increases longevity, found the opposite to be true. Daily doses of 400 international units (IUs) and above, the standard amount in vitamin E capsules, slightly decreased longevity. The dose in a typical multivitamin, 30 IUs, is well below that. But women with a vitamin K deficiency should steer clear; they may have uterine bleeding if they take too much vitamin E.

CHAPTER 4

Sleep

Here's an all-too-familiar late-night scenario: You climb into bed exhausted; before you know it, you're deep in dreamland. Then, perhaps an hour or two later, something startles you out of this much-needed rest. Maybe it's that special someone snoring at your side. Or it could be a hot flash that left your pajamas drenched in sweat. Or maybe it's anxiety about college tuition bills or an elderly parent or a problem at work. Whatever the cause, now you're wide awake and no amount of tossing and turning can get you back to sleep. You watch in despair as the numbers of your bedside digital clock flip relentlessly toward dawn. In the morning, you're bleary-eyed and irritable, snapping at everyone.

At menopause, a wide range of physiological and emotional issues can converge to rob women of the sleep they desperately need. A recent poll by the National Sleep Foundation found that 40 percent of menopausal women suffer from some type of sleep problem; 56 percent say they frequently deal with insomnia. You may think feeling rested is a luxury, but lack of sleep is a major health issue. It can make you more vulnerable to a number of diseases, including diabetes, high blood pressure, heart disease, and stroke. It also does a real number on your emotions. Many women who complain about moodiness at this stage of life don't realize that lack of sleep may be the cause.

What Can Happen

✤ More trouble falling asleep and staying asleep

✤ Becoming sleepy earlier in the evening

✤ Waking up earlier

✤ Sleep disturbed by night sweats

✤ Problems going back to sleep after awakening

✤ Less deep sleep

✤ More frequent arousals

✤ Waking up to go to the bathroom once or twice a night

Sleep problems are often ignored by women themselves or misdiagnosed by their doctors, who may not have gotten much training about sleep in medical school and don't understand how complex it is. Your sleep troubles may be directly related to hormonal gymnastics or aging, or perhaps a sleep disorder has just decided to show itself now. The more you know about the subject, the better your chances of getting a good night's sleep.

WHAT YOU NEED TO KNOW

You no longer sleep like a baby or even like a teenager (roused only by a major decibel assault). Although you once enjoyed a solid eight hours of sleep a night, you may be so exhausted now that you would happily settle for a meager five or six. Well, that dream is still possible but increasingly difficult as you age. Here's why. Sleep can be divided into two phases: rapid eye movement (REM) sleep and non-REM sleep. You alternate four or five times between these two phases during the night. Most dreaming occurs during REM sleep. The non-REM phase is divided into four stages, progressing from light to deep sleep. This pattern is called "sleep architecture," and it changes as you get older. You spend less time in deep sleep and more time in the lighter levels of sleep, where you can be awakened more easily by a barking dog or a newspaper tossed on your front porch. As you get older, you may have more trouble falling asleep and may wake up earlier, which means you get fewer total hours of slumber.

After age 50, women are more likely than men to complain about lack of sleep. That's not just because they're kvetches. Women are generally more sensitive to the mood alterations caused by lack of sleep. In laboratory studies, older women's estimates of their sleep quality were more accurate than men's. Certain sleep disorders are also more common in older women. These include sleep-disordered breathing, which is characterized by loud snoring. (Yes, women do snore, even though men usually get all the flak for it.) Women who are overweight and physically inactive are more likely to suffer from this disor-

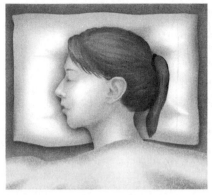

YOUNG ADULT

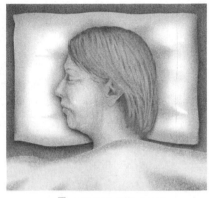

ELDERLY ADULT

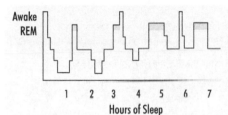

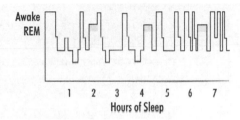

HOW OUR SLEEP PATTERNS CHANGE AS WE AGE

As we get older, we generally spend less time in deep sleep and about the same amount of time in the REM phase. Our overall physical health and emotional well-being also play a key role in how much rest we get.

der. Some scientists believe it may also be related to lower progesterone levels, since younger women who've undergone surgically induced menopause are also at higher risk.

WHAT IS INSOMNIA?

Q *Lately, I've been having a lot of trouble falling asleep no matter how tired I am. My periods are becoming irregular. Could there be a connection?*

A If you can rule out a situation that might be troubling you right now (a project at work or a family prob-

lem, for example), you should let your doctor know that you're not getting enough sleep. Chronic insomnia, or insomnia that persists for more than three nights a week over an extended period of time, afflicts about 10 percent of adults and is more common in women and older people. Women tend to find that it gets worse at menopause. Your doctor will look for an underlying physical or psychological cause, anything from back pain to a sleep disorder, to see if your sleeplessness is a symptom of another problem. But in about 25 percent of all patients who come in with chronic insomnia, doctors are unable to

When to See the Doctor

You should see your physician if you experience these
problems frequently:

❖ TROUBLE BREATHING OR LOUD SNORING (OFTEN REPORTED BY BED PARTNER)

❖ HEADACHES IN THE MIDDLE OF THE NIGHT OR MORNING

❖ HEARTBURN

❖ IRREGULAR HEARTBEAT (VERY FAST OR VERY SLOW)

❖ CONSTANT NEED TO GO TO THE BATHROOM (MORE THAN ONCE OR TWICE A NIGHT)

❖ SEVERE SWEATING

❖ A CONSISTENT PATTERN OF MORE THAN NINE HOURS OR LESS THAN FIVE HOURS OF SLEEP A NIGHT

❖ LEG DISCOMFORT THAT IMPROVES WITH MOVEMENT AND GETS WORSE IN THE EVENING

---

find anything else wrong. In these cases, it's called primary insomnia, which some researchers theorize may actually be arousal disorder. The body chemistry of these patients may predispose them to hyper-alertness when they're deprived of sleep (as opposed to the rest of us, who nod off when we're sleepy).

People who don't get enough sleep may be at greater risk for many health problems, including cardiovascular disease, obesity, depression, and viral illnesses. They're also more likely to experience moodiness as well as memory, concentration, and relationship problems, household accidents, and car crashes—not to mention a loss of productivity and alertness both at work and at home.

A HORMONAL ALARM CLOCK

Q *What would menopausal women do without Starbucks? We're all sleep-deprived! Are raging hormones to blame?*

A It's true that about half of all midlife women report trouble sleeping, but fluctuating hormone levels may start disturbing your sleep way before you hit your menopause years. Many women feel extra tired after ovulation because of rising levels of progesterone, a hormone that causes sleepiness. If the egg that's released does not get fertilized, progesterone levels fall rapidly as the uterus sheds its inner lining. This is typically when menstruating women have a few restless nights.

During the menopause years, hormone levels start to fluctuate in an erratic pattern rather than a predictable cycle. You get hot flashes and night sweats as your brain responds to this hormonal zigzagging. Although many women say the sleep disruption is minimal, others have problems for several years. Women whose ovaries are surgically removed (causing an immediate drop in hormone levels) and those at the end of the menopause transition generally report the highest rates of sleep disturbances.

Fluctuating estrogen and progesterone production may disrupt sleep because of these hormones' effect on breathing, stress reaction, mood, and body temperature (apart from hot flashes). Some animal studies indicate that estrogen and progesterone may also play a role in setting circadian rhythms (the sleep-wake cycle). In one study, researchers removed the ovaries of hamsters and found that the animals' circadian rhythms went haywire; when they were given hormone therapy, their sleep patterns returned to normal.

Do I Really Snore?

Q *For years, I've been complaining that my husband's snoring keeps me awake. Now he says I'm snoring just as loudly as he is! I've never snored before. Why would I start now?*

A Many women start snoring for the first time around the menopause transition, with the problem becoming more common and more serious as time goes on. Snoring is not just annoying and embarrassing (although it certainly is both of those things to you and your partner). It can also be a sign of sleep-related breathing disorders like apnea, which are more likely after menopause. The incidence of apnea in men also increases with age, but there may be something about the hormonal changes during menopause itself that increases the risk for women. In men, neck size and obesity are markers for apnea. The correlation isn't quite as clear for women, even though we, too, are more likely to have fat in the neck area as we get older. Until researchers understand what else could be at work here, you should let your doctor know what's going on. Apnea can cause high blood pressure and increase your risk of cardiovascular disease and stroke. Also, anyone who has breathing problems during the day could be at risk for apnea at night. Fortunately, a variety of treatments are available (see pages 76–77).

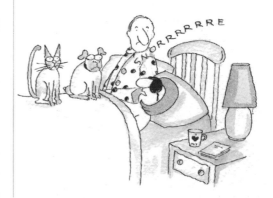

COMMON SLEEP DISORDERS

Although sleep science is relatively new, scientists have already identified more than 70 sleep disorders. Luckily, most can be treated with drugs or behavioral changes.

Apnea. This is the most common sleep disorder, afflicting about 20 million Americans. Many people think of it as a men's disease, but women are also vulnerable, particularly after menopause. You may be at risk if you snore, are overweight, have high blood pressure, or have a physical abnormality in your nose or throat.

Apnea appears in several forms. One is related to an abnormality in the nervous system that disturbs the electrical signaling to the muscles used for breathing. Another, called obstructive sleep apnea, occurs when something blocks your airways at night. Normally, as you sleep, muscles in your upper airway keep your breathing passage open as air moves through your nose, into your throat, and on into your lungs. In obstructive sleep apnea, the breathing passage can become blocked because of problems ranging from oversize tonsils to pressure caused by obesity. Many women with sleep-related breathing difficulties develop upper airway resistance syndrome, where the airway narrows but is not fully blocked. You're at risk for this if you're obese or have allergies, nasal congestion, a small chin, or tonsils. In these cases, snoring or irregular breathing may not be loud enough for your bed partner to notice, which means the problem could go undiagnosed.

When blockage or narrowing occurs repeatedly, oxygen levels in your body fall and your brain gets an emergency signal that rouses you enough to resume normal breathing. Although you'll likely be unaware of this arousal, it can devastate your sleep; some patients have hundreds of apneic episodes a night, typified by unusually long breaks between breaths followed by snorts, gasps, or snoring. You are more likely to notice headaches in the middle of the night or when you wake up in the morning, as well as severe daytime sleepiness.

Too often, it takes women years to get the right diagnosis; by then, chronic sleep deprivation may have worsened their overall health. Apnea can cause high blood pressure, and over time its symptoms can resemble those of psychiatric illnesses, especially depression.

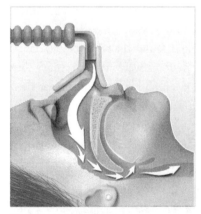

HELP AT NIGHT
Normally, air flows freely through the throat area, but during apnea the passage is blocked. A CPAP device lightly blows air into your throat to keep the passage open all night.

Some apnea sufferers become so exhausted that they fall asleep in the middle of sex.

If you're suffering from apnea, your doctor will probably suggest that you lose weight, cut back on tobacco and alcohol (which can convert regular snoring to apnea), and avoid certain drugs. You can also use pillows or other devices that help you sleep on your side. Other patients may need mechanical devices to keep their airways open, such as CPAP (for continuous positive airway pressure) and dental devices. Hormone therapy has also proved helpful. Lower levels of estrogen may weaken the cartilage of the airways, making them more vulnerable to collapse when you're sleeping. This is an area of active study.

Restless legs syndrome (RLS). Common symptoms of this disorder—painful sensations in the legs or arms, often described as tingling, creeping, or crawling—are worse when you're lying down or sitting for a long time and tend to increase in frequency and severity during the night. As the name implies, patients have a persistent urge to keep moving their legs, which makes symptoms dissipate briefly. Although the cause is unclear, RLS is known to run in families. The incidence and severity of symptoms increase with age. Some pregnant women may experience RLS, but the symptoms usually go away after birth. In other cases, RLS is associated with low iron levels or chronic diseases such as diabetes or rheumatoid arthritis. It can also be caused by chemotherapy. Eliminating caffeine sometimes helps, as does a hot bath, heating pad, ice pack, or leg massage. In any case, you don't have to suffer. Drugs used to treat Parkinson's disease work remarkably well on RLS patients.

Narcolepsy. More than 250,000 Americans are affected by narcolepsy, a condition characterized by drowsiness and daytime sleep attacks, as well as cataplexy (loss of muscle function often triggered by emotion, especially laughing). The sleep attacks, which occur even after a good night's rest, can last from a few seconds to half an hour. Narcoleptics are at high risk for car accidents since they can fall asleep at the wheel. Many people with this disorder have not been diagnosed; the average woman with narcolepsy waits 15 years before a doctor figures out what's wrong! In the meantime, women's symptoms are often mistaken for epilepsy or depression or anxiety.

Parasomnias. This category includes *REM behavior disorder,* in which sleepers act out vivid dreams—often to the distress of their bed partners, who can wake up with bruises if the dream content is violent. Most patients are middle-aged or older. *Sleep-related eating disorder* primarily affects women and often begins in the late teens and early 20s; patients raid the kitchen at night in search of high-calorie food, unaware of their actions until they step on the scale in the morning. Various medications have been used to treat these problems, but they appear to work best when combined with behavioral therapy.

HOT TIMES TONIGHT

Q *I'm 51, and my hot flashes are
so severe that I sometimes wake up
three or four times a night drenched with
sweat. At least a couple of times a week,
I have to change my pajamas before I go
back to bed. This is also a problem for
my husband—neither of us
is getting enough sleep. I
know hormone therapy is
effective in stopping hot
flashes, but I'm worried
about the health risks.*

A A lot of women
were scared off hor-
mones by the abrupt ending of the
Women's Health Initiative study in
2002. But going cold turkey overnight
may have been an overreaction. Here's
why: The women in the WHI study
averaged 63 years of age and started
estrogen-progestin therapy many years
after menopause to help determine estrogen's ability to prevent heart disease. The
results did indicate that these women
were at slightly higher risk for breast cancer, heart disease, blood clots, and stroke;
however, no one knows whether the
same is true for younger women in good
health who use hormone therapy for a
short period of time to treat acute symptoms like yours.

Before you consider any medication,
increase your exercise (but not close to
bedtime); limit alcohol, caffeine, and
tobacco; wear light clothing to bed; keep
the bedroom cool. Your doctor should
also rule out any other medical conditions that might cause night sweats, such
as thyroid disease, cancer, or chronic
infections. If your problem is still unresolved, talk to your doctor about hormone therapy. Chronic sleep disruptions
are a risk to your health; low-dose hormone therapy may be the
most effective way to stop
them. It's very much an
individual decision that
you and your doctor will
have to make in light of
your unique medical
history. (For more on this,
see Chapters 2 and 3.)

SETTING THE MOOD

I f your sleep problems have lasted more
than a week or two, get a physical to
rule out underlying medical conditions
that disrupt slumber. If you're basically
healthy, your doctor will probably suggest
that you start by improving your "sleep
hygiene." That's the lingo sleep experts
use to describe behavior that affects how
easily you fall and stay asleep. An important first step is to use your bedroom only
for sleeping and sex, not for watching TV
or paying the bills. You want to train your
brain to slow down in bed and keep daytime anxieties from spilling over into the
night. Some other tips:

A RELAXING BATH. Just before bedtime,
luxuriate in the bath. Keep your bedroom on the cool side and then snuggle

under the covers. The switch from warm to cool is relaxing and sleep-inducing.

NOISE BUSTERS. It could be your partner's snoring, a neighbor's dog barking, airplanes roaring overhead, or a toilet flushing down the hall. These sounds probably wouldn't have been a problem when you were a teenager, but as we get older our sleep is more easily interrupted by noise. Ear plugs (especially wax ones) can help. Other options are "white noise" machines, fans, or air conditioners. These last two do double duty if you're having hot flashes. If falling asleep is your biggest problem, try soothing music on the clock radio. Set it to go off in an hour and turn on classical or new age, the two genres that worked best in one study.

EXPOSURE TO SUNSHINE. This is especially important during the short days of winter. A daily dose of sunshine encourages your body's optimal production of the hormone melatonin, which will help you maintain your natural circadian rhythm so you stay alert during the day and are more likely to sleep at night.

KEEP IT DARK. Some people are extremely sensitive to the smallest amount of light at night. Even the glow from the clock radio might distract you from sleeping (turn it away from you and see what happens). Cutting down on light in the hours before bed also tells your brain it's time to sleep.

EXERCISE STRATEGY. This is a little tricky. Daily physical activity helps you sleep, but timing is everything. You should stop working out at least three hours before you go to bed. All those endorphins can keep you alert and stimulated. (Yoga is the exception.) Try heading for the gym in the morning instead. It's a great way to get you going for the day.

COMFORTABLE BEDDING. Is your mattress old or lumpy? Too hard or too soft? Invest in a new one. The right pillows can make a difference, too. There are special ones for side sleepers, back sleepers, and stomach sleepers. If you have allergies, try getting rid of your down pillows or down comforter. You could also experiment with unscented detergent and fabric softener. If hot flashes are keeping you up, buy a lightweight cotton blanket that you can toss off easily.

ROUTINE, ROUTINE, ROUTINE. Maintaining regular hours makes a big difference; it "sets" your body's clock. Make a point of going to bed and getting up at the same time every day. Even if you have a late night, get up at your usual hour. You can't always control when you fall asleep, but you can make sure that your wake-up time is consistent. If you travel to a different time zone, set a new routine as quickly as possible so you can continue to get your normal hours of sleep.

LEARNING TO RELAX

Q *My doctor said my sleep problems may have more to do with stress than with menopause and suggested I try some relaxation techniques. Which ones help with insomnia?*

A Stress can be a big barrier to a good night's sleep as well as a drag on your overall health. Think about all the demands on your time and the tough job you have balancing it all. It's no wonder that your mind is still buzzing at bedtime. It may seem a little ironic that you're stressed because you have no time and now you're being asked to find more time to relax to relieve that stress, but think of it this way: When you're not sleeping well, you're more likely to have problems with concentration and memory and you do everything less efficiently. You could actually save yourself time by taking the time to relax.

A number of techniques work, such as meditation, biofeedback, cognitive-behavior therapy, acupuncture, progressive muscle relaxation, and visualization or mental imagery. Some of these techniques can be self-taught with the help of tapes, videos, and DVDs. Others, such as cognitive-behavior therapy (a form of psychotherapy), paced respiration, and acupuncture require expert help. Your doctor may be able to suggest resources. The trick is to find several techniques that suit you and your lifestyle and then occasionally switch from one to another to keep it interesting (just as you should do for your routine at the gym). But perhaps most importantly, you have to be committed to the idea. If you're determined to learn one or more of these techniques and do them seriously and consistently, relaxation can prove very successful. Even if your whole problem isn't solved, chances are that stress reduction will need to be part of your overall sleep strategy. If you eventually decide to use some medication, these techniques can help you get off the meds sooner or reduce your dosage over time.

WINE AT NIGHT

Q *For years, a glass of wine in the evening was enough to help me relax and fall asleep. These days, I sometimes have trouble falling asleep after a drink. More often, I find myself waking up in the middle of the night and being unable to fall back asleep. Is it just me, or is it menopause?*

A It's not menopause, but it may be age. As you get older, your body doesn't metabolize alcohol as well as it did when you were in your 20s. You will have higher blood alcohol levels than a younger person, even after drinking the same amount.

Timing is also important. That glass of merlot may initially relax you, but your body will be processing it for many hours. Even a moderate amount of alcohol (12 ounces of beer, 5 ounces of wine, or 1.5 ounces of distilled spirits)

FOODS THAT MAKE YOU SLEEPY

Dairy products, seafood, meat, poultry, whole grains, and peanuts all contain tryptophan, an amino acid that your brain needs to produce the sleep-inducing neurotransmitter serotonin. Eating these foods with carbohydrates makes tryptophan more available to your brain. That's because carbs stimulate insulin, which lowers the blood level of other amino acids that compete with tryptophan. And the more tryptophan in your brain, the more serotonin. This is one reason that so many people feel like napping after turkey and stuffing on Thanksgiving (the other is eating or drinking too much). For the rest of the year, try a bedtime snack that combines a small amount of protein containing tryptophan and complex carbohydrates, like half a peanut butter sandwich on whole wheat bread or an oatmeal cookie and milk. Will warm milk make you sleep any better? Maybe, if the warmth of the liquid helps you relax, but it won't raise the amount of tryptophan in the milk. And what about alcohol? After all, a snifter of brandy after dinner has always made you a little sleepy, right? Well, as you get older, that comforting glass of brandy is more likely to wake you up in the middle of the night (and make you sweat and give you a headache).

consumed within an hour of bedtime seems to disturb the second half of sleep. You're more likely to wake up and have trouble getting back to sleep. So drinking earlier should help, right? Not necessarily. Even moderate amounts of alcohol in the late afternoon or at dinner can increase wakefulness long into the night. The alcohol itself is gone from your body by then, but the effects on the sleep-regulating mechanisms can linger for hours. Alcohol consumption also increases the chance of developing snoring and sleep-related breathing disorders such as apnea. Menopause is another risk factor for these disorders, so when you combine the two, your chances of a good night's sleep sink. Best advice: Drink very moderately and never near bedtime.

NIGHTTIME WAKE-UPS

Q *I fall asleep pretty quickly, but then I wake up an hour later and often have trouble getting back to sleep. What could be happening to make me wake up at the same time every night?*

A Some possible explanations for this problem are benign, but others are potentially serious. It could be something as simple as an outside noise that happens around the same time every night, perhaps a neighbor returning home late from work and slamming the car door. You may be more likely to hear these noises now because, as we get older, we tend to sleep more lightly. A sleep-related breathing disorder could also be waking you up. A few questions you should

From the Past

At the turn of the last century, female physicians (whose numbers were beginning to rise) often discussed the problem of sleep during menopause, especially as it related to hot flashes, in their advice books. In *Perfect Womanhood for Maidens-Wives-Mothers* (1903), Dr. Mary Melendy wrote very reassuringly about menopause as a natural transition and emphasized the importance of exercise, fresh air, nutritious food, and pleasant diversions. As for sleep, her remedy was more extreme: fasting.

think about before talking to your doctor: Do you have the same problem on vacation or in any new environment? Does your partner say you snore or have any other signs of a breathing disorder? Have you tried varying your sleep time by going to bed an hour later or earlier? Another possibility is restless legs syndrome (see page 77). Does your partner say your legs twitch at night?

In the meantime, if you wake up in the middle of the night and can't fall back asleep after 15 or 20 minutes, get up and leave the bedroom. Try reading a book or listening to relaxing music until you feel sleepy. If you're waking up because you're worried about a list you meant to write or a chore you meant to do before bed, get up and do it. That often

helps to ease your anxiety. Watching TV, especially in bed, is generally not a good idea. Getting hooked on Letterman or a movie could keep you up even longer. If you do turn on the tube, go to another room so your brain associates your bed with sleeping, not watching. Stay awake until you're really ready to fall asleep for the night in the bedroom (not on the couch with the movie still on).

RISING TOO EARLY

Q *Back in the day, I could sleep until noon. Now I go to bed late and can't stay asleep past seven. What's wrong?*

A We all feel nostalgia for those days when we slept like babies—or at least teenagers. But for most of us, those days are gone forever. As we get older, we're more likely to go to bed earlier and wake up earlier. Our sleep is more easily disturbed by light or noise that we might have been able to ignore years ago. You may find some relief with a few environmental changes. Is the early morning sun waking you? Try a darkening curtain or shade that blocks it. Ear plugs help if noise is a problem. You should also try to keep a regular schedule because it's harder to recover from constant changes in your sleep cycle. If your problem is severe and makes you excessively sleepy during the day, you might be suffering from advanced sleep phase syndrome (ASPS), which is

FOODS THAT CAN KEEP YOU UP

You've had a night out with the girls at your favorite Mexican place: a beef-and-bean burrito washed down with a Diet Coke, two scoops of chocolate ice cream for dessert, and a decaf espresso. A good dinner usually knocks you out, but now it seems to be having the opposite effect. Why is sleep so elusive? Your menu might be part of the problem. Rich and spicy foods, sugary desserts, and even beans (because they're likely to cause gas) can interfere with slumber. But the biggest offender is caffeine, which is not found in coffee or tea alone. That's why picking decaf isn't enough. Chocolate, soft drinks, juice, ice cream, yogurt, and even some over-the-counter medications contain enough caffeine to keep you alert long past midnight. Although caffeine usually reaches its peak concentration in your bloodstream within an hour after you've downed that espresso, the effects can last up to six hours or even longer in some people. Caffeine can also increase the frequency or intensity of hot flashes—another good reason to avoid it at this point in your life. Here's how some different sources of caffeine compare:

PRODUCT	SERVING SIZE	MILLIGRAMS OF CAFFEINE
Brewed coffee	8 ounces	135
Instant coffee	8 ounces	95
Decaf coffee	8 ounces	5
Tea, leaf or bag	8 ounces	50
Green tea	8 ounces	30
Instant tea	8 ounces	15
Mountain Dew	12 ounces	55.5
Diet Coke	12 ounces	46.5
Coca-Cola Classic	12 ounces	34.5
Ben & Jerry's No Fat Coffee Fudge frozen yogurt	1 cup	85
Häagen-Dazs coffee ice cream	1 cup	58
Dannon coffee yogurt	8 ounces	45
Hershey milk chocolate bar	1 bar (1.5 ounces)	10
Cocoa or hot chocolate	8 ounces	32
NoDoz, maximum strength	1 tablet	200
Dristan	1 tablet	30
Midol	1 tablet	32

relatively rare but more common in elderly people. The treatment involves readjusting your sleep clock by slowly delaying your bedtime until you're able to wake up at a reasonable hour. Sometimes, that therapy is combined with exposure to bright light at the end of the day. Your problem could also be a symptom of depression (see Chapter 8). Or you might be suffering from apnea (see page 76). Apnea is at its worst at the end of the night, when you seem to be waking up.

WHAT IF IT'S DEPRESSION?

Q *I've got a classic chicken-and-egg dilemma. I'm perimenopausal and haven't been sleeping well. I also have classic symptoms of depression: low energy, irritability, no sex drive, trouble concentrating. How do I know if depression is causing the sleep problems or lack of sleep (perhaps from hormonal fluctuations) is making me feel depressed?*

A Teasing out whether your problem is menopause or depression isn't easy because fluctuating hormones do have an effect on the neurotransmitters in your brain. Sometimes it's more one than another; sometimes it's a combination. Some women benefit from taking antidepressants and hormones together. Talk to your doctor about your specific history. Some things to look for: past bouts of depression or anxiety (whether or not they were diagnosed or treated) or emotional upheaval during hormonal events such as menstruation, pregnancy, the postpartum period, breast-feeding, or when you were taking oral contraceptives. If you have any of these in your background, you're at higher risk for depression now. Your doctor may recommend trying an antidepressant, but you should know that sleep problems are sometimes a side effect of these medications. Some women find they have to experiment with several antidepressants before they find one that works for them.

If you're still having trouble, talk to your doctor about whether you're a candidate for hormone therapy. If you have your uterus, you'll need to take a combination of estrogen and a progestogen to protect against endometrial cancer. However, progestogens can mimic or exacerbate some symptoms of depression, which confuses things. Your doctor might want to try a low-dose estrogen by itself for a few months while monitoring you closely. If you feel better, then you and your doctor can discuss what to do next. This might include adding a progestogen monthly or just a few times a year. You might experiment with different kinds of progesterone, as well as different doses to find one that works for you. Progestogens are available in pills, creams, and suppositories. There is also a device that delivers the hormone directly into your uterus, which means very little gets into your bloodstream or your brain. If you can't tolerate any type of progestogen, talk to your doctor about whether you can take a low-dose estrogen and monitor your endometrial lining with either an annual biopsy or transvaginal ultrasounds twice a year. As always, you want to take hormones in the lowest effective dose for the shortest possible time. Talk to your doctor about what this means for you.

NIGHTTIME MEDS

Q *I've tried everything to improve my sleep. I even bought a new hypoallergenic comforter because I thought I might be allergic to the down in my old one. But nothing helps. Is this the time to ask my doctor about sleep medication?*

A Before writing a prescription, your doctor might suggest a sleep technique that you didn't know about or might even send you to a sleep lab to see if you're suffering from a sleep disorder or if some other physical problem is causing you to lose sleep. However, medication may be indicated in the short term, especially if you're troubled by a stressful event such as the death of a loved one. If you do go this route, you won't be alone. According to the National Sleep Foundation, 25 percent of Americans use some kind of sleep aid every year. The most widely used are Ambien (zolpidem), Sonata, and Lunesta. Since these newer drugs more selectively target the part of your brain that governs your sleep/wake cycle, they're considered less addictive than older medications (although any sleep drug can be addictive). Older medications hit everything and can leave you groggy in the morning and affect your memory. Which medication you use depends on your sleep problem. For example, Lunesta is designed to last throughout the night. Sonata is a good choice if your problem is getting to sleep;

What to Tell Your Daughter

Your daughter's sleep patterns are changing at the same time as yours. She wants to get up and go to bed later—a shift probably dictated by biology. Unfortunately, the modern world isn't designed to accommodate the sleep needs of adolescents. Schools start so early in some places that kids arrive groggy and grouchy and certainly not ready to learn. A few districts are experimenting with later openings, which helps. School isn't the only issue; drowsy teen drivers are a major cause of accidents. Try to encourage your daughter to get at least eight hours a night. Sticking to a regular schedule and not oversleeping on weekends will help keep the adolescent body clock in sync with the timing required by school schedules. Waking late on weekends perpetuates the tendency to stay up late during the week and promotes sleep deprivation. It becomes a cycle that's hard to break.

it's also the only drug approved for use in the middle of the night if you wake up and can't get back to sleep. Another new drug, Rozerem, mimics melatonin, the hormone that tells your body when it's time to wake up and time to go to sleep. Other drugs similar to Rozerem are in the pipeline.

Because of the possibility of overuse, you should begin with the lowest possible effective dose used nightly on a short-term basis or intermittently for longer-term use. Most sleep doctors advise limited use. Follow your doctor's instructions to the letter; a few patients have reported unusual behaviors like sleepwalking and sleep eating when they take sleep aids such as Ambien (some were using a higher-than-recommended dose over a long period). You need to thoroughly discuss any treatment plan with your doctor and keep trying behavioral modifications. In the end, this is the best way to get the sleep you need.

ANTIDEPRESSANTS AND INSOMNIA

Q *When I started using an antidepressant, I figured one of the side effects would be better sleep. But the opposite seems to be happening. Why is this?*

A All antidepressants have potential side effects, and insomnia can be one of them. In fact, many medications, including antihypertensive agents, bronchodilators, diuretics, and corticosteroids, can interfere with sleep. Tossing out your pills isn't the answer. Depression and insomnia are linked (each seems to make the other worse), so you can't ignore the problem. Talk to your doctor about possibly switching to another antidepressant. If you decide to stick with your current medication, you will need to be extra careful about your nighttime routine. For example, you might need to avoid all caffeine and make sure that your bedroom is especially dark and quiet. Combining two antidepressants may also help. If your doctor doesn't have extensive experience in psychopharmacology, you might ask for a referral to a psychiatrist for a consultation.

Some people taking antidepressants may also develop restless legs syndrome (see page 77). If that's happening to you, your doctor may suggest switching antidepressants. For example, Wellbutrin (bupropion) is less likely to cause this problem than other medications.

SEX KEEPS ME AWAKE

Q *Sex right before bedtime has always been a great way for me to unwind, relax, and fall blissfully to sleep. But now, instead of wanting to drift off afterwards, sex seems to rev me up.*

A You're not alone. For some women, sex at midlife becomes *too* stimulating and can wake you up instead of putting you to sleep. Some simple changes could help. If sex now snaps you awake, go with the flow. Consider making love first thing in the morning instead of at night. Afternoon sex might also work if you can figure out the logistics. The new routine might spark romance as well. If nighttime is still the best time, try getting up after sex, moving out of the bedroom, and relaxing until you feel tired enough to go back to bed.

TRIPS TO THE BATHROOM

Q *My bladder turned into an alarm clock that goes off three or four times a night. And the more times I wake up, the harder it is to fall back asleep. Are there any remedies short of medication?*

A This is a common problem for both men and women. It's so common, in fact, that there's even a medical name for it: nocturia. Many of us can make it through eight hours at night without waking up for a trip to the bathroom when we're younger, but that ability to "hold it in" often declines with age. The culprit can be a medical problem such as a urinary tract infection, changes in the vagina at menopause, poor bladder support (especially in women who have had more than one pregnancy), or stress. Taking diuretics makes the predicament worse; so does too much caffeine, which functions as a kind of natural diuretic. An increase in both frequency and volume could be a sign of kidney disease, bladder cancer, diabetes, or high blood pressure or other cardiovascular problems. A visit to your doctor can rule out these and other

Is It True?

Fiction: Over-the-counter sleep aids are much safer than prescription medications.

Fact: While some OTC sleep medications are good for occasional insomnia, you should not take them after consuming alcohol or other drugs with sedating effects. You should also avoid them if you have breathing problems, glaucoma, or difficulty urinating. Be sure to tell your doctor everything you're taking. Also, some drugs have more ingredients than you need. For example, products like Excedrin PM and Tylenol PM contain diphenhydramine, an antihistamine that makes you sleepy (it's in Benadryl as well). But you're also getting the pain reliever acetaminophen, which is fine for occasional aches and pains but not something you should be taking every day (it could damage your liver). Moreover, these sleep aids can make you groggy and confused in the morning—not that different from the way you feel after a bad night's sleep.

conditions. If you pass the medical test, try just drinking less, especially in the late evening. Go to the bathroom just before you get into bed. And try to train yourself to hold it in longer during the day. Another option is a sling to reduce stress on your bladder at night. Ask your doctor about this.

Sleepiness Diary

Use this diary from the National Sleep Foundation to see what's keeping you from getting the rest you need. If you see a doctor about sleep problems, bring it along.

Sleepiness can interfere with your productivity, safety, and overall quality of life. This diary enables you to record how sleepy you are and how difficult it is to stay awake during your day. You can compare this to how much you slept during the night and how much you napped during your day. To record for a second week, make a copy of these pages.

WEEK OF: _____

The faces on the scale below represent different levels of sleepiness from being wide awake ("0") to falling asleep ("4"). At the times indicated on the chart, record with a "0, 1, 2, 3, or 4" for each day which face most represents how you feel at the given time.

	Mon.	Tues.	Wed.	Thurs.	Fri.	Sat.	Sun.
Morning (6 A.M. to noon) Time: _____							
Afternoon (noon to 6 P.M.) Time: _____							
Evening (6 P.M. to midnight) Time: _____							
Night (midnight to 6 A.M.) Time: _____							

The three statements in the table below represent difficulties in staying awake. For each day of the week, record how often you experienced these levels of sleepiness:

0 = Not at all 1 = Occasionally 2 = Some of the time 3 = Most of the time 4 = All of the time

	Mon.	Tues.	Wed.	Thurs.	Fri.	Sat.	Sun.
I fought off/ignored a need to sleep							
I dozed off/fell asleep without meaning to							
I needed caffeine or another stimulant drug to stay awake							

For each day below, record how much you slept the previous night and how much time you spent napping during the day in hours and minutes. Then enter your total sleep time.

	Mon.	Tues.	Wed.	Thurs.	Fri.	Sat.	Sun.
Hours/minutes spent sleeping last night	___ Hrs. ___ Min.	___ Hrs. ___ Min.	___ Hrs. ___ Min.	___ Hrs. ___ Min.	___ Hrs. ___ Min.	___ Hrs. ___ Min.	___ Hrs. ___ Min.
Hours/minutes spent napping during the day	___ Hrs. ___ Min.	___ Hrs. ___ Min.	___ Hrs. ___ Min.	___ Hrs. ___ Min.	___ Hrs. ___ Min.	___ Hrs. ___ Min.	___ Hrs. ___ Min.
TOTAL	___ Hrs. ___ Min.	___ Hrs. ___ Min.	___ Hrs. ___ Min.	___ Hrs. ___ Min.	___ Hrs. ___ Min.	___ Hrs. ___ Min.	___ Hrs. ___ Min.

Compare the hours you slept with your levels of sleepiness recorded on the sleepiness scales. While sleepiness is most often caused by not getting enough sleep, for some people it may be the result of a sleep disorder or other condition. If you're concerned about this, share your charts with your doctor when you talk about your sleep.

MATERNAL WIRING

Q *I used to be able to fall asleep easily, but that ability went out the window when I had children. I always thought I would make up my ever-increasing sleep debt when the kids were finally out of the house (which they are now). Instead, I still sleep fitfully and wake up at the slightest noise. Have sleepless nights become a bad habit?*

A In general, women are more likely than men to be awakened in the middle of the night by family members, whether they're small children with nightmares or teenagers coming home late. In a study by the National Sleep Foundation, 21 percent of women said they were frequently awakened by others, compared to only 12 percent of men. This "maternal wiring" could be nature's way of making sure you hear your baby when he cries. Most women without other physical or emotional problems tend to return to their pre-baby sleep habits after a while. For some, however, such light sleeping can indeed become a habit, and years later they may find themselves overly sensitive to every little sound in the house. Age also changes the quality of sleep. As you get older, you generally spend less time in deep sleep. Stress, anxiety over your "empty nest," or some undetected medical problem can exacerbate this tendency. Work on improving your sleep habits, especially by keeping your bedroom dark and quiet. A "white noise" machine could also limit distracting sounds. If none of these works, you need to talk to your doctor to see if there's a medical explanation for your light sleeping.

LATE HOURS AT THE GYM

Q *I really want to stick to a fitness routine, but now the only time I can get to the gym is after dinner. Will this make it easier to get to sleep?*

A Working out can definitely help you get better sleep, but not if you exercise within three hours of bedtime. Your body gets pumped up and ready for action, so you have trouble cooling down and relaxing. Try splitting up your routine and limiting aerobic exercise to earlier in the day, especially during the workweek. If you can't make it to the gym, incorporate extra activity into your regular routine by parking farther away, taking the stairs instead of the escalator, or walking instead of driving when you can. Another idea is to put aside a quarter-hour every morning and walk seven and a half minutes away from your house and then seven and a half minutes back. If you like going to the gym at night, consider yoga or other exercises that relax you. These will interfere less with your sleep and might even improve it!

DOING WHAT COMES NATURALLY

Many women are attracted to supplements and herbs to solve sleep problems because they just don't like the idea of taking drugs. But this is often a false distinction. Everything from herbals to prescription drugs qualifies as chemical intervention. The fact that one is sold in a health food store and another requires a prescription is no guarantee that the former is safer or more effective. In fact, the Food and Drug Administration does not require proof of these dietary supplements' effectiveness or safety before they are sold in stores. What's inside a bottle of supplements may not necessarily match what's on the label. You're also less likely to know much about correct dosage, interactions, and side effects. While scientists are showing more interest in studying alternative medications, little high-quality research has been done in this area. With that said, the most popular alternative sleep aids include:

MELATONIN. The bottles in the health food store contain a synthetic version of the natural hormone produced in your pineal gland, a pea-size structure in the middle of your brain. Levels of natural melatonin rise and fall during the day, dropping when you're exposed to sunshine and rising at dusk. Melatonin helps to regulate your sleep/wake cycle. In the last decade, synthetic melatonin has become a popular treatment for jet lag and insomnia. In clinical studies, researchers have found that as little as .10 milligram makes it easier for subjects to go to sleep no matter what time of day. Most doctors seem comfortable with occasional low doses for this purpose. But many are more reluctant when it comes to recommending regular use for insomnia, mainly because few studies have been done and the results have been mixed. Even the smallest commercially available dose—1 milligram—is more than three times the amount normally found in adults. That's why some countries, including Canada, don't permit melatonin to be sold over the counter.

VALERIAN ROOT. Used in Europe for many years and approved in Germany to treat sleeplessness and nervousness, valerian root enjoyed a resurgence as a natural sleep aid after L-tryptophan was taken off the market in 1990; it's usually sold in pill form because the raw root smells and tastes terrible ("dirty socks" is the typical description). You may have to use it for a week or more before you feel its effects. A review of research done on valerian root has concluded that its benefits are inconsistent. Some studies have shown it to be effective; others have shown little or no difference between this substance and a placebo. In 1998, the U.S. Pharmacopeia (USP), which establishes drug and dietary supplement standards, issued a monograph discouraging its use. While there is no known toxicity, side effects with long-term use include headache, restlessness, sleeplessness, cardiac disorders, muscle spasms, and vision problems. Not much is known about its interaction with other drugs. Pregnant or breast-feeding women shouldn't use it.

KAVA (*PIPER METHYSTICUM*). Herbalists have long recommended kava, a member of the pepper family typically sold as a tea or dietary supplement, for treatment of insomnia, mild anxiety, and stress. Several studies of kava have indicated that it reduces depression and other typical menopausal symptoms in postmenopausal women. In 2002, however, the FDA issued a warning to consumers and physicians about kava after it was linked to rare but severe cases of liver toxicity, including cases of hepatitis, cirrhosis, and liver failure, in Germany, Switzerland, France, the United Kingdom, and Canada. American health officials have specifically warned against using kava if you take any prescription drugs, drink alcohol frequently, or have existing liver problems. Those taking the supplement are advised to have a liver function test before starting and to repeat the test twice a year. Health officials say the substance is also addictive and has a variety of known side effects, including stomach upset, headache, sedation, and restlessness. Chronic heavy users have been

known to develop yellowish skin and a scaly skin irritation known as kava dermopathy, which may appear with eye irritation. Some European countries and Canada have removed kava products from store shelves after concluding that there were not enough data proving it safe and effective. This substance is also marketed as kava kava, ava, awa, intoxicating pepper, kew, rauschpfeffer, sakau, tonga, wulzelstock, and yangona.

CHAMOMILE (*ANTHEMIS NOBILIS*). Most commonly available as a tea, chamomile is often recommended to promote relaxation and reduce gastrointestinal distress. Weak teas will make you feel relaxed; stronger teas will make you sleepy. Few human studies verify its effectiveness (one small study looked at chamomile as a possible cure for colic in infants), but it does exhibit a sedative effect on lab animals. In high doses, however, chamomile can induce vomiting. Asthmatics should avoid it because it tends to make symptoms worse. It can also prompt reactions in anyone allergic to ragweed, daisies, and chrysanthemums. In addition, chamomile can amplify the sedative effect of other herbs or drugs and delay blood clotting. If you get it on your hands, avoid touching your eyes; it stings. Chamomile is also sold as German chamomile, Hungarian chamomile, *Matricaria chamomilla*, and Roman chamomile.

CHAPTER 5

Sex

Maybe you're one of the lucky ones. You're in your 40s or 50s and your sex drive has never been stronger. You and your partner are always in tune. In fact, you're regularly mistaken for newlyweds because you can barely keep your hands off each other. But now a few words for the rest of us.

Remember the good old days when all you had to worry about was getting pregnant? That's not much of an issue anymore, but there are many other barriers to the sex life you want. You're not in the mood a lot of the time. Most nights, you just wish your partner would roll over and go to sleep. When you do feel like a little action, it takes forever to get warmed up. Sometimes sex is more painful than pleasurable. And it's not all about you. As men get older, erectile dysfunction becomes more common.

But don't give up. The first thing to remember is that there is no quota for sex. Whatever *seems* right to you and your partner *is* right for you—

whether it's twice a day, twice a week, or every other month. Next, know that many couples discover that sex can be even more fun once they negotiate their way around the obstacles. If you and your partner feel happy with yourselves and each other, good sex will follow—at any age.

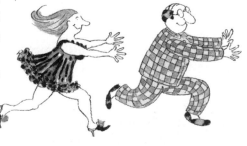

IMPROVING
YOUR ODDS

Sex is a highly individual experience all through life, and that's especially true around the time of menopause. Some women enjoy sex now more than ever. They're more experienced. They know what they like and are willing to ask for it. They may have less stress and more time. As their hormone levels fluctuate, they may even experience a surge of "free testosterone" that increases their sex drive. And after menopause they don't have to worry about getting pregnant.

But women's hormones can also work against them. During the menopause transition, some women experience a real drop in sexual desire and never seem to be in the mood anymore. Others may have trouble achieving orgasm as regularly as before, or perhaps they just feel less sexual. Menopausal symptoms— hot flashes, vaginal dryness, sleeplessness, moodiness, excessive and erratic bleeding—can also make women feel pretty unsexy. Other issues that can play a role include how they feel about getting older, physical fitness, the availability and health of a partner, medications, and stress.

Translation? If you value your sex life, you may have to try more things and work harder to maintain it. The best advice doctors give about menopause and sex is this: Use it or lose it. Women who continue to have regular sex during the menopause transition have fewer problems than those who cut back or stop. Part of the reason is physiological. The more sex you have, the more you encourage blood flow to the genital region, which helps to keep the tissues healthier. Vaginal lubrication is more plentiful in women who have intercourse on a regular basis. Pelvic muscles that are used regularly are more likely to be strong and responsive. In addition, having sex regularly encourages you to keep thinking of yourself as a sexual being.

Some researchers theorize that the body may respond to high levels of sexual activity by producing more hormones. Australian sex researcher Lorraine Dennerstein has always been fascinated by the small subset of women

What to Tell
Your Daughter

Although you may never have heard of it, the fastest-spreading sexually transmitted disease in the country is human papillomavirus (HPV), otherwise known as genital warts. Half the women and men in the United States have already been exposed to it, and it's believed to be responsible for 99 percent of the world's cervical cancers. A new vaccine that protects against the most worrisome strains of HPV is now recommended for females aged 9 to 26. Research is under way on its effectiveness for older women.

When to See the Doctor

Call if you experience any of these symptoms:

✤ A GREENISH YELLOW VAGINAL DISCHARGE WITH AN UNPLEASANT ODOR (IMMEDIATE ATTENTION REQUIRED IF ACCOMPANIED BY FEVER AND ABDOMINAL PAIN)

✤ PAINFUL SWELLING AROUND THE VAGINA OR LABIA

✤ PERSISTENT VAGINAL YEAST INFECTIONS, CHARACTERIZED BY A WHITE CURD-LIKE DISCHARGE, POSSIBLY ACCOMPANIED BY REDNESS AND ITCHING AROUND THE VAGINA AND LABIA

✤ PAIN OR BLEEDING DURING OR AFTER INTERCOURSE

who have sex every day. She's found that no matter which treatment group these women are randomized into during clinical trials, they never report any vaginal problems. Other sex researchers have found similar results. This doesn't mean that every woman going through the menopause transition has to have sex every day, but it does show that a positive attitude about maintaining a good sex life can help a lot.

It's also important to realize that both men and women tend to feel less sexual desire as they get older. Over time, you may find that it takes you longer to feel aroused or to reach orgasm. Caressing may need to become more direct and focused. If you can recognize and embrace these changes, you will learn to expect and accommodate them. This may mean expanding your definition of foreplay to include things like taking warm baths before sex as a kind of pregame activity, as well as allowing more time to set the mood with candle-light, romantic movies, sexy lingerie, fantasy, or massage. You may also want to experiment with positions, locations, and timing of your sexual rendezvous.

It's encouraging to note that when the magazine *More* (aimed at women over 40) surveyed 1,328 of its readers, more than half (53 percent) of those in their 30s said their sex lives were better than when they were in their 20s.

One more thing: If a midlife or mature woman's sex life isn't satisfying, it usually has more to do with the health of her partner than with her own physical or psychological problems. When women were asked by researchers conducting the Duke Longitudinal Study why they stopped having sex, the top three answers given (representing 74 percent of the responders) related to the health of their partner, including a man's inability to maintain an erection. If you run into problems, talk to your doctor about where in your area you can get the help you need.

What Can Happen

❖ Sex gets better for some, but a third to a half of peri- and postmenopausal women experience one or more sexual problems, including complaints about loss of desire, ability to achieve arousal or orgasm, and pain during sex.

❖ You may need more time and stimulation to get aroused (the same is true of men), and your body may produce less lubrication in response to sexual cues.

❖ Orgasmic heights may diminish or may take longer to achieve. Sensitivity of the clitoris can increase or decrease. In most cases, responsiveness is not as quick as it once was. Uterine contractions during orgasm may become less intense.

❖ Your entire genital area becomes drier and skin becomes thinner and less elastic as estrogen levels decline. During a pelvic exam, your doctor may check for signs of vaginal atrophy or bleeding even if you aren't complaining of symptoms.

❖ Your vulnerability to vaginal infection increases as pH level changes and vaginal walls thin with estrogen loss. Detection of infections may be tricky because of changes in vaginal discharges.

❖ Urinary tract infections become common. (For more information on urinary infections and related issues, see Chapter 7.)

❖ Many of the sexual problems experienced during these years have to do with the partner's inability to perform sexually or lack of a partner.

❖ Pregnancy is still a possibility if less than a year has passed since your last period. Contraception is a must.

AGE VS. MENOPAUSE

Q *I don't feel as much desire as I did when I was younger. Is this age or hormones?*

A The jury's still out on this one. Surveys indicate that women of all ages complain of sexual problems. For many women, it takes years to figure out how to have an orgasm. In the National Health and Social Life Survey, about a third of the women aged 18 to 59 said they had experienced loss of desire for at least a few months some-

time in the last year. After age 60, the proportion of women complaining about desire issues starts to climb.

LACK OF DESIRE

Q *I'm noticing a drop in sexual desire, but I don't want to use hormones, drugs, or herbs. Are there any alternatives?*

A Sexual desire involves a lot more than hormones, as you no doubt came to realize long ago. The quality of your relationships, your upbringing,

READ ALL ABOUT IT

Just spending more time thinking and reading about sex can help a lot. If you need inspiration, try expanding your horizons. Maybe your bedtime reading needs to change. Try a romantic novel or erotic literature written for women (such as *Slow Hand: Women Writing Erotica* or the *Herotica* series). If you're unsure about the latter, go to an online bookseller and read an excerpt before you buy the book. Consider signing up for a couples course or workshop, like Hot Monogamy (see the directory of programs at www.smart marriages.org). There's a wide array of self-help books written by therapists and doctors; almost all of them include a few sections with specific ideas, exercises, and games to add spark to your sex life. (See Appendix II for recommendations.) The Internet offers lots of areas for sexual exploration—everything from women's health websites to chat rooms to sex toy stores to hard-core pornography. While some of the things you'll find online may be degrading, repulsive, and upsetting, there's also a lot of good information. (If you start with mainstream women's health sites and follow their links, you should be able to wade in slowly.) The Internet also allows you the freedom and privacy to do the kind of exploring that you might otherwise find too intimidating or embarrassing. Be sure you do your surfing and ordering from home, however. Many businesses have the ability to check the sites you've visited on your office computer.

---

how you feel about your body, the amount of stress you have, whether you're depressed, and how much sleep you're getting all play a huge part. Try to assess how long you've had this problem. Is it constant, or does it come and go? For some perimenopausal women, hormone levels can zigzag from month to month, causing temporary problems that may disappear on their own, only to reappear again. If that's not your situation, make a list of what's going on in your life that may be dampening your enthusiasm for sex. If you have a partner, talk openly about your concerns and ask for feedback. Remember that when you don't discuss these things, your partner may misinterpret your lack of interest as rejection.

You can also consider doing some of those things that you should be doing anyway, like losing a little weight, cutting back on fatty foods, or drinking less alcohol. These steps may help a lot. And then there's exercise, which increases blood flow throughout your body, including the genital area. If sleep deprivation is on your list, try some of the relaxation techniques discussed in Chapter 4. Take the time and trouble to set up romantic interludes. (That's the fun idea in the lot.) Rethinking your priorities may mean putting a romantic weekend get-away at the top of your to-do list.

Another option is a consultation with a certified sex therapist or counselor who can tailor a program to your situation and recommend effective exercises to help you increase intimacy. Some thera-pists encourage overstressed women (in otherwise healthy relationships) whose libidos are flagging to simply "do it." They believe that even if you're not in the mood, the act of having sex is likely to put you *more* in the mood. On the other hand, if you think depression, anx-iety, or relationship problems are the barrier, consider therapy.

Make sure that your disinterest in drug therapy doesn't keep you from talk-ing about this problem with your doctor. There are lots of medical issues beyond hormones that could be at work here—everything from chronic fatigue syn-drome to depression to a serious vitamin or mineral deficiency. After going over your medical history for clues and mak-ing sure that none of your medications is the culprit, your doctor may refer you to a specialist for more help. Be sure to bring along some notes so you can discuss what you've tried on your own.

SEARCHING FOR AN EXPERT

Q *How do I find a doctor who's an expert in female sexual issues?*

A Because female sexual medicine is a fairly new clinical area, you may need to do some searching before you

Is It True?

Fiction: Estrogen is the female hormone and testosterone is the male hormone.

Fact: Endocrinologists, doctors who specialize in hormones, have noted that women actually produce more testosterone than estrogen in their lifetimes and that men make more of both than women do.

find the right specialist. It's usually a good idea to start with your internist and ob-gyn. If they have no expertise in this field (which is likely, since most medical colleges do not include much on sexual medicine even now), they're in a good position to know the specialists in your area. Depending on your spe-cific complaint, they may refer you to a specialist in sexual medicine, an endo-crinologist, urologist, psychologist, psy-chiatrist, social worker, or sex therapist. If it's a sex therapist, make sure she's certified by the American Association of Sex Educators, Counselors and Therapists (AASECT). You can find members in your area via their website (www.aasect.org). Generally speaking, they will want to make sure there's no

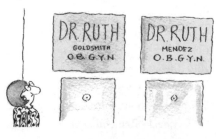

medical or physical basis for your problem. Before you go to your first appointment, draw up a list of your symptoms and questions, as well as any medications (both prescription and over-the-counter) that you're taking.

GOLFING BUDDIES

Q *My ob-gyn plays golf with my husband, and I feel very uncomfortable talking to him about my lack of sexual desire. I really want to address this problem, but I just can't get myself to bring it up.*

A During a recent medical conference, we met a doctor who works at a luxury spa. She told us that many of the women who make appointments with her to discuss their sexual problems do so because they don't want to take them to their doctor back home. So you are not alone. But you don't have to travel hundreds of miles to solve your problem! If you really don't feel comfortable talking to your ob-gyn about this, you can make an appointment with another doctor—an internist or one who specializes in sexual disorders or menopausal symptoms. Maybe you'd feel more comfortable talking to a female doctor. Keep in mind, however, that if you decide to do a consultation elsewhere, you'll need to tell your regular doctor about whatever new medications (prescription or herbal) you choose to take. It's dangerous to hold back this kind of information out of embarrassment.

WHAT'S SEX THERAPY ABOUT?

Q *What should I expect from a visit to a sex therapist?*

A There are lots of misconceptions about sex therapists, including the notion that you might be asked to take off your clothes and make love right in front of them while they critique your technique. Sex therapy is actually a form of psychotherapy (talk therapy). Most practitioners are psychologists, psychiatrists, social workers, or nurses who have undergone special training to help singles or couples deal with sexual issues that are hampering their relationships. The therapist typically begins a consultation by taking a detailed history that includes your past and present relationships and your religious beliefs, values, and upbringing, as well as reviewing your sexual, physical, psychological, and emotional health. The point of this therapy is to help you (and your partner) find ways to give and receive physical pleasure in order to strengthen your emotional relationship, not to turn you into a sex machine or encourage you to do things that violate your moral or religious beliefs. Typically, the therapist will give you "homework" that might consist of new and (hopefully) more effective ways to relate to your partner or to increase your sexual or sensual feelings. You might also be asked to do some reading or watch some instructional DVDs. Medical insurance often covers this type of therapy.

FUN AND GAMES

Q *I've heard that sex toys can help your love life, but I have no idea what I'm looking for or where to buy any of these things. And I'm too embarrassed to ask. Any suggestions?*

A Sex therapists say that many women react with disgust or dismay when they recommend sex toys or vibrators as a way to boost stimulation. But the simple fact is that your physiology is changing, and you may need a few new tricks and toys to keep things interesting. This doesn't mean you have to do things that make you uncomfortable, but one of the sexiest things you can bring to the bedroom is an open mind and a sense of humor. You might want to start out with something pretty simple, like chocolate body paint and a pair of brushes, or the Kama Sutra Weekender Kit. If you've never used a vibrator (and feel self-conscious about trying one), you may find some comfort in knowing that lots of women use them. In a recent survey, *More* magazine found that 45 percent of the respondents used vibrators and sex toys. Many of these products are made to stimulate both your vagina and your clitoris, sometimes at the same time. There are also products small enough to slip onto your finger and others designed for the very discreet. Some look like fountain pens (the Vibra Pen) or makeup tubes (the Lipstick vibrator and the Stowaway) and even a nail polish bottle (Incognito). Others are very quiet (an important asset if you still have kids at home). You can use them alone or with your partner. Some, like erection rings, are designed for men to wear during intercourse and provide direct stimulation to the clitoris. Remember to clean all toys and vibrators thoroughly before and after each use.

From the Past

*I*n the 19th century, menopausal women were warned that sexual activity would exacerbate their symptoms and might actually trigger fatal illness. In her book *The Meanings of Menopause,* Ruth Formanek says doctors in the 1800s advised midlife women to "avoid amorous thoughts that might be evoked by viewing lascivious pictures, reading love stories, and anything that might cause regret for charms that are fled, and enjoyments that are ended forever." Some physicians of that era even warned midlife women that menopausal symptoms were a kind of payback for wild living, defined as sexual passion, immodest dress, eating stimulating foods, prurient reading, contraception, or masturbation. All of the above were said to increase the sufferings of the menopausal woman because nature compelled "the payment of her violated laws, by means of malignant disease or years of invalidism."

Where do you buy this kind of stuff? In many parts of the country (especially California, the Midwest, and the South), you can buy these items at Passion Parties, the modern equivalent of Tupperware parties. The company estimates that about 10,000 Passion Parties are held every month in America's living rooms. Besides sex toys, lubricants, and lingerie, one of their most popular items is white chocolate passion pudding.

If you're concerned about maintaining your privacy, there are lots of sex toy purveyors online. Try browsing several sites until you find one you like. (This could even be a form of foreplay. See Appendix II for some web addresses.) Remember to check out these sites from home, not from the office. (Assume your company monitors your online activities.) Many online and mail-order companies ship this type of merchandise in the equivalent of a plain brown wrapper and use a tame version of their name (like the initials of the store) on your credit card statement. Local drugstores often sell vibrators in the sports medicine area. Typically, they're marketed as "massagers," but some are more clearly labeled. Vibrators come in a variety of price ranges (some as cheap as $12) and strengths. If yours feels too vigorous, try using it on top of your underwear or look for something with variable settings.

HORMONE THERAPY AND LIBIDO

Q *I think my body must be totally screwed up. A few months ago, I started having hot flashes, sleeplessness, and moodiness, but my interest in sex actually increased. I started on a low-dose hormone therapy a few weeks ago to deal with the hot flashes, and it worked. The symptoms are gone but so is my libido. Aren't increased hormones supposed to zip up your sex drive?*

A A woman's sex drive is not necessarily an easy thing to understand—even when it's your own. The sexual seesaw you're on has an explanation. When you're nearing menopause, your hormone levels don't go straight downhill; instead, they go through twists and turns and ups and downs that would make a roller coaster jealous. Some of these convolutions result in hot flashes and night sweats. They can also bring the heightened libido you were experiencing.

To be more specific, the culprit in your scenario is a protein called sex hormone binding globulin (SHBG), which binds itself to both the estrogen and testosterone circulating in your body. SHBG levels fall as estrogen levels decrease. The theory is that when this happens,

PASSION TUPPERWARE PARTY

SEX TOYS

there's less around to bind with testosterone, which means you have more "free" testosterone in your system and your libido gets a jump start. But when testosterone levels are up—and estrogen is down—you can get the mixed signals of desiring more sex but not wanting to follow through because of vaginal dryness. By adding an oral estrogen to the mix, your SHBG and estrogen levels rise and the amount of free testosterone in your body falls, taking your sex drive with it. One study found that adding supplemental estrogen can also prompt a woman's body to produce less testosterone from the ovaries and the adrenal glands, which simply adds to the problem. Talk to your doctor about the possibility of switching to a non-oral estrogen, which can boost hormone levels in your bloodstream and help with the hot flashes without a rise in your SHBG levels. If that doesn't do it, talk to your doctor about whether you should add some testosterone to your current regimen. Before you decide to try this, make sure you read up on the risks and benefits of testosterone treatments (see page 107).

WHERE'S MY ORGASM?

Q *I seem to be having a harder time reaching orgasm these days. What's changed?*

A While orgasms can become less intense as you get older and may not last as long, there's no evidence that women become incapable of experiencing orgasms as they age. If you were once able to reach orgasm during intercourse (only about 30 percent of women can normally do this) and now find that you can't, try more direct stimulation of the clitoris. You may be able to incorporate this into foreplay by trying different positions or slipping a vibrator between you and your partner as you're having intercourse.

If the problem persists, think more broadly about underlying causes. If you're having trouble becoming adequately aroused, consider a consultation with a sex therapist who can offer a variety of exercises and techniques to resolve the problem. If you think the problem may be related to what's going on in your relationships or other stressors in your life, consider individual or couples therapy. Some antidepressants (including those recommended as alternative treatments for hot flashes) can have sexual side effects. You may need to switch medications or add Wellbutrin (bupropion) to remedy the situation. If the problem is painful penetration (dyspareunia), see page 113. If you've gone without sex for a time and are now trying to reignite your engine, you may need something akin to a tune-up to get yourself ready. Moisturizers, water-based lubricants, masturbation (with or without a vibrator), local estrogen treatments, and a genital exercise program that includes Kegel exercises (see pages 118–19) all may help.

RETHINKING SEXUAL DYSFUNCTION

For decades, most of the people doing research on women's sexual behavior were men who assumed that women experienced sex the same way they did. In other words, they thought that healthy women always felt an undercurrent of sexual tension and desire and were always looking for an opportunity to act on those feelings, and those who didn't feel that way were somehow dysfunctional. But in recent years a group of researchers led by Rosemary Basson have challenged the conventional thinking on female sexual behavior. They assert that while a woman may feel plenty of sexual excitement with a new lover, women in long-term relationships typically aren't thinking about sex all the time; instead, they're motivated by a need to maintain or improve the relationship. So, while men's sexual progression is usually illustrated as linear (desire leads to arousal leads to orgasm), these researchers visualize the female sexual progression as a circle, with one phase affecting all the others. A woman's need for closeness with her partner prompts her to become sexually engaged, which in turn leads to arousal, desire, and finally sexual satisfaction.

If a woman doesn't want to have sex anymore, and it doesn't bother her, is there anything wrong with her? The new answer is "no." If a woman can no longer achieve an orgasm but considers herself sexually satisfied, should she seek treatment? Again, the answer is "no." Instead, the term *dysfunction* should be reserved for persistent sexual problems revolving around desire, arousal, orgasm, or pain *only if they cause personal distress.*

According to this reassessment, what's going on in a woman's head has more to do with her perception of being sexually aroused than with whatever is happening between her legs. Low hormone levels, vascular problems, severed nerves, depression, or exhaustion can affect her sex life, but so can sexual "context": how she feels about her life or her partner; how she's doing physically, psychologically, socially, and emotionally; what medications she's taking; how much sleep she's getting; her sexual history, losses, culture, morals, and upbringing.

This reassessment is prompting doctors to collect a comprehensive patient history—and to listen more closely to what their patients are telling them. This doesn't mean that solutions will be easy, but women today have a better chance of improving their sex lives than ever before.

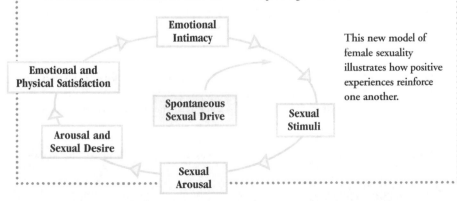

Emotional Intimacy

Emotional and Physical Satisfaction

Spontaneous Sexual Drive

Sexual Stimuli

Arousal and Sexual Desire

Sexual Arousal

This new model of female sexuality illustrates how positive experiences reinforce one another.

TESTOSTERONE 101

You probably think testosterone is the stuff that makes men get into fights at ball games. But this hormone is flowing through your blood, too. When you were a preteen, your adrenal glands began pumping out hormones called androgens, which signaled the hypothalamus and pituitary gland in your brain that it was time to start production of estrogens, testosterone, and progesterone in your ovaries. That's the beginning of puberty. On a typical day in adulthood, you actually produce more testosterone than estrogen; however, as ovulation approaches each month, estrogen production surges ahead. Testosterone may also play a role in regulating a woman's mood, energy, memory, spatial orientation, muscle tone, and, of course, sex drive. Its effect on breast cancer is unclear.

Here's a rundown on what we know and don't know about testosterone in women:

Where it comes from. Your adrenal glands and ovaries produce most of the androgens in your body. Other sources include skin and muscle cells (as a result of a naturally occurring chemical conversion). Your brain also produces a small amount of these hormones.

How much is enough? We know that men's bodies make up to 20 times more testosterone than women's bodies do. However, how much testosterone any one woman needs is unclear. As a result, many doctors discount the relevance of measuring their female patients' testosterone levels.

Raging libidos. Between the ages of 20 and 45, a woman's testosterone levels fall by about 50 percent. This is primarily due to reduced testosterone production by the adrenal glands and ovaries before the onset of menopause. Natural menopause has little effect on testosterone levels. So while your ovaries are producing a lot less estrogen as you move through the menopause transition (by the end, it's down by 90 percent), they keep producing testosterone. This means that many women actually experience a relative increase in the ratio of testosterone to estrogen during the menopause transition. For some, that translates into a boost in sex drive.

Not tonight, honey. Some women find that sexual desire seems to vaporize during the menopause transition. Again, testosterone could be the reason. If the ovaries or the adrenal or pituitary glands get damaged or malfunction, you produce less testosterone. Some medications can have a similar effect. During a long perimenopausal transition, women may experience an erratic libido as their estrogen and testosterone levels yo-yo up and down. One month, they may feel downright frisky; the next month, the thrill is gone. Some women choose to ride this out; others end up seeking oral contraceptives or hormone therapy to smooth things out.

When the change is abrupt. The loss of testosterone is felt most acutely after removal of the ovaries. Six weeks later, a woman's testosterone levels are half what they were before the surgery. If the surgery occurs after age 45, there may be almost no testosterone in her bloodstream. For these women, testosterone is often just one of many factors affecting their libido. Dealing with the aftermath of surgery, cancer, depression, or other difficult issues can compound the problem.

Individual differences. The impact of hormonal decline on any one woman's sex life varies greatly. How sexy you feel at any particular time may have more to do with what else is going on in your life and whether you have a healthy partner. If you start experiencing problems with your sex life, you and your doctor should carefully evaluate your medical history and any stresses that might be complicating your life. You may benefit from testosterone therapy, but this should be among the last things you try.

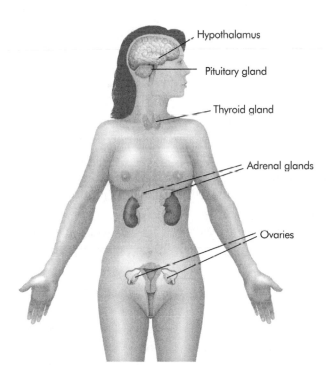

- Hypothalamus
- Pituitary gland
- Thyroid gland
- Adrenal glands
- Ovaries

WHERE FEMALE ANDROGENS COME FROM

During your reproductive years, most of your testosterone comes from your adrenal glands and your ovaries; androgens are also produced by your brain and by skin and muscle cells (through a natural chemical conversion). In your menopausal years, testosterone continues to be produced by all the same players, but in diminishing amounts as time goes by.

Why Not Viagra?

Q *Viagra seems to work so well for men with sexual problems. Does it work for women?*

A In 2004, after years of research, Viagra's manufacturers announced that they were ending their attempts to develop a female version. The hope was that, in women, the drug sildenafil would relax the smooth muscles around the clitoris so that it would become more easily engorged, heightening sensitivity and desire. (In men, it relaxes the smooth muscle tissue around the penis so that it can become engorged.) While it did increase vasocongestion, or genital engorgement, many women did not associate the physical changes they experienced with subjective feelings of sexual arousal and desire. A variety of studies have indicated that often there is no difference between the vasocongestion experienced by women complaining of low arousal and those who say they have no sexual problems at all. In the Viagra studies, the sildenafil was no more effective than the placebo in boosting libido.

Although the FDA hasn't approved Viagra for females, some women have been known to sneak one of their partner's little blue pills and feel that it works for them. Was it their heightened expectations or the drug itself that made the difference? It's impossible to know for sure, but we do know that the placebo effect is pretty powerful when it comes

to sexual response. If you're thinking of experimenting with it yourself, talk to your doctor first to make sure it's safe for you. Keep in mind that the FDA specifically warns against using these types of medications if you take drugs containing nitrates (usually for heart disease). There can be negative interactions with grapefruit and grapefruit juice. There are also some reports of heart attacks, sudden death, stroke, and sudden blindness associated with men taking Viagra; it's not clear if these events were related to ingesting the medication or were the result of engaging in sex and if the same risks pertain to women.

If you have arousal issues and are interested in increasing vasocongestion without these kinds of risks, talk to your doctor about using the Eros Clitoral Therapy device. This FDA-approved mini-vacuum effectively increases genital engorgement with no side effects. (There's a detailed description of this device on page 129).

Easing the Transition

Q *I'm now in the early stage of perimenopause, and I'm noticing that my sex drive is all over the place. Some weeks, I'm hotter than ever. Other weeks, I couldn't care less. I assume my hormones are fluctuating like crazy, but I also assume that this will be going on for a while. Is there any medication I can take while I'm in the transition?*

A It's harder for doctors to help during the transition for exactly the reason you outlined—your hormones are a moving target. But if this is a significant problem for you, talk to your doctor or consult with an endocrinologist about whether a small dose of estrogen (or estrogen and testosterone) would help even things out for you. Sometimes small doses can fool a woman's body (specifically the hypothalamus and pituitary gland) into thinking the ovaries are responding better to their signals than they actually are and thus reduce the frantic signaling to produce more hormones. As always, try to use the smallest dose possible for the shortest time necessary. If you still have a uterus, talk to your doctor about what you need to do to protect or monitor your endometrium.

SHOULD I TAKE TESTOSTERONE?

Q *I know that hormones should never be the first consideration, but what about a shot of testosterone to boost my low libido?*

A Research does show that testosterone can prompt a modest increase in sexual desire, particularly among women who have had their ovaries removed. If you and your doctor decide it's worth a try, the next problem is figuring out what to take. Most of the testosterone products available—shots, patches, creams, pills, or pellets injected under the skin—were developed for men. Once the decision is made, your doctor has to rely on experience to estimate the right dose, because there are no formal guidelines.

In recent years, drug companies have worked to develop products for women, but so far none has been approved by the Food and Drug Administration. A testosterone transdermal patch called Intrinsa was turned down, in part because of bad timing. Only a short time before the Intrinsa hearing, the Women's Health Initiative study of estrogen therapy had been stopped short because of safety concerns. Moreover, critics of the drug argued that most of the women who participated in the randomized clinical trials had only one more sexual encounter a month than the women taking a placebo; they also expressed concern about the drug's proven side effects (acne and unwanted hair) as well as the lack of information about its effects over the long term. Supporters of Intrinsa were quick to point out that Viagra received approval even though its known side effects were much more serious (it can cause heart problems and prolonged erections). Viagra didn't have long-term safety and efficacy data, and neither did the two other products that have since been approved for erectile dysfunction. (In fact, research is rarely done on the long-term safety and efficacy of drugs before they are approved by the FDA.) And while the gains in sexual desire were modest, many of the Intrinsa study's participants were happy with the results and wanted to stay on it. More research is required before the manufacturer goes back to the FDA. Other testosterone products for women are in various stages of development, and it seems inevitable that one of them will win government approval at some point in the future.

In the meantime, doctors can continue to prescribe either products designed for men or Estratest, a combination of estrogen and testosterone developed as a treatment for hot flashes but often prescribed for low libido in women. While it's long been assumed that testosterone, like other hormones, likely increases a woman's risk of cancer, a new study indicates that older women taking this drug (most of whom were longtime hormone users) had two and a half times the breast cancer risk of those who had never taken hormones. (Estratest has never been approved by the FDA for the treatment of hot flashes or low libido; it remains on the market during the appeal process.) The North American Menopause Society (NAMS) recently issued a position statement urging doctors to consider all other possible causes of sexual dysfunction before prescribing testosterone; however, if a woman and her doctor want to give it a try, it should always be paired with estrogen and both hormones should be prescribed at the lowest effective dose for no more than six months. NAMS also recommended that preference be given to testosterone patches and creams over oral products.

If you decide to pursue this, it's probably best to seek out a specialist in sexual medicine (typically an ob-gyn or an endocrinologist) because the dosing for these products is tricky. You'll need regular monitoring to make sure you're not getting too much. If your dose is too high, you could develop excessive facial hair and a receding hairline, among other masculinizing traits. Be sure you use these hormones exactly as prescribed. This is especially true of testosterone creams; these are often mixed by compounding pharmacies (which make up individual products for customers). Some patients wrongly assume that if a little dab helps a little, a lot will help a lot. And instead of mind-blowing orgasms, they end up with a mustache. This is potent stuff.

What Else Is Out There?

Q *From what I've learned, it looks like my options with testosterone aren't great. What about DHEA?*

A DHEA (dehydroepiandrosterone) is a hormone that's sold in health food stores and vitamin aisles at the grocery store. In the body, it's made by the adrenal glands and can be converted into testosterone and estrogen. Research on its ability to relieve sexual complaints has shown mixed results. While DHEA is available over the counter, most doctors believe it's a mistake to self-prescribe hormone treatments. As with all other dietary supplements, its quality and safety are not overseen by the FDA and its purity can vary. The amount of testosterone that DHEA produces in your body can also be highly variable, which makes it hard to get the dosage right. While little is known about the consequences and safety of long-term use, some doctors recommend a daily dose of 50 milligrams to patients who complain of a lack of desire and have low levels of androgens in their blood because of malfunctioning adrenal glands. Questions have been raised about its effect on breast cancer and heart disease. DHEA is not available for sale in Canada, and major medical groups such as the North American Menopause Society and the American College of Obstetricians and Gynecologists do not recommend its use. However, for the woman who's tried everything else without success and desperately wants to get passion back into her life, this may be a risk worth taking.

EASY BLISS

Q *I thought it would be harder to achieve orgasm around menopause, but it's gotten easier for me. Am I weird or what?*

A About 27 percent of the midlife women surveyed in the TREMIN Research Program on Women's Health said orgasms were easier, while about 32 percent said they had more difficulty. The physical changes your body is undergoing may have a lot less to do with how you're functioning sexually than with how comfortable you are with your body, your partner, and what you've learned about how to achieve pleasure. The TREMIN researchers concluded that future studies should "explore more fully" why some women's sexual responses increase as they get older.

THE THRILL IS GONE

Q *I'm postmenopausal, and I never think about sex anymore. In fact, I don't care if I ever have sex again. My feeling is that this is the way it's supposed to be. Am I wrong?*

A Many people are satisfied with less sex as they age; the number of sexual encounters they have does not correlate with their level of sexual satisfaction. In fact, a significant number of people who aren't having sex at all are content with this situation. However, while some women aren't bothered by their own diminishing desire, their partners can interpret it as a kind of rejection. For other women, decreasing desire is a profound loss; without it, they feel like strangers in their own bodies. Some women without partners worry that they'll never really connect with someone again. And others assume that sexual desire is supposed to disappear as we age.

Overall, we know that there is a gradual decline in sexual responsiveness and interest as time goes by. But many people remain sexually active well into their 70s, 80s, and 90s. A *Consumer Reports* survey found that more than about 75 percent of women in their 50s were still strongly interested in sex. Nearly 70 percent of women in their 60s and nearly 60 percent of women in their 70s answered the same way. But if you're one of the women who are happy to see sex go, you're not alone. It doesn't mean

there's something wrong with you. It also doesn't mean you'll always feel that way. An important element of the definition of sexual dysfunction is whether it causes you distress. And that's a question every woman has to answer for herself.

VAGINAL WOES

During the menopause transition and in the years afterwards, hormonal changes can leave the vaginal walls dry, thin, and less elastic. This, in turn, can interfere with your sex life at a time when you're looking for a little fun.

CULTURAL DIFFERENCES

Scientists who study the sex lives of midlife women tend to focus on those who are Caucasian and middle-class because they're the easiest to recruit. But are all women really the same? In recent years, the federally funded Study of Women's Health Across the Nation (SWAN) has attempted to find out by recruiting thousands of baby boomers (42 to 52 years old when the study started in the mid-1990s) who were racially and culturally diverse. One issue on the table was whether premenopausal women had more interest in sex than perimenopausal women did, and if there were any differences based on race and culture. The study found that a woman's proximity to menopause didn't predict her level of sexual desire, satisfaction, arousal, or

physical pleasure, or the importance of sex in her life. What did make a difference was her overall attitude toward sex and aging, as well as her cultural background. For example, African-American women reported having intercourse more often than the other groups, while Hispanic women complained that they now felt less physical pleasure and had more trouble getting aroused. Chinese women reported feeling more pain during intercourse than Caucasian and African-American women did and had problems with desire and arousal. Japanese women also had more arousal issues. Of course, not all Japanese women (or Caucasian, African-American, Chinese, or Hispanic) are the same, but this research is a welcome step toward understanding the diversity of women.

Luckily, there are vaginal lubricants that you can buy over the counter. Check the labels, and stick with the water-based lubricants. Choices include Astroglide, K-Y Personal Lubricant, Lubrin, Moist Again, and Replens Intimate. Some online companies even offer samplers of a variety of vaginal lubricants if you want to try out several different types or are embarrassed to buy these products in a drugstore. Avoid oil-based products like petroleum jelly or baby oil; they may irritate delicate skin and can encourage bacterial growth in your vaginal area.

There are also personal moisturizers, such as Replens, K-Y Long-Lasting Vaginal Moisturizer, and Astroglide Silken Secret. These products have an adhesive component that enables them to provide relief longer than the vaginal lubricants; they're designed to restore that familiar feeling of moist, comfortable skin for days or even up to a week at a time. Aquaphor ointment is another alternative recommended by dermatologists. Moisturizers that you use on your face and body should not be used in your vaginal area, especially if they contain alcohol or perfume. Vinegar douches should also be avoided. Some women use products with vitamin E, but dermatologists warn that it's often ineffective and can result in contact dermatitis (a skin rash caused by contact with an irritant), particularly in women with sensitive skin.

No solid studies have demonstrated the effectiveness of alternative remedies such as belladonna, bryonia, lycopodium, dong quai, or motherwort. There is only limited evidence that adding flaxseed and soy flour to your diet may reduce symptoms. (See Appendix I for more details on different therapies.)

LOW ON LUBRICATION

Q *I still get my period every month, but I don't have anywhere near the vaginal lubrication that I used to have when I got sexually aroused. What can I do?*

A It's fairly common to have menopausal symptoms when you're still menstruating. If you've been paying close attention to your body, you may have already noticed subtle changes in your monthly blood flow or the length of your periods. Reduced lubrication during sexual arousal is often the first symptom of perimenopause that women notice.

Start by using a vaginal lubricant during sex, but make sure it's water-based; oil-based products are not safe to use with a diaphragm or condom. You may want to take a few extra seconds to warm the lubricant in your (or your partner's) palm before applying. Make sure you cover your vaginal area as well as the top of the penis or condom for maximum effectiveness. You may also want to consider a lubricated condom. Having more sex can also help. Women who have intercourse regularly seem to generate more lubrication than those who do it less frequently.

A SENSITIVE VAGINA

Q *Now that I'm postmenopausal, my whole genital area feels hot, dry, and itchy all the time. I use a lubricant when I'm having sex, but it's not enough.*

A You're experiencing one of the most common menopausal symptoms. This misery can be caused by many things, so let's go down the list.

First of all, the lower level of estrogen you now have in your body can make the genital area feel drier and more sensitive (a condition called vulvodynia). The first thing to consider is whether something might be irritating your skin, such as panty liners, perfumed soap, douches, synthetic underwear, panty hose, or latex condoms. Even if these items weren't a problem in the past, they may be a problem now that you're more sensitive to irritants. Excessive exercise or sweating or high levels of stress or trauma could be adding to your problem.

Another possibility is that menopause may have thinned your vaginal walls and raised the pH levels in your vagina. Either condition can make you more vulnerable to infection. Don't assume you can diagnose this yourself. Lab work may be needed to determine the exact problem. It's a good idea to avoid feminine hygiene sprays and scented deodorants designed to camouflage vaginal odors that sometimes are the first warning sign of infection. Ask your doctor whether a product like RepHresh, which helps bring your vaginal area into pH balance, might be helpful in reducing future infections. You should also ask if any of the medications you're taking could be adding to your vaginal dryness. If you're experiencing dry eyes and mouth as well as a dry vagina, mention this to your physician. It could be an early sign of Sjögren's syndrome, a chronic autoimmune disease that's most commonly diagnosed in women over 40.

If no special problems are detected, your doctor is likely to recommend a personal moisturizer. But if the problem persists, a local vaginal hormone treatment might make sense for you. There

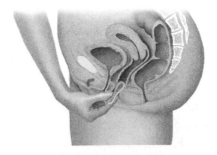

THE VAGINAL RING This form of treatment is simple to use. Just choose a comfortable position, either lying down or standing with one foot on a stool or chair, and push the ring into the vaginal opening. If it slips, push it in again.

are a variety of products that deliver estrogen vaginally via rings, tablets, and creams (see Chapter 2 for more details). Unlike the oral estrogens that get absorbed systemically (and may increase the risk of blood clots), these local hormones slip into your bloodstream without passing through your liver. They are usually effective in restoring vaginal lubrication and elasticity.

If you prefer the oral preparations, go with the lowest effective dosage for the shortest duration necessary. Results from the randomized controlled Women's Health Osteoporosis Progestin and Estrogen trial indicate that doses of 0.3 and 0.45 milligram of oral conjugated equine estrogen with or without a progestin were effective in treating vaginal symptoms. (By comparison, the dosage used in the WHI study that caused increased cardiovascular risks in older women was 0.625 milligram.) While there are no long-term data yet to prove it, many researchers hypothesize that lower-dose hormone treatments may be associated with less increased risk and fewer side effects.

YOGURT TREATMENT

Q *Some friends from Russia insist that putting yogurt inside your vagina helps to restore pH balance while you're going through menopause. This seems more natural than taking some sort of medication. Is there any chance that it will work?*

A Eating yogurt or taking acidophilus capsules orally may help, but inserting yogurt or cultures of lactobacilli into your vagina as a topical cream won't do anything but create a great environment for the growth of bacteria. Yogurt is also not recommended as a moisturizing treatment for itching, irritated vaginal skin.

ALLERGIES DOWN UNDER?

Q *I know this sounds more than a little crazy, but my vaginal area seems much drier and more irritated in the spring and fall—at the same time my allergies are acting up. Could these two problems be connected somehow?*

A They could be, especially if you're using antihistamines to help clear up your drippy nose and weepy eyes. One of the properties of antihistamines is that they have a drying effect on all the mucous membranes in your body, not just the ones that are located in your nose. This means your genital area can be affected by them. Other things that can have a similar effect include diuretics, caffeine, and alcohol.

You can try using a vaginal moisturizer or water-based lubricant to help relieve the problem. If that doesn't have the desired effect, talk to your doctor about changing your allergy treatment or possibly using a local hormone treatment occasionally to reduce your seasonal symptoms.

PAINFUL SEX

Q *I've always thought my sex life would improve after menopause because I wouldn't have to worry about an accidental pregnancy. Instead, I find it's increasingly painful to have sex.*

A About one in five women will experience painful intercourse (dyspareunia) at some time in their lives. After menopause, it's typically related to the effect of hormonal changes on the vaginal walls. In other words, where there was once accommodation, there's now an uncomfortable friction. Some women, particularly those who go for extended periods without having intercourse, experience an actual narrowing of the vagina, which is why this problem often becomes apparent in women whose partners have recently begun taking Viagra or a similar treatment after years of erectile dysfunction.

What you do about the pain depends on its cause and severity. Water-based vaginal lubricants and personal moisturizers can make a big difference in mild cases. If the problem persists or is more severe, make an appointment with your doctor, who will want to find out if the irritation is caused by an infection, sexually transmitted disease, or allergic reaction. (If the doctor is going to do an internal exam, ask for the narrowest speculum to reduce your discomfort.) If the pain feels like it's coming from deep inside your pelvis, mention this to your doctor. (It could be a symptom of a wide variety of things, from a simple cyst to a muscle tear or even ovarian cancer.)

If the problem really is dyspareunia, you can use either vaginal or systemic estrogen therapy to restore your vaginal health. They're equally effective. Vaginal therapy is available in vaginal tablets, rings (Estring), and creams. If the pain is severe, your doctor may decide to start you on a pretty hefty dose of estrogen to speed recovery before lowering it for maintenance. Most women feel better within a few weeks; a few may require long-term treatment in order to maintain vaginal health.

A review of these treatments found that women tended to prefer the vaginal ring over other delivery systems because it's easy to use with little discomfort. Women who use creams tend to have more side effects (uterine bleeding, breast pain, and more of a buildup of the endometrial lining). Women who prefer pills can get relief with low doses of oral medication (both 0.3 milligram and 0.45 milligram of conjugated equine estrogen have been proven effective). Pills, like other systemic treatments, have the added advantage of reducing hot flashes. Systemic treatments are also available in patches, creams, and a ring (Femring).

Assuming you want to resume sexual activity once you feel better, your doctor may suggest that you use well-lubricated vaginal dilators (available online or from any good medical supply store). Progressive muscle relaxation techniques may also help (instructions are easily found on the web at sites like www.mayoclinic.com/health/relaxation-technique/SR00007). Once the skin tone is restored, remember to maintain it with personal moisturizers. And don't forget to use lots of water-based lubrication during sex.

WHAT'S THE RUB?

Q *I use my vaginal estrogen right before I go to bed, but I can't help wondering if the estrogen might rub off on my husband when we're making love. I know that using testosterone can cause masculine traits in women; could vaginal estrogen feminize my husband?*

A A doctor told us about one couple she'd seen who accidentally (and repeatedly) used vaginal estrogen as a lubricant. The husband experienced feminization (that is, he grew mini breasts) from being exposed to large doses of the estrogen cream. But once his wife stopped using the cream before sex, everything went back to normal. (By the way, something similar happens to women when they have intercourse with a man who has just applied a topical androgen like AndroGel.) Occasional low-dose exposure probably won't make any difference. To be on the safe side, try using the estrogen cream earlier in the day or simply wait until after sex.

YEAST INFECTIONS

Q *I've always been susceptible to yeast infections when I use antibiotics, but now I'm getting the same symptoms regularly, even when I'm not on antibiotics. Is this somehow related to menopause?*

A Yeast infections can be caused by lots of things: antibiotics, sexual intercourse, spermicides, douches, or a weakened immune system. You're also at higher risk of developing them during periods of hormonal change such as pregnancy, when you're breast-feeding, and the menopause transition. That's because erratic hormone levels can alter the healthy environment of the vagina and cause the bacteria and fungus that normally exist there in small quantities to increase rapidly. While some women with a yeast infection experience no symptoms at all, many notice an itching, burning sensation that sometimes gets worse during urination or intercourse; increased redness and swelling; and a white odorless discharge that resembles cottage cheese.

If this were the first time you experienced a yeast infection, you would have needed to see your doctor for lab work to confirm the diagnosis, since a number of medical conditions mimic these symptoms. But since you've had recurrent yeast infections and recognize the symptoms, you're probably used to treating the problem with over-the-counter medications. Keep in mind, however, that a recent study found that only a third of women accurately diagnosed what they thought was a yeast infection; 20 percent had more than one infection, and the rest had something else. Getting an accurate diagnosis is particularly tricky if you're already using medication to cure a yeast infection, so if you're in doubt, get tested before you start an over-the-counter treatment. (Otherwise, you could end up treating a variety of infections for weeks.) Persistent vaginal infections can also put you at higher risk of acquiring HIV and postoperative infections. A good rule of thumb is to see your doctor if there seems to be something a little different about your symptoms (such as a yellow or green discharge or one that has an odor) or if they persist after the treatment course is complete.

One more quick piece of advice: Next time you get a prescription for an antibiotic, be sure to mention that antibiotics tend to give you yeast infections. Sometimes a different medication can be prescribed. If not, your doctor may suggest that you start treating the infection that's coming before the first symptoms appear.

STARTING TO DATE AGAIN

Q *I'm in my mid-50s and recently started dating after a long, difficult divorce. Out of nowhere, I've suddenly started noticing a lot less lubrication during foreplay and intercourse, as well as an unusual discharge and pelvic pain.*

A Your problem could be a combination of things. Vaginal atrophy brought on by abstinence plus a yeast infection is one possibility. A sexually transmitted disease (STD) could also be part of the mix. It's easy to forget that even when you can no longer get pregnant, you're still vulnerable to STDs. Either way, don't try to diagnose this one at home. Go to the doctor and get yourself checked out; the problem is unlikely to go away on its own.

TAKING A BREAK

Q *I don't have a regular partner right now, but that doesn't mean I never want to have one again. Besides lubricants and moisturizers, what can I do to keep my vaginal area healthy?*

A Not having a partner is the most common midlife sexual problem, and many women hope it's only temporary. Like every other area of your body, your genitals need exercise and stimulation to stay healthy. By increasing blood flow to this area, you encourage continued responsiveness and prevent your vaginal walls from narrowing and the tissue from thinning (doctors call this vaginal atrophy). In the most severe cases, the vagina can literally close up. And an abandoned clitoris may have a hard time responding if one day you decide to call it out of a long retirement.

A little experimentation on your part will help determine what works best for you. One of the most obvious (and

healthy) things you can do is to mastur-
bate, either manually or with a vibrator.
Kegel exercises are also helpful. Many
women are advised to do these exercises after childbirth to prevent a leaky
bladder, but they're also great for keeping your vaginal muscles in good working order. The contracting action is the
same one you use to pull in a slipping
tampon or to stop a stream of urine. (See
pages 118–19.)

Some women find it easier to exercise
their vagina when they have something
around which to clench their vaginal
muscles. Amazing as it may seem, there
are a variety of vaginal workout tools.
Plastic dilating rods, often used by
women who have undergone radiation as
a means of stretching the vagina and preventing the formation of scar tissue, can
also be used for exercising and tightening
the vagina. Simply lubricate the rod,
insert it halfway into your vagina, then
clench your vaginal muscles around it for
5 to 10 minutes at a time. Depending on
your situation, you may need to do this
two or three times a week. Other options
include vaginal barbells, weights, and
cones. One popular version is called
Betty's Barbell, designed by sexologist
Betty Dodson. Another is called the
Kegelcisor. You can find many of these
items at medical supply stores or online at
sites featuring sexual aids. If you've had
problems with pelvic floor prolapse or
find Kegel exercises difficult to master,
consider consulting a physical therapist
for guidance on how to use these muscles.

METHODS OF CONTRACEPTION

No matter how many menopausal
symptoms you have, until you go a
year without a period you should assume
that you can still get pregnant. If that
isn't in your plans, now is not a time to
get casual about contraception. Half of
all pregnancies that occur in women 40
and older are unplanned, and the older
you are when you get pregnant, the
greater the chance of complications for
you and the baby. (This may explain
why one study found that 65 percent of
the pregnancies that occur in "older"
women end in abortion.) If you're perimenopausal, it may be time to rethink
the kind of contraception you and your
partner have been using up to this point.

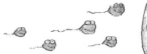

There are lots of choices, and some do
multiple things. But some forms of contraception may be riskier now. Here's a
rundown of your options:

ORAL CONTRACEPTIVES. If you haven't
used oral contraception in a few decades,
you may still be under the impression that
their use is considered dangerous for
women over 35. Not so. Since the late
1980s, oral contraceptives have been
available in much lower doses. Most prescriptions today contain 20 to 35 micro-

HOW TO KEGEL

When it comes to exercise, you're a star. You run. You've signed up for strength training. You even take a tai chi class. But are you Kegel-ing?

Kegel (pronounced "kay-gul") exercises were designed to strengthen your pelvic floor muscles. Not only do they keep your sexual muscles in shape, but they can improve your sexual response. They're also great for avoiding or reducing bladder and bowel incontinence and reducing the risk of developing pelvic organ prolapse.

The first step is locating the muscles that stretch between your pubic and tail bones at the base of your pelvis and help support many of your internal organs. First imitate the muscular movement you would make to pull up a slipped tampon with no hands. Then put a finger or two inside your vagina and contract the muscles around them; you've located more muscles. (These are also the ones you use to interrupt a stream of urine or stop yourself from passing gas.)

You need to master two basic exercises. Begin by relaxing your body. As you exhale, squeeze, lift, and slowly draw up your pelvic floor muscles to a count of 10, then relax them for an equal amount of time. Some women visualize an elevator going slowly up and down as they do this, but essentially you're tensing the muscles around your vagina and anus. Repeat 10 to 15 times a day to start. If your muscles are weak, it may be difficult to hold them for more than three counts. Eventually,

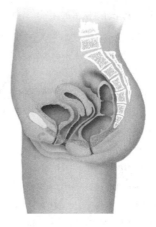

PELVIC FLOOR MUSCLES
This side view illustrates how pelvic floor muscles help to support many internal organs.

grams of estrogen. (For comparison, in the 1970s, a common dose was 100 micrograms; in the 1960s, 175 micrograms.) In 1989, the Food and Drug Administration dropped its warning for women over 40 (except for those who smoke or have special health problems) and approved the pill's use until the onset of menopause, even at age 55.

An oral combination of estrogen and a progestogen not only prevents pregnancy but also helps to manage perimenopausal symptoms such as erratic and excessive bleeding, hot flashes, vaginal bleeding, and bone loss, and may even lessen the chances of bone fracture during the postmenopausal years. Additional benefits include keeping

work up to a count of 10 and add more repetitions. The second exercise is similar. You do the same tensing, lifting, and drawing up, but it's faster. Squeeze for two counts, then release for two counts, 10 to 15 times.

You can add repetitions each month as you gain strength. The quality of each repetition is more important than the quantity. Eventually, you want to do somewhere between 50 and 100 a day.

You're probably rolling your eyes right now—one more thing you have to do every day! But you can "squeeze them in" 20 here, 20 there, over the course of your day. Some studies show that you're more likely to do them correctly at home, at a set time, like first thing in the morning. Any position works: standing up (knees slightly bent, feet shoulder-width apart), lying down (head on pillow, knees bent, feet a little apart), or sitting down (use a hard, straight-backed chair). If you're sitting, your feet should be flat and your knees slightly apart, or stretch out your legs and cross your ankles. These exercises should be performed without tensing the muscles of your thighs, buttocks, or abdomen—and don't hold your breath.

As you get proficient, you can do them anywhere: while you're stuck in traffic, standing in the checkout line, or even while you're having sex. Talk about multitasking.

If you're not sure you're doing them right, ask for help. (Doing them wrong can actually cause harm, such as pressure on the bladder.) Someone at your doctor's office may be able to give you guidance. Or consider a consult with a physiotherapist, who may use biofeedback (special equipment gives you visual feedback so you know which muscles you're contracting), electrical stimulation (a small vaginal probe is inserted to stimulate the muscles to contract), or vaginal weights (small cone-shaped weights inserted into the vagina and held there against gravity; as you improve, heavier weights are used). These techniques occasionally have adverse effects, so be sure to have a professional guide you.

periods on a predictable schedule, reducing the need for a hysterectomy related to fibroids and other bleeding problems, and dramatically reducing the risk of ovarian or endometrial cancer (lifetime use decreases ovarian cancer risk by 80 percent and endometrial cancer risk by 40 percent or more) with no increase in the risk of breast or cervical cancer. Oral combination contraceptives may also protect against benign breast tumors and pelvic inflammatory disease. But they are not for everyone. If you're over 35 and you're obese, or you smoke, or you have a history of blood clots, stroke, hypertension, or diabetes, the risks of using oral contraceptives will rise with your age. The pill also carries increased

THE MORNING-AFTER PILL

As the name implies, this form of contraception is for those times when your usual method fails for some reason—you miss a series of pills, a condom breaks, or you have unprotected sex. In most cases, combinations of estrogen and a progestin are ingested within 72 hours of intercourse. Another dose usually follows 12 hours after the first. A pregnancy test is sometimes included. This method is only about 75 percent effective and doesn't work once a fertilized egg has been implanted. Morning-after pills will not terminate a pregnancy or prevent STDs. Side effects can include cramping, vomiting, headaches, and nausea. A progestin-only version called Plan B is 89 percent effective and is less likely to cause nausea. Because other forms of contraception are much more reliable, morning-after pills should not be used as a regular form of birth control.

risk for those with breast, endometrial, liver, or any other estrogen-dependent cancer; a history of cerebral vascular or coronary artery disease; abnormal uterine bleeding of unknown cause; jaundice (from a previous pregnancy or earlier oral-contraceptive use); active liver disease; and migraines with an aura. Don't take them if you may be pregnant.

The risk of developing a blood clot, which is related to the estrogen content of the pill, is increased in women with a genetic defect in the clotting system.

Heart attack or stroke happens, rarely. Other side effects include nausea, headaches, and breast tenderness, but these tend to diminish with continued use. Irregular bleeding and spotting may also occur with lower-dose formulations. If that occurs, you may want to talk to your doctor about bumping up your dosage. Some women experience weight gain on oral contraceptives, but studies indicate that just as many women lose weight on them. Most oral contraceptives put you on a monthly cycle (three weeks of hormones, one week off). There is also a newer product, Seasonale, that extends your cycles so that you have only four periods a year. This pattern may be especially appealing to women who are having a lot of bleeding problems. As long as you're taking oral contraceptives, you'll get regular bleeds even if your body has reached menopause. For this reason, most doctors recommend that women stop taking oral contraceptives around age 50. One final thing to remember: Oral contraception offers no protection against sexually transmitted diseases.

TRANSDERMAL PATCH. OrthoEvra, a skin patch that offers a week's worth of contraception, contains norelgestromin (a progestogen) and ethinyl estradiol. Over the course of a month, the patch is replaced three times and then left off for a week. It's easy to use and helps to regulate erratic menstrual bleeding. However, the FDA has placed a warning on this product because women who use it are exposed to about 60 percent more estrogen than those who use a standard-dose (35-microgram) birth-control pill. The FDA said it was not known whether women using this product were subjecting themselves to higher risks of side effects such as blood clotting problems, but in general higher doses are associated with higher risk. It offers no protection against STDs.

VAGINAL RING. Nuvaring, a plastic ring containing ethinyl estradiol and etonogestrel, works for three weeks once inserted in the vagina. Women take a one-week break before inserting another ring. Besides providing cycle control, this contraceptive prevents vaginal dryness. It's not yet known if it protects against osteoporosis or gynecological cancer. It offers no protection against STDs.

INJECTIONS. Lunelle is a once-a-month hormone injection containing medroxyprogesterone acetate (a progestogen) and estradiol cypionate (an estrogen). Women who use it reduce their risk of ovarian cysts and tumors. It also protects against cancer and endometriosis and helps to regulate menstrual flow. It offers no protection against STDs. Side effects are similar to those of oral combination contraceptives. Pregnancy can occur if an injection is not given within 33 days of the last one.

PROGESTIN-ONLY CONTRACEPTIVES. Women who can't use estrogen-based contraceptives because of medical risk factors can consider progestin-only formulations. The depot, or long-lasting, form of medroxyprogesterone acetate (DMPA) is a 150-milligram intramuscular injection, given every three months. Some unscheduled bleeding and spotting may occur, and half of its users stop having monthly periods after four treatments. Ovulation may not resume for 12 to 18 months after the treatments stop. Because DMPA suppresses production of ovarian estradiol, it also has a negative effect on bone mineral density. Because of this, some doctors pair DMPA with low-dosage estrogen patches or pills (like those used for menopausal hormone therapy). There are also progestin-only oral contraceptives ("mini-pills"), which require strict adherence to a daily schedule to be effective since their dosage is so low. There is some risk of irregular bleeding and spotting with these pills as well. Occasionally, women also stop having periods. Progestin-only patches are not sold in the United States but are available in other countries.

SPERMICIDES. Easily available over the counter, spermicides are preparations (creams, foams, suppositories, gels) designed to kill sperm on contact once they've been placed in the vagina near the cervix. Make sure you read the directions carefully for proper use and optimal effectiveness. Spermicides do not offer any protection against sexually transmitted diseases, and they can irritate some delicate skin types.

BARRIER METHODS. These contraceptives (male condoms, female condoms, cervical cap, diaphragm) work by blocking the sperm's access to the female egg and are very effective if you use them correctly *every time* you have sex. Latex condoms are the only contraceptive method that offers proven protection against most STDs if used for vaginal, oral, and anal sex. Because of this, some people combine condom use with other contraceptive methods.

INTRAUTERINE DEVICES (IUDS). Placed in the uterus for 5 to 10 years at a time, IUDs are one of the most popular contraceptive devices worldwide, although less than 1 percent of American women use them. (This type of birth control fell from favor in the United States after the banning in 1974 of an IUD called the Dalkon Shield, which was associated with a high rate of infection and painful insertion. At that time, these devices did not need to undergo government inspection; FDA approval is now required for all IUDs sold on the American market.) The two devices that are now available in the United States are the copper IUD (ParaGard T 380A), which can remain safely in the uterus for up to 10 years, and the levonorgestrel-releasing intrauterine system (Mirena IUS), which lasts about 5 years. Both devices must be inserted by a physician. Side effects of the copper IUD include increased cramping and greater blood flow, so it may not be a good choice for women who have painful or unusually heavy or prolonged periods under normal circumstances; a levonorgestrel-releasing device, which tends to reduce both blood flow and painful cramping, is a better choice in those cases. Many women experience some breakthrough bleeding and spotting right after an IUD is inserted, but these side effects tend to lessen over time. While many women have lighter regular periods, others continue to experience some light erratic spotting and some stop having periods altogether (amenorrhea). There are some risks with this procedure. A small percentage of women experience a punctured uterus during placement, and some devices are expelled from the body during the first few months. You can reduce the chance that either of these events will occur by scheduling your appointment with a doctor who has been specifically trained in IUD insertion. If you don't know, ask.

WHAT ABOUT STERILIZATION?

Q *My husband and I have three kids, and we're in agreement that our family is now complete. What are the pros and cons of surgical procedures that will ensure the impossibility of another pregnancy?*

A If you're sure you don't want to get pregnant again, sterilization offers the most protection against a future pregnancy, and it doesn't have to involve surgery. The no-incision method is performed with an instrument called a hysteroscope, which is passed through the vagina and cervix to insert two small metallic coils (Essure micro-inserts) in the fallopian tubes. The scar tissue that eventually forms there blocks the tubes and prevents future pregnancies. With good follow-up care, this method has proven 99.8 percent effective. The simplest surgical method of sterilization is a vasectomy for men. The female equivalent is the tubal ligation, which involves tying off and cutting (or cauterizing, clipping, or banding) both fallopian tubes. While not 100 percent effective, it's pretty close. The failure rate is estimated at 4 to 8 per 1,000 surgeries. In rare cases, an ectopic pregnancy (a life-threatening pregnancy outside the uterus) can occur. Women who have been sterilized and experience pelvic pain and vaginal bleeding should call their doctor immediately. While reversal is possible for men, it's more difficult for women (microsurgery to repair a tubal ligation is not covered by insurance and is successful only about half the time). As with any surgery, there are some risks associated with anesthesia and infection. None of these methods offers any protection against sexually transmitted diseases. Tubal sterilization does not end menstruation, and there is some question as to whether it increases the risk of heavy or painful periods after the procedure. As a group, women who have undergone tubal sterilization are more likely to have had a hysterectomy during

their lifetime than other women. Sterilization may reduce the risk of ovarian cancer.

THEY'RE NOT TALKING

Q *None of my friends has ever even mentioned sterilization. How common is it?*

A This is one of those things that many people don't talk about, yet 50% of women aged 40 to 44 who practice contraception have been sterilized (many because of a hysterectomy). Another 20 percent have a partner who has had a vasectomy.

LOSING LIBIDO

Q *I was on birth-control pills 20 years ago, before I had my kids. When I went off them, I noticed that I felt much sexier. Now I've reached menopause but am still having a lot of menopausal symptoms. I'm thinking about going on hormone therapy. If I do, will I lose my libido again?*

A There are similarities between birth-control pills and hormone therapy, especially combination hormone therapy (necessary if you still have a uterus). However, birth-control pills—even modern formulations that generate fewer side effects—have much higher levels of hormones in them.

That said, the slightly complicated reason that you felt less sexy on birth-control pills may still pertain to hormone therapy.

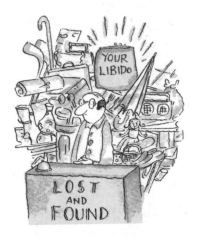

When you increase your estrogen intake by taking a birth-control pill or *oral* hormone therapy, the levels of a compound called sex hormone binding globulin (SHBG) increase, too. In your body, SHBG's job is to latch onto circulating estrogen and testosterone. The result is that there's less "free" testosterone to turn on your sex lights.

To bypass that problem, talk to your doctor about the possibility of using one of the non-oral estrogen options (creams, gels, patches), which will increase your estrogen level but do little to your SHBG. Or, if you prefer a pill, talk to your doctor about whether an estrogen-testosterone combination would work for you. (You'll need to add a progestogen to this mix.) Another option would be to add a little supplemental testosterone to your estrogen-progestogen combination. Make sure you discuss all of the benefits as well as the risks of these different combinations with your doctor.

DOES WITHDRAWAL WORK?

Q My husband and I have been practicing withdrawal as a means of contraception. How reliable is this?

A Withdrawal is not at all reliable as a method of contraception. Even if you and your husband are super careful when you're having sex, semen can seep out of the penis before full ejaculation occurs. Moreover, this method offers no protection against sexually transmitted diseases.

I'VE GOT RHYTHM

Q Contraceptive devices are against my religion, so I've been using the "rhythm method." It's worked so far. Can't I just continue using it?

A Natural family planning, or the "rhythm method," offers some advantages. It's inexpensive and requires no drugs, surgeries, or special devices. But research shows that rhythm is not as reliable as other contraceptive methods. And even if you've been using this method successfully for years, it can become much less reliable during the perimenopausal years. Because your periods may no longer follow predictable patterns, ovulation may occur sooner or later than usual. You can go months without a period and then, without warning, get one again. That means, as you know, that you can get pregnant again, too.

SPECIAL PROBLEMS

BLEEDING DURING SEX

Q *I'm several years past menopause, and lately I've been bleeding whenever I have sex. Could this be a sign that I have cancer?*

A Many women experience some bleeding during the years after menopause. Because yours occurs during or after sex, it may be related to thinning, irritated vaginal skin caused by the drop in your estrogen level. Vaginal bleeding is particularly likely if you haven't been having sex very often or haven't been moisturizing or lubricating your vaginal area on a regular basis. It could be related to fibroids, polyps, or any hormone therapy you might be using. It's also possible that it's an early sign of malignancy . . . or nothing at all. The bottom line is that you must promptly report any post-menopausal bleeding to your doctor. If the source of the trouble turns out to be your thinned vaginal walls, there's a range of solutions—from moisturizers to localized hormone therapy—that can solve your problem.

THE DEPRESSION-SEX LINK

Q *About two months after I started taking Paxil to help with my menopausal blues, my general mood got a lot better. But I wasn't "in the mood" anymore, if you know what I mean. Could these things be related?*

A While depression itself can have a big effect on how you feel about sex, so can antidepressants, particularly popular selective serotonin reuptake inhibitors (SSRIs) such as Paxil (paroxetine), Prozac (fluoxetine), Celexa (citalopram HBr), Lexapro (escitalopram oxylate), Luvox (fluvoxamine maleate), and Zoloft (sertraline hydrochloride). Effexor (venlafaxine), tricyclics (such as amitriptyline), and monoamine oxidase inhibitors (such as phenelzine and tranylcypromine) can also cause this problem. Now that you're feeling better, your doctor should review your medical history to ensure that your medication is causing the problem and then give you some options. The simplest is to wait and see if it goes away. Sometimes, as you adjust to a drug, the symptoms decrease or become more tolerable. But this happens only 30 percent of the time, and six months could go by before you notice a difference. Lowering your dose may do the trick, or taking "drug holidays" on the weekends may help. (This latter idea requires you to schedule sex, however.) If neither works, your doctor may suggest trying another drug. Antidepressants that have been shown to have fewer sexual side effects include Wellbutrin (bupropion), Remeron (mirtazapine), and Serzone (nefazodone). Edronax and Vestra (both containing reboxetine), available in Europe. If you want to stick with the antidepressant you're already using, talk to your doctor about the possibility of adding Wellbutrin. This

ERECTILE DYSFUNCTION AND YOU

The inability to get or maintain an erection may not seem like something you should have to worry about, but a lot of women do. National surveys indicate that about a third of all men (ages 18 to 59) complain of sexual problems, including erectile dysfunction and premature ejaculation. Interestingly, prevalence rates track very closely to age: 40 percent of 40-year-old men said they suffered from erectile dysfunction; 70 percent of 70-year-olds said the same thing. If this happens to your man, don't take it personally. It's not related to how attractive he finds you. It's all about blood flow and hydraulics.

Three drugs have been approved to treat this condition: Viagra (sildenafil), Levitra (vardenafil), and Cialis (tadalafil). Viagra takes effect in about 30 minutes and is good for up to four hours. Levitra should be taken one to four hours before sex and may be restricted to one dose every 72 hours. Cialis can be taken half an hour before sex and may last up to 36 hours. This point is worth remembering. Many women complain that they feel pressure to get in the mood as soon as their partner pops his pill. Cialis may give you more flexibility. It's also helpful to know that none of these treatments results in an automatic erection. The penis still needs to be sexually stimulated to become engorged.

While these drugs are effective, they don't work for everyone. An estimated 30 to 40 percent of erectile dysfunction appears to be resistant to these treatments.

combination often works well for women, and some small studies indicate that it can even enhance sexual response. (That's a side effect you won't mind so much!)

Some antidepressants, like tricyclics, tend to increase drying in the vaginal area. This side effect can be made more tolerable by using more lubrication or extending foreplay. If nothing else works, your doctor may suggest trying supplemental testosterone. Because finding solutions to sex problems caused by pharmaceuticals can be time-consuming and complex, you might want to ask for a consultation with a psychiatrist to find the best solution.

If you've had a series of depressive episodes and your doctor wants you to stay on antidepressants for the long term, it's crucial to keep searching for a good solution. Sexual side effects eventually prompt many women to stop taking these drugs, causing more frequent and severe depressive episodes. Another incentive to keep your depression under control: Research has established that depression is associated with a higher risk of chronic illness, like dementia and heart disease. It's worth the trouble to find a long-term solution.

THAT OLD LOVIN' FEELING

Q *Does induced menopause also mean a rapid loss in sexual desire? At least with natural menopause, you have time to get used to your changing body.*

A Your sex life after surgery may be affected by many factors: a loss of desire because of the abrupt decline in androgens after removal of the ovaries, pain (or even fear of pain), and stress over health issues. If you've had a hysterectomy, your vagina may have been affected. After chemotherapy, you're often exhausted and sometimes nauseated, so it's more difficult to feel romantic desire. However, if you had a hysterectomy because of excessive, uncontrolled bleeding, the surgery may make the prospect of sex more appealing than it's been in a long time. (For much more on this, see Chapter 6.)

HYSTERECTOMY AND SEX DRIVE

Q *A few years ago, I had a hysterectomy involving just my uterus. Since my ovaries are still intact, I didn't expect any change in my hormone levels or my sex life. Right after the surgery, I felt a little blue and figured that was affecting my interest in sex. But after all this time I seem to have less and less desire for intimacy. Will it ever get better?*

A Some women do get depressed following a hysterectomy, but yours could also be a physical problem. About one-third of all women who undergo a hysterectomy involving just the uterus experience a shutdown of one and sometimes both ovaries a few years after the procedure. With that comes a significant drop in hormone levels, which could be affecting your sex drive. Typically, the effects are felt more strongly over time. In some cases, early menopause can begin something you may not be aware of since you haven't been menstruating since the operation. It's a little tricky making this diagnosis, especially if you're experiencing perimenopause and its typical fluctuating hormone levels. Talk to your doctor about getting these levels checked. Keep in mind that, as a group, women who go through surgical menopause are more likely to experience hormone deficiency syndrome than women who go through it naturally, and may need higher doses of estrogen and testosterone to correct the problem.

While your experience is not uncommon, it doesn't happen to everyone. A study published in the *Journal of the American Medical Association* found that most women who got the surgery due to excessive bleeding, pelvic pain, fibroids, or endometriosis said they were having more satisfying sex after their hysterectomy than before.

LEAKING DURING INTERCOURSE

Q *This is so embarrassing, I can't believe I'm even bringing it up, but I've started urinating during intercourse. Talk about dampening the mood!*

Perhaps you can take comfort in knowing you're not alone. Some women start having this problem after childbirth; others experience it after a hysterectomy or menopause. (The drop in your estrogen level may be partly responsible.) The problem is usually related to improper closing of the urethral sphincter or a weakening of the pelvic floor. Technically, what you're experiencing is known as stress incontinence; some women experience the same momentary loss of muscle control when sneezing, laughing, or coughing. One solution is to strengthen the muscle that controls urine flow. Kegel exercises can help. If that doesn't make a difference, consult your doctor or a urologist. Sometimes, surgery is the answer. (See Chapter 7.)

SEX ENHANCER?

Q *I've heard that the antidepressant Wellbutrin can enhance your sex life. If I'm having trouble with arousal, can I try that instead of hormones?*

A In a few small short-term studies conducted on people who had sexual difficulties but no depression, Wellbutrin (bupropion) was shown to be effective. A tiny single-blind study (20 women) done at the University of Alabama found that about 70 percent of women taking 150 or 300 milligrams of Wellbutrin per day said they felt more overall sexual satisfaction after taking the drug and experienced more

intense orgasms. A double-blind placebo-controlled study of premenopausal women diagnosed with hypoactive sexual desire disorder (HSDD), conducted at multiple hospitals, had similar results. Why it works in some cases and not in others isn't known, and more study is needed. If you're interested in giving this a try, talk to your doctor. Like any other drug, Wellbutrin has side effects of its own (it shouldn't be used by those with a vulnerability to seizures or with a history of eating disorders and can also cause sleeplessness and weight loss). If you're a smoker, bupropion is effective in helping people who want to stop smoking; for this purpose, it's sold under the brand name Zyban.

ORGASM AND HYSTERECTOMY

Q *My hysterectomy (during which my uterus and cervix were removed) seems to have had no effect on my sex drive, but I don't seem able to climax during intercourse the way I once did. Is this a physical or psychological problem?*

A The sensations that trigger orgasm vary from woman to woman. For some, the feeling of a penis tapping against the cervix has that effect. Others find that their orgasms aren't as intense without the shudder they used to experience in their uterus. It's also possible that some of the nerves involved in vaginal orgasm were severed during the surgery. Try being a little more experimental sexually. Most women find more than one way to trigger orgasm, and different can be better.

You should also consider how you felt emotionally about this surgery. Are you mourning the loss of your fertility? This could be the way your body is dealing with it. If so, consider talking to a therapist if the problem persists.

DRYNESS AFTER CANCER

Q *I was pushed into menopause early because of chemotherapy related to breast cancer. Can I use a local vaginal estrogen therapy to deal with dryness there, or will it increase my chance of a recurrence?*

A There's no evidence-based answer to your question. Doctors don't know whether local vaginal estrogens have an effect on breast tissue. As a result, you may get different advice from different doctors, depending on how severe your symptoms are, what stage of cancer you're dealing with, and what kind of treatment you're currently getting. Some oncologists will just say no. But many will permit their patients to use a very low-dose vaginal estrogen like the tablet Vagifem two or three times a week for symptom relief. If you still have your uterus, make sure you and your doctor discuss your need for endometrial protection.

If your doctor says no to all types of hormone therapy, try reducing your symptoms with water-based moisturiz- ers made specifically for the vaginal area and make sure you use lots of lubrication with intercourse.

EROS TO THE RESCUE

Q *As part of my cervical cancer treatment, I had radiation. I'm on hormone therapy now, but my body isn't responding to sexual overtures. Is there anything more I can do about this?*

A Radiation is an effective cancer treatment, but it can leave a variety of sexual problems in its wake. Scar tissue can develop, and the vagina can become less responsive and pliable even with hormonal treatments.

There are some encouraging results, however, from a very small study (15 women) done at the University of Chicago, University of Illinois, and Northwestern University into ways to improve the sexual response of women who had undergone radiation for cervical cancer. The study participants used an FDA-approved handheld suction device called Eros to stimulate their genital area four times a week for three months. The 13 women (average age: 43) who stuck with the program found that they moved from the bottom 10 percent in terms of their sexual functioning to the normal range by the end of the study. They told researchers that the device improved their sexual response (lubrication, genital sensitivity, clitoral sensation, and orgasm) as well as their overall satisfaction.

Follow-up gynecological exams verified improved elasticity, color, moisture retention, and less bleeding and ulceration. Clinical trials found no side effects, but there were no long-term follow-ups. The device is available by prescription only, so talk to your doctor if you're interested in trying it yourself. You either can use it as the study participants did, or just prior to sexual activity as a form of foreplay.

CHEMOTHERAPY AND SEX

Q *The chemotherapy I'm getting for cancer has put me on the express train to menopause. It's been a difficult time for me, but I figured I could continue to rely on sex being an outlet for all the stress I'm dealing with these days. Where has my libido gone?*

A Chemotherapy can do a number on your libido for a whole lot of reasons. You may not be getting enough sleep because you're worried about your illness. You are at higher-than-normal risk for suffering from significant menopausal symptoms like hot flashes and night sweats. Plus all the physical changes you've experienced (surgery, hair loss, weight gain) may leave you feeling less confident about your allure. Some women also experience significant changes in their vaginal area during this time—more dryness and irritation, more infections, maybe even pain during intercourse. This can be particularly true of women who have been abstinent

for a while. The chemicals used for your therapy tend to irritate the vaginal and uterine lining. The clitoris can also be affected; it may not be as responsive to touch and vibration. You'll be able to reach orgasm, but it may take longer to get there.

It's not unusual for those with cancer to develop depression as well. Another double-edged sword: Depression suppresses your libido, and some of the most popular antidepressants can, too. Make sure you mention this problem to your prescribing doctor. Sometimes a prescription addition or substitution can improve your sex drive and depression at the same time.

Part of your troubles could be hormonal. While some women experience no change in their ovary function after chemotherapy, others may find that their ovaries shut down. When estrogen and testosterone levels drop, your sex drive may also fall. This is not necessarily a permanent problem. In some cases, the ovaries are temporarily stunned by chemotherapy but start working again several months later.

What can be done if hormone depletion is to blame depends on the specific type of cancer you have. Hormone therapy is usually not recommended for those with an estrogen-sensitive form of breast, ovarian, or uterine cancer. A random controlled trial to determine if breast cancer survivors could take hormone therapy had to be closed down early because of an increase in breast cancer, but another study didn't show an increase. Two alternative treatments may be worth considering. ArginMax, a combination of vitamins, minerals, and other dietary supplements developed by a doctor at Stanford for cancer survivors who can't take hormones, showed positive results in two small studies that measured its effectiveness. There's also Zestra, a genital massage oil made of borage seeds and evening primrose oil (see Appendix I).

RADIATION AFTEREFFECTS

Q *I'm scheduled for radiation as part of my cancer treatment. When faced with a life-and-death scenario, the future of my sex life isn't my top priority. But is it inevitable that it's going to be affected?*

A It depends on your cancer and exactly what will get radiated. Ovaries that have been radiated stop producing hormones. That's why so many cancer patients find themselves dealing with menopause so quickly. In addition, radiation can take a toll on the suppleness of your vaginal tissue. Vaginas that are radiated can develop scar tissue and become less elastic and responsive. It's worth having a conversation with your doctor about your alternatives *before* the radiation treatments begin. In some cases, a woman's ovaries and vagina can be protected from taking a direct hit. Sometimes, doctors are able to move ovaries and their blood supply out of the line of fire during treatment and then move them back afterwards.

DOCTOR ISSUES

Q *My husband is about 12 years older than I am, and we've always had a great sex life. But now that I'm a few years past menopause, I'm not responding sexually the way I used to and I miss that part of my life. I have brought this up with my doctor several times, thinking he'll suggest that I try testosterone or something. Instead, he always brushes it off and moves on to something else.*

A Unfortunately, this isn't all that unusual. Your doctor may not know a lot about sexual dysfunction; perhaps he doesn't want to admit it. He may think you're experiencing the natural course of aging and that nothing can be done about it. Maybe he has a general leeriness about prescribing hormones except to address specific physical ailments, like hot flashes or super-dry vaginas. But it could also be that your doctor doesn't think it's a good idea to rev up the libido of a woman with an older husband; he may fear that you and your husband will end up with mismatched sex drives and he'll be to blame. Still, your questions deserve answers. You may want to try one more time to discuss the issue directly with your doctor; press him for an answer. But if you don't get satisfaction, it may be time to try another doctor—perhaps a specialist in sexual medicine.

Sexually Transmitted Diseases

Maybe there's a new love in your life. Or maybe you're dating for the first time in years. Either way, it's important to realize that if you're sexually active, you're nearly as vulnerable as a teenager to sexually transmitted diseases. With 20 different varieties now identified, there's no doubt that STDs are serious business. Some cause cancer. Some can be fatal. While more treatments are available than ever before, some remain incurable.

Your best line of protection is knowledge. Have the courage to ask your partner some relevant questions before you start a new sexual relationship. Be willing to get tested yourself and to be candid about the results; otherwise, you risk infecting others or being reinfected yourself. Any unusual symptoms in the genital area, including mild itching, burning, soreness, rashes, bumps, or discharges, should be checked out by your doctor even if they seem to disappear after a while. Regular checkups are a smart move no matter how sexually active you are, because early treatment often gives best results.

There are other things you can do to boost your chances of staying disease-free. Avoid douching after sex; this practice not only washes away some of your body's protective bacteria, but also makes you more vulnerable to many sexually transmitted diseases. Do use condoms, which offer the best protection against HIV/AIDS and most STDs. Keep in mind, however, that condoms have a way of leaking or breaking, and they only protect what they cover. You *can* catch an STD even if you use one.

Viruses
Human papillomavirus (HPV). The current estimates are that half of all American women and men have been exposed to HPV, making it the fastest-spreading sexually transmitted disease in the United States. HPV is believed to be responsible for 99 percent of all cervical cancers, and it may play a role in other genital cancers as well. One in four women is expected to develop precancerous cells in her cervix at some point in her life because of this virus. That's why getting an annual Pap smear (which detects most precancerous cells in the cervix) should be a high priority for you. When caught early, it can be treated.

The HPV virus is related to the virus that causes common skin warts. It has few symptoms except small, hard bumps in the vaginal area, on the penis, or around the anus that cause no pain. These bumps can grow and take on a cauliflower appearance if left untreated. Remedies include topical medication or cryosurgery (freezing with an ice-cold probe); recurrent warts may need to be treated with interferon injections. (For more information about the new HPV vaccine and cancer, see Chapter 13.)

HIV/AIDS. You may think of HIV/AIDS as a gay disease—but think again. Women now account for 26 percent of newly diagnosed AIDS cases, a fourfold increase since 1986. Most women get infected by having unprotected heterosexual sex, sometimes with a partner they've had for years. In some cases, this is related to cultural or religious taboos that discourage men from acknowledging their bisexual or homosexual activity to female partners. African-American women have been disproportionately affected, especially in communities where many men have spent time in prison. The AIDS virus is potentially deadly because it attacks the body's ability to fight off infection. Initial symptoms include extreme fatigue and fever; lesions often appear as well. As time goes on, the AIDS victim becomes increasingly vulnerable to pneumonia and cancer, which can lead to death. While there is no cure, adherence to a strict drug regimen can slow and sometimes control the progress of the virus. Condoms are the best protection against transmission, but for good results you have to use them correctly every time you have sex. Before starting a new sexual relationship, be sure your partner has been tested. And get tested yourself. Early detection is crucial to good survival rates.

Herpes. About 60 million Americans (one in five) have genital herpes, which is spread by the herpes simplex virus (HSV) through sexual contact. Flu-like symptoms may be experienced after 2 to 10 days, followed by the appearance of open sores or painful blisters in the genital or mouth area. It can be difficult for women to detect the disease because the sores may erupt inside the vagina. Typically, the blisters disappear after a few weeks. Recurring or severe outbreaks can be treated with prescription medication. Drugs are available to treat the symptoms and to reduce the risk of transmission. Condoms are of limited help.

Hepatitis. There are three types of this disease, which attacks the liver. Type B can be spread through the exchange of body fluids (semen, saliva, blood, vaginal secretions, sweat, tears) and is far more contagious than HIV/AIDs. Type C is typically spread blood to blood; IV drug users and those working with blood products are the most at risk, but it can be spread through unprotected sexual contact. Type A is spread mostly through contaminated water and food or fecal-oral contact but also through unprotected sex.

Types B and C can be fatal if serious liver damage occurs or the liver becomes vulnerable to cirrhosis or cancer. While many cases of hepatitis go away on their own, a minority infected with hepatitis B and a majority infected with type C become lifelong carriers and can infect others. Symptoms, if they occur, are similar in all three types and include yellowish eyes and skin, dark yellow urine, unusually light stools, exhaustion, fever, diarrhea and flu-like stomach, and muscle and joint pain. There is a vaccine for types A and B, but none for C. A simple blood test verifies the diagnosis. Some people with types B and C can be helped with interferon injections combined with antiviral drugs.

BACTERIAL INFECTIONS
Chlamydia. The most common of the bacterial STDs, chlamydia can be successfully treated with antibiotics. The problem is that this stealthy bacteria often infects with no noticeable symptoms. In some cases, however, it can cause abnormal genital discharge and/or a burning during urination. If left untreated, it can cause pelvic inflammation disease (PID),

which can lead to infertility or an ectopic pregnancy (a doomed pregnancy outside the uterus, often in a fallopian tube).

Syphilis. Another STD that can infect without noticeable symptoms, syphilis may develop into something deadly. An infected person may notice a painless open sore around the vagina, on the penis, near the mouth or anus, or on the hands. Untreated, it next appears as a rash that quickly disappears. As time goes on, the infection attacks the central nervous system and the heart. Penicillin is the usual treatment.

Gonorrhea. This STD typically announces its presence with an unusual discharge from the vagina or penis or with painful urination. Untreated, it can cause pelvic inflammation disease, which can lead to

PREVENTING STDs IN WOMAN-TO-WOMAN SEXUAL RELATIONSHIPS

◆ Prevent transfer of any body fluids, including menstrual blood and vaginal fluids, from cuts or other openings.

◆ During oral sex, cover the partner's vaginal area with a barrier impermeable to fluid to avoid contact with vaginal secretions.

◆ Use a latex barrier between vaginas during vulva-to-vulva sex.

◆ Avoid sharing sex toys. Either clean them in hot, soapy water or use a new condom before switching users.

—North American Menopause Society

infertility or an ectopic pregnancy. It can be treated with penicillin or other antibiotics.

Trichomoniasis. Caused by a microorganism that lives in men's reproductive systems without any symptoms, trichomoniasis is spread through sexual contact and is a common cause of vaginal infections in women that can lie dormant for years. (They're sometimes diagnosed after an abnormal Pap smear.) They can also cause an active infection characterized by a heavy gray or green foul-smelling discharge, sometimes accompanied by itching, swelling, or redness. Some women may also experience painful intercourse or symptoms that duplicate those caused by a urinary tract infection: burning during urination or a constant urge to urinate. Both male and female partners must be treated to eliminate the chance of recurrence. Condoms offer some protection.

PARASITES

Pubic lice. Sometimes called "crabs," these creatures are the most common STD caused by parasites. While infestations typically occur during sexual contact, they can result from sharing clothing or objects such as toilet seats or blankets. Lice survive by sucking blood from their hosts, causing an itchiness, inflammation, and redness that call attention to their presence. Upon close inspection, these tiny animals can actually be seen moving around; with a magnifying glass, the eggs they lay at the base of pubic hairs are also visible. Washing the genital area after sex may get rid of them, but eradication may require medications, some available over the counter, others by prescription.

CHAPTER 6

Bleeding

Growing up, many of us affectionately referred to our periods as Aunt Flo. But during perimenopause Flo becomes one of those relatives who drop in unexpectedly, stay well beyond their welcome, and sometimes become a real pain. Erratic bleeding patterns are very common during perimenopause, but what's erratic for one woman may just be a version of normal for others.

One woman may have fewer cycles over time, each shorter and lighter than the one before until they disappear altogether. Then her sister may go from having regular monthly periods to menopause practically overnight.

And her best friend may experience the other extreme: heavy, messy, and scary bleeding problems; going through a pad or tampon every hour; having to think carefully about what color pants to wear; making the bed with layers of extra absorbent pads. Some women will bleed for 20 days in a row, get a break for 5 or 10 days, and then start their cycle again. Others never know when they're going to gush and pass blood clots, and their blood flow seems uncontrollable. No wonder bleeding problems are among perimenopausal women's biggest worries and loudest complaints.

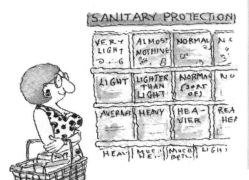

WHAT YOU NEED TO KNOW

Most women are acutely aware of even the smallest change in their cycle and can usually recall menstrual events from years before, especially if they occurred during a major event in their lives. Women also have a tendency to worry about these changes. Too often, we assume that any change is a sign of disease, especially cancer. While it's smart to be vigilant and mention changes in menstrual flow (spotting between periods, for instance, or very heavy flows) to your doctor, these events shouldn't inspire panic. There are many more versions of "normal" menstruation than we once thought. Discovering what's really normal has been the primary goal of the TREMIN Research Program on Women's Health, which has followed several thousand women (including several generations of the same families) since 1934. TREMIN researchers were the first to establish that every healthy woman did not have a 28-day cycle, as scientists once insisted was true. To do that, the incredibly patient founder, Dr. Alan E. Treloar, followed 2,702 women for 30 years and tabulated most of the data by hand before converting the information to punch cards in the 1960s. His research also proved that cycle variability is at its most extreme at the start, when girls begin menstruating, and at the end, just before menopause is reached (see Chapter 1). Women between the ages of 20 and 40 have the most consistent cycles.

What to Tell Your Daughter

We don't have a full picture, but the available pieces of the puzzle indicate that you may inherit menstrual cycle length and duration, as well as the age at which you reach menarche, from the women in your family. Extremely short and extremely long cycles may also run in families. Finally, a few studies indicate that the length of your menstrual cycle, measured when you're between ages 20 and 25, may predict when you'll reach menopause. Women whose cycles are shorter than usual (complete in 26 days or less) tend to reach menopause earlier than women whose cycles stretch out to 33 days or more.

WHAT'S NORMAL?

Q *What defines normal bleeding at perimenopause?*

A About 90 percent of women will see some changes in their bleeding patterns over the four to eight years before they stop menstruating. It's normal to skip periods, to have lighter periods or heavier periods, or to have a flow that lasts less than two days and more than four. The duration of the cycle often shrinks for a while (to 21 to 23 days) before expanding to longer and longer intervals until it stops altogether. It's also normal to have 28-day cycles all the way through peri-menopause until bleeding stops for good.

A study of 380 perimenopausal women found that 28 percent of the subjects noticed changes in both the amount and duration of their periods; 23 percent experienced changes in the amount of menstrual flow; 9 percent only saw changes in the frequency of their periods; and 13 percent went for three or more months without a period. All these changes are normal for peri-menopause.

Scientists have found that women typically lose about an eighth of a cup to a quarter-cup of blood and other discharge every cycle. Some women lose more, some less.

Is It True?

Fiction: Everybody's periods are pretty much the same.

Fact: There's much more variety than we thought. It might surprise you to learn that some women get a period every 11 days; others, every 100—less than four times a year. Some women lose so little blood every month that it's barely measurable, while others lose more than two cupfuls every cycle.

WHAT'S ABNORMAL?

Q *So, what defines abnormal bleeding at perimenopause?*

A Any of the following bleeding patterns qualify as "abnormal" and should be mentioned to your doctor: heavy bleeding and gushing, particularly when accompanied by clots; bleeding that lasts more than seven days in a row; cycles that begin less than 21 days apart or more than 35; any spotting or bleeding between periods; bleeding that begins during or after you've had sex; any change in your bleeding pattern, such as a period that stretches out an extra two days.

The take-home message about irregular bleeding is that you need to hit the right balance here. Pay attention to all changes and mention them to your doctor, but don't automatically assume that any change is a sign of cancer. It probably isn't, but why not find out for sure?

TOO LITTLE

Q *Is there such a thing as bleeding too little?*

A Women on oral contraceptives tend to have scanty periods, but if your flow is really short (less than four days) and light and you're not on the pill, you should mention this to your doctor, no matter what your age. It could be a sign of thyroid disease, inflammation of the uterine lining, or other conditions.

ACCORDING TO SCALE

To help women describe their symptoms more accurately, TREMIN researchers developed the Mansfield-Voda-Jorgensen Menstrual Bleeding Scale:

1. Spotting. A drop or two of blood, not even requiring sanitary protection (though you may prefer to use some).

2. Very light bleeding. You would need to change the least absorbent tampon or pad one or two times per day (though you may prefer to change more frequently).

3. Light bleeding. You would need to change a low- or regular-absorbency tampon or pad two or three times per day (though you may prefer to change more frequently).

4. Moderate bleeding. You would need to change a regular-absorbency tampon or pad every three to four hours (though you may prefer to change more frequently).

5. Heavy bleeding. You would need to change a high-absorbency tampon or pad every three to four hours (though you may prefer to change more frequently).

6. Very heavy bleeding or gushing. Protection hardly works at all; you would need to change the highest-absorbency tampon or pad every hour or two.

The TREMIN researchers test-drove this scale by randomly recruiting 31 women aged 35 to 55, all of whom were still menstruating and none of whom were using hormones. These women agreed to meticulously save and preserve all their used menstrual products—even stained toilet paper—from three complete cycles. They were also asked to use the six-point scale at the left to estimate how much blood they had lost. At the end of each cycle, a technician collected the samples so the researchers could measure their content. When all 1,489 products were processed, the data showed that the majority of the women's own ratings closely correlated with their actual blood loss. This was particularly true of the women who were the heaviest bleeders.

If you're experiencing heavy bleeding, or if you just want to keep better track of your flow, TREMIN recommends using the same menstrual calendar used by their participants (see opposite). You can download it for free by going to www.pop.psu.edu/tremin/tremin-docs.htm and clicking on the 2000–2001 calendar card. (This calendar doesn't line up with days of the week, so it can be used during any year.)

THAT'S HEAVY

Q *What does heavy bleeding mean, exactly?*

A Anything more than a third of a cup meets the definition of a heavy flow. In the most extreme cases, however, the loss can be more than two cups per cycle. (Yikes!) While some women literally catch their menstrual fluid in an inserted measuring cup (environmentally friendly, reusable menstrual cups are alternatives to pads and tampons, and some brands have measuring lines on the interior), most

The TREMIN Women's Health Calendar

1. Circle first and last dates of menstruation and join with a line.

2. Using the Mansfield-Voda-Jorgensen Menstrual Bleeding Scale, enter a code number above each menstrual date to designate amount of bleeding.

JANUARY
1 2 3 4 5 6 7 8 9 10 11 12 13 14 15 16 17 18 19 20 21 22 23 24 25 26 27 28

FEBRUARY
29 30 31 | 1 2 3 4 5 6 7 8 9 10 11 12 13 14 15 16 17 18 19 20 21 22 23 24 25

MARCH
26 27 28 29 | 1 2 3 4 5 6 7 8 9 10 11 12 13 14 15 16 17 18 19 20 21 22 23 24

APRIL
25 26 27 28 29 30 31 | 1 2 3 4 5 6 7 8 9 10 11 12 13 14 15 16 17 18 19 20 21

MAY
22 23 24 25 26 27 28 29 30 | 1 2 3 4 5 6 7 8 9 10 11 12 13 14 15 16 17 18 19

JUNE
20 21 22 23 24 25 26 27 28 29 30 31 | 1 2 3 4 5 6 7 8 9 10 11 12 13 14 15 16

JULY
17 18 19 20 21 22 23 24 25 26 27 28 29 30 | 1 2 3 4 5 6 7 8 9 10 11 12 13 14

AUGUST
15 16 17 18 19 20 21 22 23 24 25 26 27 28 29 30 31 | 1 2 3 4 5 6 7 8 9 10 11

SEPTEMBER
12 13 14 15 16 17 18 19 20 21 22 23 24 25 26 27 28 29 30 31 | 1 2 3 4 5 6 7 8

OCTOBER
9 10 11 12 13 14 15 16 17 18 19 20 21 22 23 24 25 26 27 28 29 30 | 1 2 3 4 5 6

NOVEMBER
7 8 9 10 11 12 13 14 15 16 17 18 19 20 21 22 23 24 25 26 27 28 29 30 31 | 1 2 3

DEC
4 5 6 7 8 9 10 11 12 13 14 15 16 17 18 19 20 21 22 23 24 25 26 27 28 29 30 | 1

DECEMBER
2 3 4 5 6 7 8 9 10 11 12 13 14 15 16 17 18 19 20 21 22 23 24 25 26 27 28 29

JANUARY
30 31 | 1 2 3 4 5 6 7 8 9 10 11 12 13 14 15 16 17 18 19 20 21 22 23 24 25 26

FEBRUARY
27 28 29 30 31 | 1 2 3 4 5 6 7 8 9 10 11 12 13 14 15 16 17 18 19 20 21 22 23

of us need help putting those amounts in perspective.

Excessive bleeding is the most common reason for having a hysterectomy. There is concern that many of these surgeries may actually be unnecessary, more a result of miscommunication between doctor and patient than a major health problem. For instance, women who usually have light periods have a much different idea of "heavy bleeding" than do women who bleed heavily every cycle. That's because every woman assumes her flow is average and adjusts her descriptions of "heavy" or "light" from there.

Too Much

Q *How unusual is heavy or prolonged bleeding during the menopause transition?*

A Not unusual at all. About 10 million American women deal with excessive menstrual bleeding every year, and half of them are in the 40-to-50-year-old age group. But while it's common, heavy bleeding often has a powerful impact on these women's lives;

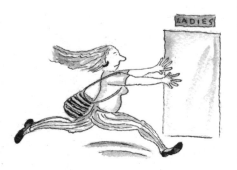

40 percent say they have difficulty working outside the home because their periods are so unpredictable and heavy that they live in constant fear of having a public accident. It can also put women at risk for anemia, since iron is released in the blood flow.

CAUSE AND EFFECT

Irregular bleeding can be caused by a hormonal imbalance, a normal part of perimenopause. But abnormal bleeding can be a sign of infection, pregnancy, thyroid or liver problems, polyps, cysts, fibroids, or cancer. It can also be related to using a variety of medications, contraceptives, or supplemental hormones. That's why it's important for you to talk to your doctor about everything you're experiencing and anything that concerns you.

When to See the Doctor

If you experience any of these symptoms, check with your physician:

❖ VERY HEAVY BLEEDING THAT LASTS MORE THAN FIVE DAYS OR INCLUDES CLOTS

❖ INTERMITTENT SPOTTING THAT DOESN'T FOLLOW A MONTHLY PATTERN

❖ BLEEDING WITH PAIN OR FEVER

❖ BLOOD IN YOUR URINE OR PAIN WHEN URINATING

❖ ABRUPT CESSATION OF PERIODS (YOU COULD STILL GET PREGNANT)

❖ BLEEDING DURING AND AFTER SEX

❖ ANY UNEXPECTED BLEEDING FROM THE UTERUS OR VAGINA

❖ UNUSUALLY SHORT OR LIGHT FLOW IF YOU'RE NOT ON THE PILL

HORMONAL IMBALANCE. As you move closer to menopause, your ovaries won't be producing as much estrogen as they once did. You may have more cycles that do not include the release of an egg for fertilization. As a result, your ovaries may be producing a continual stream of estrogen but no progesterone. The lack of progesterone may prompt your uterine lining to become much more overgrown than normal. Rather than the predictable periods you get when estrogen and progesterone are a tag team, estrogen-alone can result in crazy cycles and heavy, prolonged blood loss. These are not only annoying, embarrassing, and restrictive, but may also make you more vulnerable to endometrial cancer. That's one of the main reasons you need to mention irregular or heavy bleeding to your doctor.

GYNECOLOGICAL CANCERS. Only occasionally does irregular or heavy bleeding signal cancer of the uterus or cervix, but this is the main warning sign these cancers give. Regular pelvic exams, combined with Pap smears, ultrasounds, and biopsies as needed, can lead to early diagnosis of gynecological cancers. (For more information, see Chapter 13.)

PREGNANCY. You can get pregnant until you reach postmenopause. Heavy bleeding can be a sign of a miscarriage or an ectopic pregnancy. If there's any chance you could be pregnant, you need to get this checked out immediately.

What Can Happen

❖ As you move through perimenopause, expect your periods to come closer together before they begin to move farther apart and finally stop altogether.

❖ Approaching menopause, you can expect your periods to become more erratic. There are lots of versions of normal, and some women experience no changes until the very end.

❖ You might experience heavy bleeding, which is more common than once thought and can be difficult to manage. If your doctor recommends a hysterectomy, get a second opinion. There are many available treatments.

❖ There's always a small chance that irregular bleeding is a warning of gynecological cancer, which increases in women between 45 and 60. Mention it to your doctor and be prepared to answer detailed questions.

❖ If you take oral contraceptives or certain forms of hormone therapy, you may experience "withdrawal bleeding" when you stop taking estrogen. This is not the same as a normal menstrual period since ovulation is not involved.

INTRAUTERINE DEVICES (IUDs). If you have one and it's causing heavy bleeding, you need to consult with your doctor about a different method of birth control.

This list will help you understand the terms your doctor might use:

◆ **Amenorrhea.** Your periods have stopped, temporarily or permanently.

◆ **Hypomenorrhea.** Decreased flow appears at regular intervals.

◆ **Hypermenorrhea.** Your periods are heavier but appear at regular intervals.

◆ **Oligomenorrhea.** Your periods are coming less frequently.

◆ **Dysmenorrhea.** Your periods have become painful.

◆ **Metrorrhagia.** Bleeding is occurring between menstrual periods.

◆ **Polymenorrhea.** You're getting a period every 21 days or more frequently.

◆ **Menometrorrhagia.** Your periods are often heavy and irregular.

◆ **Menorrhagia.** Very heavy, prolonged (but regularly occurring) periods.

FIBROIDS. No one knows what causes these common noncancerous tumors to grow in the muscles of the uterus, and there's no way to prevent them. Fibroids generally appear between the ages of 30 and 50; since estrogen seems to spur their growth, they shrink naturally after menopause. Although most of the time they cause no symptoms, about 25 percent of women are made aware of them because of prolonged heavy periods accompanied by cramps, painful intercourse, and back pain, as well as bladder and bowel problems. Hormonal treatments such as oral contraceptives have not proved to be reliable. In the past, one of the only ways to deal with fibroids was to surgically remove them with a hysterectomy. Although they're still one of the most common reasons women have hysterectomies, there are many new less drastic treatments.

A *myomectomy* removes fibroids but leaves the uterus intact. That's good for women who want to maintain their fertility; the downside is that in about 20 to 40 percent of cases the fibroids recur. There is also a small chance that the surgery will cause scarring (adhesions) that can complicate fertility. Doctors determine which type of myomectomy to use based on the nature, size, and location of the fibroids. One type removes fibroids through the navel and abdomen with a laparoscope, basically a long, thin tube with a light. A second type removes them with a hysteroscope, a thin instrument similar to a telescope that enters the uterus through the cervix. A third, called an abdominal myomectomy or a laparotomy, involves an incision in the abdomen and can be used for all fibroids. A laparoscopic myomectomy with mini-laparotomy lets surgeons remove larger fibroids than a laparoscope alone could handle; the abdominal incision is usually three inches or less.

Uterine fibroid embolization is a newer and somewhat more controversial treatment for fibroids. A doctor who specializes in interventional radiology makes a

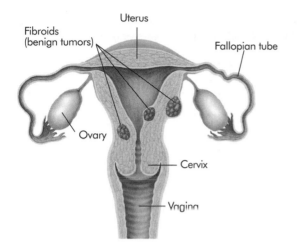

Fibroids
(benign tumors)

Uterus

Fallopian tube

Ovary

Cervix

Vagina

**WHERE FIBROIDS
GROW** Fibroids can grow
in three different locations:
between the muscles of the
uterine wall (intramural); under
the uterine lining and into the
uterine cavity (submucosal);
or from the uterine wall to the
outside of the uterus.

**UTERINE FIBROID
EMBOLIZATION** In
this controversial treatment,
a catheter is threaded
through an artery and used
to block the blood flow to a
problematic fibroid.

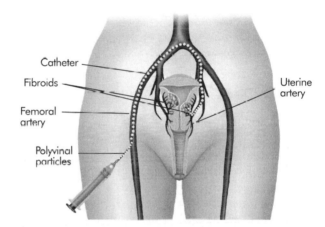

Catheter

Fibroids

Femoral
artery

Polyvinal
particles

Uterine
artery

small nick in the groin area and inserts a catheter into the artery. The catheter brings tiny plastic particles about the size of grains of sand into the artery supplying the fibroid. This cuts off the blood flow and shrinks the tumor.

Myolysis involves using lasers, electrical currents, or freezing to destroy fibroids during a laparoscopy. While leaving the uterus intact, this procedure can complicate future pregnancies and is generally not recommended for women who still hope to conceive. There are no studies on its long-term effectiveness compared with myomectomy.

Medication is another option. If a woman is close to menopause or has fibroids that need shrinking before surgery, doctors may treat her with gonadotropin-releasing hormone (GnRH) agonists, which temporarily shrink fibroids by blocking estrogen production. The treatment lasts up to six months before the fibroids return. The abortion pill RU-486 is also being studied as a treatment for fibroids.

At the Doctor's Office

Working with your doctor to figure out unusual bleeding is the first step toward treating it effectively. Before your appointment, make sure you're ready to answer these questions:

◆ Can you describe your normal flow and your recent experience?

◆ How often are your periods occurring?

◆ What color is the flow? Are there any clots?

◆ Are you experiencing any pain with the bleeding?

◆ Are you experiencing any spotting or intermittent bleeding between periods?

◆ Are you using contraceptives?

◆ What medications are you using?

◆ Is the bleeding problem hurting your ability to function?

It's very helpful to bring along a calendar with your periods marked (beginnings and endings), as well as notations on any unusual occurrences such as the passing of clots or changes in length or volume. Your doctor might also ask you to take your temperature on a daily basis to determine if you're still ovulating.

After reviewing your medical history, your doctor will probably give you a pelvic exam. Depending on your specific situation, one or more of the following tests and procedures may be recommended:

◆ A pregnancy test.

◆ Blood work (including tests for blood counts and hormone levels).

◆ An ultrasound of your uterus and/or ovaries.

◆ An endometrial biopsy.

◆ A hysteroscopy. In this procedure, a flexible scope with a light is inserted into the vagina and through the dilated cervix, permitting a view of the uterus. Anesthesia (local, regional, or general, depending on the situation) is administered beforehand. Sometimes the scope is used strictly for diagnosis, but it can also be used as a surgical tool if necessary.

◆ Dilation and curettage (D&C). This involves widening the cervix (dilation) and scraping the uterine lining (curettage), usually to resolve bleeding problems.

◆ A laparoscopy. In this procedure, a thin telescope-like instrument with a light is inserted into the abdomen through a small incision near or through the navel as part of an outpatient procedure. General anesthesia is usually given before it begins, although

Embarrassed to Ask

Q *I've read that abnormal bleeding is the most common symptom of endometrial cancer, but doesn't every perimenopausal woman have abnormal bleeding? How do I know when to mention it to my doctor?*

I'm afraid he'll say, "Of course you have abnormal bleeding, you're going through menopause," and I'll feel like an idiot.

A You're right that irregular bleeding is typical during perimenopause *and* that it's a common warning

occasionally regional or local anesthesia is used instead. Several more quarter-inch to half-inch incisions may also be made to move organs in and out of view of the scope. This procedure enables a doctor to look inside the abdomen for the cause of a problem, such as heavy bleeding. A hysteroscopy might also be done at the same time. Like the hysteroscopy, the laparoscopy can be used for both diagnosis and to perform surgery if necessary.

◆ A hysterosalpingography (HSG). This is a specialized type of X-ray designed to detect problems in the fallopian tubes and uterus. Most typically, it's used to determine if a woman's fallopian tubes are blocked, but it can also be used to detect growths or scarring within the uterus. After a local anesthetic is administered to the cervix, a special liquid is placed inside the uterus and through the fallopian tubes for viewing on an X-ray screen. Because the fluid may cause the uterus and fallopian tubes to stretch, it can be painful and prompt cramping. Pain medication is usually given beforehand. This procedure cannot be done on a day when heavy bleeding is taking place. You will need someone to take you home afterwards. Make sure you use an absorbent pad, because the draining fluid can stain clothing. Pain relievers and antibiotics are typically given as part of the follow-up treatment.

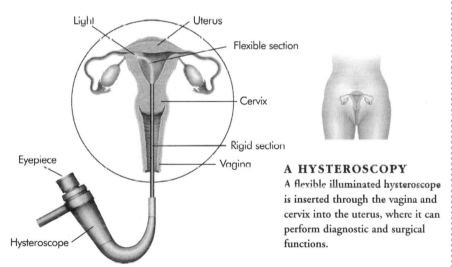

Light

Uterus

Flexible section

Cervix

Rigid section

Eyepiece

Vagina

Hysteroscope

A HYSTEROSCOPY

A flexible illuminated hysteroscope is inserted through the vagina and cervix into the uterus, where it can perform diagnostic and surgical functions.

sign of gynecological cancer. The fact that you're in perimenopause does not mean you can't also have cervical, ovarian, vaginal, endometrial, or uterine cancer, too. In fact, many of these cancers become most prevalent between ages 45 and 65. But it's also true that most irregular bleeding is *not* a sign of cancer. Only your doctor can assure you that your current bleeding pattern is no big deal. Depending on your particular situation, your doctor will likely do a pelvic exam and run some blood tests, and maybe request a biopsy or an ultrasound. You may also be asked to wait a few weeks or months to see if the abnormal pattern continues before you have more tests.

If a biopsy or ultrasound indicates that you're unlikely to have cancer, take that as reassuring news; however, if the abnormal pattern returns or continues, it's your job to keep bringing it up to your doctor. Some cancers take years to develop to the point where they can be detected. If abnormal bleeding continues, you may need to be repeatedly retested. About a third of premalignant growths are discovered on the second, third, or fourth round of testing. The trick here is to be vigilant without assuming the worst. Chances are, this is nothing to worry about—but you want to keep this issue on your doctor's radar screen.

Finally, you should be able to bring up any concern with your doctor without fearing ridicule. If you don't feel comfortable doing that, it's time to think about finding a new doctor.

WHY NOT TAMPONS?

Q *Why aren't there more products on the market to deal effectively with really heavy bleeding?*

A You could have found extra absorbent tampons on the drugstore shelves in the 1980s. But some women who wore them for extended periods of time developed toxic shock

syndrome. As the name implies, these women went into shock and some even died. The products were soon pulled from the shelves, and no safe, effective alternative has been developed so far. To deal with excessive bleeding, many women use multiple tampons and sanitary napkins to get the protection they need. But be aware that high-absorbency tampons are still associated with toxic shock. (Symptoms include high fever, chills, dizziness, vomiting, diarrhea, fainting, and a rash that resembles a sunburn.) If you suspect you're suffering from toxic shock, remove your tampon immediately and call your doctor. Because of continuing concern about toxic shock, it's recommended that you use the *least* absorbent tampons required to deal with your situation.

If you're interested in alternative methods of dealing with your menstrual flow, choices include natural sponges that can be rinsed out and reused, a disposable menstrual cup that's inserted high up in the vagina like a diaphragm (you can have sex while it's in place), and a reusable rubber cup placed lower inside the vagina. Both cups collect menstrual fluid (rather than absorbing it) and need to be emptied several times a day. While the reusable cups are relatively expensive ($20 to $40) compared with a box of tampons, they can be used for about 10 years and they're great for the environment.

IS IT ALL BLOOD?

Q *What exactly is in menstrual fluid? Is it really all blood?*

A Although the color of blood dominates, what you see is actually a combination of cervical mucus, cells from the uterine lining, and vaginal secretions, as well as blood.

DEALING WITH ANEMIA

Q *I've been having very heavy flows for months now, and I'm feeling really worn down. A friend said I need to take iron pills for this. That sounds incredibly old-fashioned.*

A Women who have very heavy menstrual flows are at higher risk of developing anemia, a disorder caused by insufficient red blood cells. Symptoms of anemia include headaches as well as feeling very tired or dizzy.

Rather than diagnose this on your own, see your doctor and get a blood test. Then discuss the best way to deal with it. You may want to take iron pills, but you may also want to change your diet. Red meat, prunes, enriched cereals, and dried beans and peas are all good food sources. Eating these foods with others rich in vitamin C will increase their absorption. Calcium, on the other hand, reduces absorption. In severe cases of anemia, a transfusion may be necessary. While you're at your doctor's, don't forget to discuss ways to reduce your very heavy flow.

WHAT IF IT'S HORMONES?

What are your treatment options if hormonal imbalance is at the root of your problem with unpredictable periods that are also long and heavy? Depending on your overall health and what your pelvic exam and lab work show, your doctor may suggest that you take a hormonal contraceptive in pill form or delivered via a vaginal ring, a transdermal patch, an injection, or an intrauterine device. Which one you choose depends on your medical history as well as your preference and your doctor's. The patch needs to be changed weekly and provides a comparatively high dose of hormones. The ring is easy to use; you simply take it out and reinsert it every few months. (See Chapters 2 and 3 for more information on the patch and the ring.) Many women prefer pills because that's what they're used to.

CONTRACEPTIVE PILLS. Low-dose pills, approved for nonsmoking women under 55, regulate irregular bleeding and protect against pregnancy, hot flashes, and bone loss. The pill can also lower your chances of developing endometrial or ovarian cancer. However, oral contraceptives can increase your risk of venous thromboembolism, a type of blood clot. While this risk is very low in healthy women in their 30s and 40s, it rises with body mass and age. The pill is not recommended for women with a history of blood clots, heart or vascular problems, jaundice, or an estrogen-dependent cancer (such as breast or endometrial cancer). Your doctor will probably also discourage use of oral contraceptives if you're obese or if you have high blood pressure, diabetes, or migraines with an aura. Some women on the pill have nausea and breast tenderness, but both tend to decrease with use. Some women say they get headaches and gain weight on the pill, but researchers haven't found that cause and effect.

Generally, you should take the lowest effective dose. Comparative studies indicate that lower-dose estrogen pills (20 milligrams) cause less breakthrough bleeding than slightly higher formulations (35 milligrams). If one type of oral contraception doesn't work or causes too many side effects, talk to your doctor about trying a different product or dose. If you want to bleed as little as possible, ask about the extended-cycle pill that will allow you to go four months without a period.

While many doctors recommend hormonal contraceptives to help control heavy bleeding, you should know that they are not approved by the FDA for this purpose.

PROGESTOGEN TREATMENTS. A levonorgestrel-releasing intrauterine system (IUS) is another way to provide contraception and manage prolonged heavy bleeding and excessive cramping. The IUS can be inserted into your uterus during an office visit. Once inside, it tends to slow down the growth of the uterine lining. Many women experience some initial irregular bleeding and spotting, but these side effects usually go away fairly quickly. Once your body adjusts to the IUS, you'll most likely have light cyclical periods or light irregular bleeding. Some women stop having a period while on the IUS.

Progestin-only treatment is another option for women who can't use estrogen-based contraceptives. Each injection lasts about three months. Irregular periods and spotting are common during the first year of use. Monthly periods may stop (temporarily) in about half the cases. If you stay on this treatment for a long period of time, be sure you talk to your doctor about possible bone loss.

If you're also experiencing hot flashes or lubrication problems and you can use estrogen, a very low dose can be added to your progestogen regimen.

There are also high-dose progestin, low-dose estrogen pills for smokers and other women who should not use oral contraceptives because of diabetes, high blood pressure, obesity, or migraine headaches. This treatment sometimes causes spotting or breakthrough bleeding initially and may eliminate periods for months at a time (amenorrhea).

Cyclic oral progestogens, which you take for 12 to 14 days a month, can also produce predictable periods. If you have hot flashes, a low-dose estrogen might be added.

GnRH AGONISTS. Gonadotropin-releasing hormonal agonists can fool your body into thinking it's reached menopause. Typically, doctors restrict use of GnRH agonists to six months because of the bone loss and hot flashes they can cause. However, if you've developed anemia, they may be considered.

Nonhormonal Treatments

If you don't want to use hormones, here's an overview of some other options:

Rest. If you have an occasional single day of heaving bleeding, sometimes getting extra rest will reduce your flow.

Over-the-counter nonsteroidal anti-inflammatory drugs (NSAIDs), such as ibuprofen and naproxen, might do the trick. They can be effective in reducing both blood loss (by 20 to 50 percent) and painful cramping. If you need to use these drugs longer or more often than the label recommends, check with your doctor.

An *endometrial ablation* destroys a thin layer of the endometrium to stop excessive bleeding. This is a surgical procedure, but no incisions are made; surgical devices are inserted through the vagina and dilated cervix. (See page 150.) The success rate is high, but occasionally heavy bleeding returns; in some cases, normal periods, light periods, or spotting may occur afterwards. As with any surgical procedure, endometrial

ablation has its risks (infection, the dangers of anesthesia, a uterine puncture), and there is little information about its long-term effects. But unlike hysterectomies, ablations are performed on an outpatient basis, and recovery is usually much faster.

If you're considering an endometrial ablation, you'll want a doctor who is experienced in this field. Be sure to discuss your anesthesia and pain relief options before the surgery. While there's very little chance that you can get pregnant after this procedure has been performed, you should continue using birth control just to be sure. Pap smears and regular pelvic exams should continue as well.

TAMOXIFEN AND BLEEDING

Q *I've got breast cancer and am taking tamoxifen to reduce my risk of recurrence. The nurse told me that I need to be particularly good about reporting unusual bleeding. Why?*

A Abnormal bleeding can be a symptom of endometrial cancer, and taking tamoxifen (Nolvadex) slightly increases your risk for this type of uterine cancer. Tamoxifen is a selective estrogen receptor modulator, which means it acts like estrogen in some parts of the body and not in others. This drug offers some protection against estrogen-responsive tumors because it can slip into the estrogen receptors on cancer-prone molecules in the breast, prevent-

ENDOMETRIAL ABLATION: KEEPING THE UTERUS

There are several specific types of the surgical proccedure called endometrial ablation, including:

Fluid-filled thermal balloon ablation. In this procedure, a deflated balloon is inserted into a woman's uterus through the cervix and then filled with a heated liquid. As the balloon expands and comes into contact with the walls of the uterus, heat and energy are used to destroy its lining. This technique is not recommended for women who have a large or irregularly shaped uterus. Nor is it an option for women who've had a classical cesarean or certain other abdominal surgeries involving the uterus.

Electrical ablation. This procedure utilizes a thin wire loop or rollerball tool that conducts electrical current to destroy the uterine lining. The doctor monitors the surgery with the aid of a hysteroscope. Once in place, it releases a gas or liquid to expand the uterus, making it easier to perform the surgery.

Lasers. These high-intensity light beams can vaporize or otherwise destroy targeted tissue. They can also be used to stop bleeding at its source. A hysteroscope is usually used in this surgery as well.

Cryoablation. Similar to the above procedures, cryoablation uses freezing agents to destroy the uterine lining.

Microwave ablation. Microwaves are produced by a probe inserted into the uterus.

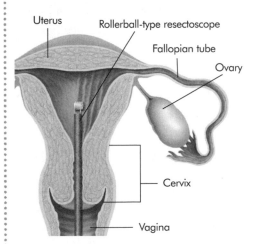

Uterus
Rollerball-type resectoscope
Fallopian tube
Ovary
Cervix
Vagina

EXAMPLE OF ENDOMETRIAL ABLATION A rollerball-type tool is used to destroy the uterine lining in order to reduce or eliminate excessive bleeding.

ing estrogen from docking there. The result: less estrogen available to fuel a recurrence of breast cancer. However, tamoxifen acts like estrogen in the uterus and can promote overgrowth of the lining. When women weigh the relative pluses and minuses, most decide that the protection tamoxifen offers against a recurrence of breast cancer is worth it. But this means that women taking it need to be particularly vigilant about reporting any abnormal vaginal bleeding to their doctor and having it checked out.

Because of all this, you may want to talk to your doctor about a similar drug, raloxifene, which offers anticancer protection without increasing the risk of endometrial cancer. But it has its own side effects (see Chapter 13).

MISSING DOSES

Q I've been using the pill for birth control for most of my adult life and recently missed a bunch of doses because I've been traveling a lot. Since then, my periods have been erratic, really long, and very heavy. I'm also getting hot flashes. Did I accidentally bring on menopause? And can I go back on my pills?

A Missing those birth-control pills didn't push you into menopause. The pills were actually masking your symptoms. When you missed some days, you got a glimpse of where you are in the menopause transition.

Most doctors advise women to go off oral contraceptives sometime between the ages of 50 and 55, the typical age of menopause. If you're on the brink of menopause or have already reached it, your doctor will probably want you to discontinue your pills because they have a higher hormone level than you need at this point and you no longer require protection against an unplanned pregnancy. If you have significant symptoms and you're still perimenopausal, your doctor may encourage you to go back on the pill. If you have significant symptoms and you've moved on to menopause, your doctor will discuss a variety of lifestyle and pharmaceutical options, including short-term low-dose hormone therapy.

INTERFERENCE WITH SEX

Q This heavy bleeding that I'm experiencing right now is really getting in the way of my sex life. Any suggestions?

A Anytime you have a symptom that interferes with your ability to have a normal life, you should bring it to the attention of your clinician. A lot of women assume that whatever level of bleeding they're experiencing is normal and just has to be endured—or that the only alternative is a hysterectomy. Depending on what's causing the bleeding, your doctor should have an array of solutions. In some cases, medications, including low-dose oral contraceptives, or an intrauterine device (IUD) can slow your flow and keep your periods regular until you reach menopause. There are also surgical interventions, such as an endometrial ablation (see pages 149–50), that are less drastic than a hysterectomy. If this is a long-term problem, you need a long-term solution, because heavy bleeding can lead to anemia. But what do you do in the short run? You may want to start with a frank talk with your partner about how you both feel about making love when you're bleeding. Some women assume that it's a turnoff, but that's often not the case. If you discover that it doesn't bother either of you, protect the bed with a washable mattress pad and dark sheets, plus a couple of layers of old (preferably dark) towels. If vaginal lubrication has become an issue for you, menstrual blood flow offers the advantage of providing constant moisture. Afterwards, some couples like to climb into a hot shower together. If you want to find a way to have intercourse without dealing with the mess, you can insert a diaphragm or a disposable menstrual cup (the brand name is Instead; it's available at drugstores or online) to catch your flow. The diaphragm offers the extra advantage of contraception; the menstrual cup does not. If intercourse isn't a must, you can insert a tampon or two and find more creative ways to make each other happy. If you

prefer pads, consider using a vibrator on top of your underwear to achieve clitoral orgasm. Will having sex make the bleeding worse? It varies. One study of 120 perimenopausal women found that those who had intercourse during menstruation tended to have heavier periods than those who didn't. One final word: If you have multiple sex partners, keep in mind that you're more susceptible to pelvic infection when you're bleeding.

A Gusher

Q *I've been having a heavier-than-normal flow during the transition, but last week I just gushed blood. I found the whole thing very frightening. Will this keep happening?*

A Although it's a common experience among perimenopausal women, gushing is still scary and kind of stunning when it happens to you, partly because you can't control the flow. It's especially unnerving when it catches you completely unprepared or when you're wearing light-colored clothing. It's not known exactly why these excessive flows occur or which women will continue to have the problem. Mention this episode to your doctor, especially if blood clots were passed. If it happens more than twice, your doctor can suggest ways to control excessive bleeding, including oral contraceptives and progesterone treatments. You should also be checked for anemia.

BLEEDING AFTER SEX

Q *I'm postmenopausal and haven't bled for years. But now I bleed every time I have intercourse.*

A While it's possible to have another period a year or two after you thought you had reached menopause, the fact that your bleeding happens only with sex suggests that its source may be vaginal rather than uterine. As estrogen levels drop, vaginal skin gets thinner and more fragile. If you haven't been using lots of lubricants or personal moisturizers or haven't been having sex very often, your vagina is likely to get irritated when it's put back into action. But since there are lots of things that can cause bleeding after menopause, it would be smart to get it checked out. If it turns out to be related to a dry vagina, talk to your doctor about the range of solutions, including short-term use of a local hormone therapy. (See Chapter 2.)

HYSTERECTOMIES: WHEN AND WHY

The diagnosis could be fibroids, endometriosis, uterine prolapse, or even uterine cancer. Your doctor recommends a hysterectomy—an operation to remove your uterus. Some women find this news traumatic, and not only because they're facing major surgery. To them it means losing their womb—the essence of what makes them female. Other women react differently, happy to be free of pregnancy worries and debilitating bleeding. Whatever your own reaction, you're not alone. Hysterectomies are the second most common major operations for women (after cesareans). While the number of hysterectomies in the United States has declined to 600,000 a year from its peak of 740,000 in 1975, the Department of Health and Human Services estimates that about a third of American women will have had a hysterectomy by age 60—one of the highest hysterectomy rates in the world.

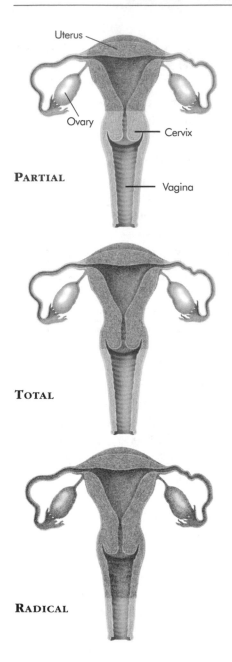

PARTIAL

Uterus

Ovary

Cervix

Vagina

TOTAL

RADICAL

WHAT HAPPENS IN A HYSTERECTOMY In a partial hysterectomy, only the uterus is removed. The cervix and ovaries may be removed as well in total and radical hysterectomies, respectively.

That said, hysterectomies are controversial; many doctors think the operation should be performed only when alternative treatments haven't worked. In the past, most women would have had their ovaries routinely removed when they had a hysterectomy, especially if they were close to the age of natural menopause. Now that decision is more complex. Depending on the reason for the hysterectomy, at least one of the ovaries can be left intact, allowing a natural path to menopause. But age may still play a role in the decision. Some doctors recommend removing the ovaries of patients who are close to menopause since this greatly reduces the risk of ovarian cancer and even breast cancer. Other doctors disagree. Hysterectomy is rarely an emergency procedure; you have time to get the answers you need to make your decision. Make sure you get a second opinion. Some questions to ask:

• Are there any alternative treatments for my problem?

• How will the surgery be performed?

• What are the risks?

• Do my ovaries need to be removed? If so, will I take hormones?

• Will I have a scar?

• How long will I be in the hospital? When will I be able to get back to work?

• What side effects can I expect?

• Will the operation affect my sex life?

Types of Hysterectomies			
	POINT OF ENTRY	AVERAGE HOSPITAL STAY	AVERAGE RECOVERY TIME
Total abdominal	Abdominal (4-to-6-inch incision)	3 to 6 days	6 weeks
Vaginal	Vagina	1 to 3 days	4 weeks
Laparoscopic-assisted vaginal (LAHV)	Vaginal/navel (tiny incisions in abdomen)	1 to 3 days	4 weeks
Laparoscopic supracervical	Tiny incisions in abdomen/navel (less than ¼ inch)	1 day or less	6 days

Traditionally, a hysterectomy meant just one thing: a large incision across your abdomen and a long recuperation period. Today, there are other options. Which one your doctor chooses depends on the problem you're treating. A *total hysterectomy* involves removal of the uterus and cervix. The ovaries and fallopian tubes may or may not stay in place. If the ovaries are removed, you enter menopause immediately. In a *partial hysterectomy*, the portion of the uterus above the cervix is removed. Fallopian tubes or ovaries may or may not be taken out. It's also an easier operation. After a partial hysterectomy, a regular Pap smear is still required. A *radical hysterectomy* is the most extensive surgery and generally recommended only to treat some uterine or cervical cancers. This type of hysterectomy involves removal of the uterus, cervix, upper vagina, and some of the pelvic lymph nodes. The ovaries and fallopian tubes may stay in or be removed.

Surgeons approach the uterus from the abdomen or the vagina. In an abdominal hysterectomy, the surgeon cuts through the skin and connective tissue to get at the uterus. Recovery may take many weeks because of the time needed to heal the incision. This is the most invasive type of hysterectomy and also the most common—it's generally used for large fibroids, severe endometriosis, pelvic infections, and some cancers. A vaginal hysterectomy involves a circular incision around the cervix. It's commonly used to treat prolapse and early cancers. In a laparoscopically assisted vaginal hysterectomy, the surgeon inserts a laparoscope (a thin telescope with a light) through a tiny incision in the navel and abdomen. An even less invasive procedure is a laparoscopic supracervical hysterectomy, which lets the surgeon use the laparoscope and small surgical instruments to separate the uterus from the cervix and then carefully remove it. Preserving the cervix may help reduce the risk of pelvic floor prolapse, incontinence, and other possible complications of a total hysterectomy.

YOUNG AND OLD

Q *I thought only older women had hysterectomies, but a friend of mine who's 42 is about to go into the hospital to have her uterus taken out. Isn't that unusual?*

A Actually, your friend is exactly the average age of women who undergo a hysterectomy. More than 75 percent of all women who have a hysterectomy are between 20 and 49 years old. Problems like fibroids and endometriosis affect younger women, not women who are past menopause.

RISK ASSESSMENT

Q *I know a hysterectomy is major surgery, but does that mean it's dangerous? What are the risks?*

A Any surgery carries risk; your doctor should explain all this to you. Don't agree to the surgery until you understand everything. Now to the particular hazards of hysterectomies, which are actually among the safest operations performed today. Let's start with the worst but rare possible outcome. In the absence of cancer or pregnancy, the

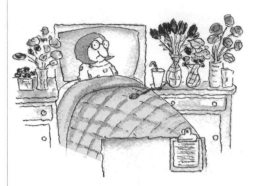

overall death rate from hysterectomies is 6 to 11 deaths per 10,000 women. The most common complication is fever from an infection. Other possible problems include hemorrhage, injury to nearby organs, and a blood clot in the lungs. In general, a vaginal hysterectomy is less risky than abdominal surgery.

Long-term effects include possible premature ovarian failure, pelvic pain, and diminished sexual interest and response. At greatest risk for depression after a hysterectomy are women under 35, those who haven't had a child, those who want children, and women who lose ovarian hormonal functions after the operation.

Remember, these are all *possible* problems. You could sail through surgery without experiencing any of them. But it's important to know all the pros and cons before you make a decision.

OTHER CHOICES

Q *What about medication or less invasive surgery as an alternative?*

In some cases, you may be able to put off surgery. If you have fibroids, many doctors adopt a "wait and watch" approach since there's no reason to treat these benign growths unless they're causing significant pain or discomfort. Both fibroids and endometriosis often stabilize or diminish as you get close to menopause and your estrogen levels drop. In the meantime, you may be able to take medications that interfere with the effects of estrogen. Minor uterine prolapse can be treated with a pessary, a device that's inserted to support the uterus mechanically. Strengthening and exercising the pelvic muscles also helps. (For details on how to Kegel, see pages 118–19.) Whatever your situation, it's important to ask your doctor to explain the different approaches and what might work for you.

A LITTLE FLATTENING

Q *I'm scheduled for a hysterectomy, and I'm wondering if I could get a tummy tuck at the same time. I wouldn't feel so bad about losing my uterus if I could come out of this with a flat stomach!*

A If you've been wanting to get this kind of work done, we think this is a great way to make lemonade out of lemons. You'll need to talk to your ob-gyn and your plastic surgeon about whether you're a good candidate for this. The doctors will have to coordinate their surgery schedules, but it's not unusual to combine nonemergency procedures that require anesthesia. We have a friend who did this (and had a little liposuction on her thighs at the same time). Just be aware that while your medical insurance will pay for the hysterectomy, it's very unlikely to cover the cosmetic surgery.

OVARIES IN OR OUT

Q *I'm 48 and about to have a hysterectomy to treat large fibroids. My doctor says I should have my ovaries removed to prevent cancer, but there's no ovarian or breast cancer in my family. Is this necessary?*

A It's a controversial issue. Some doctors think it's smart to remove the ovaries of a woman close to menopause or past it in order to protect against ovarian cancer, which is very difficult to detect at an early stage when it's still treatable. But other doctors contend that not only is this cancer rare, but women without ovaries can develop it if it's already present in other cells. A younger woman who loses her ovaries would have an increased risk of heart disease and osteoporosis. The loss of testosterone produced by the ovaries might also affect a woman's sexual pleasure, as well as deprive her of a natural source of estrogen (through testosterone conversion) after menopause. Your doctor should explain exactly why taking out the ovaries is important in your case. If you don't like the answers, don't agree to the surgery. Get a second opinion.

Finally, be prepared. We know of a number of women whose doctors had agreed to leave their ovaries intact but who woke up from surgery to find them gone. This can happen because something troubling was found that hadn't been detected before. But you need to have a clear discussion with your doctor about all the possibilities.

LIBIDO LOSS?

Q *I'm getting a hysterectomy but keeping my ovaries. My sex life should improve, right?*

A Sexual response is very individual, but surveys indicate that most women who get the surgery after years of dealing with excessive bleeding, pelvic pain, fibroids, or endometriosis report that sex is better after a hysterectomy. Still, some women miss the uterine shudders they used to get with their orgasms; for others, the penis tapping their cervix was an orgasmic trigger. On rare occasions, some of the nerves that help you produce an orgasm can get severed during surgery. If this happens, you can try experimenting with new positions or methods of stimulation, including a vibrator. You may find something that works as well or better. If not, think about a consulta-

tion with a gynecologist who specializes in sexual function, or ask your doctor for a referral to a sex therapist. It may also be a good idea to see a therapist if you think there might be a psychological component to any loss of libido. For example, some women mourn the loss of their fertility.

In a minority of cases (about 30 percent), a hysterectomy disrupts blood flow to the ovaries and several years after surgery one or both ovaries start shutting down. Sometimes this sends you into menopause earlier than normal. The subsequent drop in hormone levels could make you feel like every night is "Not tonight, honey." This loss of sex drive tends to get stronger over time. Because you're no longer menstruating, you don't have the usual signal that menopause is starting: irregular periods. If this is your situation, talk to your doctor about taking estrogen and testosterone to get you through this transition. Women who go through surgical menopause are more likely to experience hormone deficiency syndrome than women who go through it naturally and may need higher doses of estrogen and testosterone to correct the problem.

KEEPING THE CERVIX

Q *I don't understand why it's such a big deal to keep my cervix. That seems a little like saving the door after the house is torn down.*

Although there's some disagreement about this, many doctors feel that leaving the cervix reduces the chances of developing urinary incontinence and pelvic floor support problems. The cervix may also improve your chances of maintaining sexual arousal and the ability to reach orgasm. As long as you have your cervix, you may have some bleeding periodically and you may still need an annual Pap smear.

REMOVAL OF FALLOPIAN TUBES

Q *If your ovaries are removed, do you keep your fallopian tubes?*

A There's no reason to keep them. If the ovaries are taken out, the fallopian tubes are generally removed as well because their only role is to carry eggs to the uterus.

FALLEN UTERUS

Q *My doctor says my uterus is sagging and I might need surgery someday. What's happening inside me?*

A As you get older, muscles that support your vagina lose tone and sag downward, and your bladder or rectum can be pulled down as well. It's a very common occurrence, and most women aren't bothered by it very much. In some women, however, the sagging is so severe that they feel a heavy or dragging sensation in their pelvic area and have problems controlling urination or bowel function. Sometimes one of the

organs protrudes through the vaginal opening. This is a major reason for doing Kegel exercises (pages 118–19). A pessary may keep the uterus in place. In the most serious cases, a hysterectomy can provide relief. You need to decide if your discomfort warrants that step.

PAP SMEARS

Q *I had a hysterectomy because my fibroids were becoming larger and more painful. I still have my cervix. Do I need a Pap smear every year?*

A A Pap smear is an important screening test for cervical cancer. However, you may now fall into one of the three groups of women who generally don't need the test: young women who aren't sexually active, women over 70 who have had normal Pap smears in the past, and women who've had a hysterectomy for benign conditions such as fibroids. You still need regular pelvic exams. One caveat: You'll need a Pap smear if you've ever had an abnormal smear or if you had a hysterectomy because of a cancerous condition.

POSTMENOPAUSAL BLEEDING PROBLEMS

Any uterine or vaginal bleeding occurring after menopause (except when it's associated with hormone therapy) needs to be checked out by a doctor. It could be nothing. Research into menstrual cycles indicates that a small percentage of women will get another period or two even after a break of one or two years. Because postmenopausal women may still be producing a little estrogen but no progesterone, some doctors will prophylactically give them a dose of a progestogen, just to be sure that any remaining endometrial lining is sloughed off. By doing so, they hope to reduce the risk of cancer developing there. While there have been no clinical studies to determine if this is an effective method of reducing the incidence of cancer, many doctors think there's little chance that it would do any harm and may well be preventive. But it could also be caused by something like an infection, a sexually transmitted disease, or vaginal dryness. A postmenopausal woman with a narrowed cervix (cervical stenosis) may develop an accumulation of pus or menstrual fluid or blood in her uterus (hematometra). A variety of treatments, including antibiotics and cervical dilation, may be needed to resolve the problem.

Unexplained bleeding could also be a warning sign of a gynecological cancer. While there's no need to panic, it does call for a pelvic exam and possibly an ultrasound or biopsy. If nothing unusual is found, be reassured. But if the bleeding continues, you'll need to follow up with your doctor and be retested. A significant number of premalignant growths are found after repeated testing.

CHAPTER 7

Aches and Pains

Our hearts and minds are ready for excitement and adventure. So why do our bodies rebel? Even if you're exercising regularly and doing everything you can to maintain a healthy weight, you may find yourself struggling with some of the common midlife complaints that we talk about in this chapter, starting with headaches and moving on to mouth and gum problems, thyroid trouble, shoulder injuries, breast pain, arthritis, a leaky bladder, and sore feet. None of these ailments is immediately life-threatening, but any one of them can get in the way of all the things you want to do. It's more than a little discouraging to finally have time and money for that trip to Hawaii only to find that your aching knees don't want to go along.

Men have many of the same complaints as they get older, so we can't blame menopause for everything. Aging inevitably changes our bodies. We're also dealing with new stresses, such as caring for sick parents, coping with changes at work, and adjusting to the empty nest. All of these can make us more vulnerable to illness.

Still, there are some surprising connections between the hormonal roller coaster many of us are riding and migraines, creaky joints, and even urinary tract infections. Scientists are only beginning to unravel these links; there's much to learn about how estrogen interacts with all the different mechanisms in your body. For now,

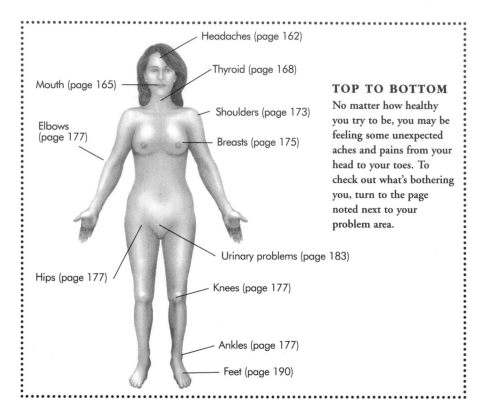

Headaches (page 162)

Thyroid (page 168)

Mouth (page 165)

Shoulders (page 173)

Elbows (page 177)

Breasts (page 175)

TOP TO BOTTOM
No matter how healthy you try to be, you may be feeling some unexpected aches and pains from your head to your toes. To check out what's bothering you, turn to the page noted next to your problem area.

Urinary problems (page 183)

Hips (page 177)

Knees (page 177)

Ankles (page 177)

Feet (page 190)

perhaps just knowing that it's not all in your head may be a comfort (unless you're talking about migraines, of course). And realizing that there's help out there—that you don't have to just grin and bear it—is a huge relief.

HEADACHES

L et's start at the top with the king of all headaches: the migraine. Often accompanied by throbbing pain, nausea, vomiting, sensitivity to light, and tension in shoulder and neck muscles, migraines can occur on one or both sides of the head. Bright lights and noise often make the pain worse. You will probably hear the two most prevalent kinds of migraines described as "classic" and "common." Classic migraines are preceded by an "aura," a vision disturbance that can last for 20 minutes; the headache usually comes on within an hour after the aura. Common migraines have no aura and may start more slowly and be more debilitating. Both kinds can last from a few hours to days and typically occur in clusters once or twice a month, although many migraine sufferers are afflicted only once or twice a year.

Estrogen has long been linked to migraines. Before puberty, boys are slightly more subject to migraines than girls are. Among adults, women have

When to See the Doctor

Call your doctor if you experience any of the following:

❖ A SUDDEN AND SEVERE HEADACHE WITH FEVER, STIFF NECK, OR VOMITING

❖ A HEADACHE THAT CAUSES CONFUSION OR LOSS OF CONSCIOUSNESS

❖ PERSISTENT HEADACHES THAT REQUIRE MEDICATION MORE THAN TWO DAYS A WEEK

❖ UNEXPLAINED WEIGHT GAIN OR LOSS

❖ PERSISTENT FATIGUE

❖ NERVOUSNESS OR ANXIETY FOR NO REASON

❖ A CRUNCHING SENSATION IN A JOINT OR THE SOUND OF BONE RUBBING ON BONE

❖ STEADY OR INTERMITTENT PAIN IN A JOINT

❖ BLOOD IN YOUR URINE AND PAIN WHEN URINATING

two to three times more migraines than men. But estrogen is not the only culprit. Other triggers include certain foods (red wine, cured meat, alcohol, chocolate, and onions, to name a few), stress, lack of sleep, and smoke or other odors.

MENSTRUAL MIGRAINES

Q *I've always gotten migraines around the time of my period. When I was pregnant, the migraines disappeared. Can I expect to be migraine-free after menopause?*

A Relief could be on the way. After menopause, women's migraines tend to taper off. Many women have migraines during menstruation but not during pregnancy. (Others, however, find their attacks are unchanged or even worse during pregnancy.) Scientists think

declining estrogen levels are responsible. Perimenopausal women seem particularly vulnerable, especially if they have a history of frequent headaches when they're menstruating. Less than 10 percent of female migraine sufferers have headaches only at the time of menstruation, according to the National Headache Foundation.

THAT AWFUL PAIN

Q *My migraines are certainly related to triggers (in my case, stress), but what actually causes the pain? It feels like my head's going to split.*

A The pain of migraines comes from the swelling of blood vessels around the brain in response to falling levels of the chemical messenger serotonin. Serotonin levels can be affected by many things, including blood sugar, certain foods . . . and estrogen levels. Family history may also play a role; there's good evidence for a genetic predisposition to migraines. However, scientists still don't understand exactly why or how all these things come together to produce a migraine in any single individual.

HORMONES AND MIGRAINES

Q *If there's a connection between estrogen and migraines, does that mean I should or shouldn't take oral contraceptives or use hormone therapy to deal with menopausal symptoms?*

A The answer really depends on your overall health history, the severity of your migraines, and your most common triggers. You need to discuss all of these with your doctor before you make a decision. Some recent studies suggest that combined oral contraceptives increase the risk of stroke in women with migraines. The risk appears to be greater for women who have classic migraines. If you're a smoker who gets migraines, your doctor will probably say you should avoid oral contraceptives.

Women who go through natural menopause seem to have fewer headaches than women who have had induced menopause. Low-dose estrogen therapy can help some women. Doctors think women with migraines may do better with hormone patches than with oral

estrogen. (For more on the risks and benefits of menopausal hormone therapy, see Chapter 2.)

TREATMENTS

Q *I know there are pills I can take for my migraines, but I'd like to try some nonpharmaceutical remedies first. What works?*

A To stop migraines before they start, keep a diary to pinpoint your triggers and then avoid them. If, say, stress is a trigger, practice relaxation techniques like meditation or yoga. Getting enough sleep is also important. But don't try to tough it out too long. Most people have lots of migraine triggers, and it's pretty hard to avoid all of them. It's also important to catch a migraine early; if you wait too long, it will be much more difficult to stop. Mild migraines often get better with over-the-counter painkillers like acetaminophen, aspirin, and ibuprofen. If you're taking these more than a couple of times a week, you need to see your physician for more help.

A class of drugs called serotonin agonists or triptans (which act on a subgroup of serotonin receptors) is often where doctors start. Some brand names are Imitrex, Maxalt, Zomig, and Relpax. These medications can cause tingling in your fingers or tightness in your throat and chest (which may feel like a heart attack). You shouldn't

DO YOU HAVE MIGRAINE ON THE MENU?

Keep a food diary to see if any foods trigger your headaches. Some possibilities include:

◆ Aged, canned, or cured meat

◆ Aged cheese

◆ Alcohol, especially red wine

◆ Avocados

◆ Beans, including broad, lima, and Italian

◆ Chocolate

◆ Meat tenderizer

◆ Monosodium glutamate (MSG)

◆ Nuts and peanut butter

◆ Onions

◆ Papaya

◆ Peas

◆ Pizza

◆ Yogurt

take them if you have a history of cardiovascular disease or uncontrolled high blood pressure. Another group of drugs are ergots, which come from a rye fungus. They constrict blood vessels and stimulate serotonin. Brands include Migranal Nasal Spray (which works best at the start of a headache), Ergostat, and Cafergot, which includes caffeine. These also have possible side effects, including nausea, vomiting, and leg cramps, and should not be used by people with cardiovascular disease, high blood pressure, or kidney or liver disease. If you use any of these drugs, it's important to follow your doctor's instructions. Using them too infrequently, for example, may actually increase the frequency of migraines.

MORNING HEADACHES

Q *I seem to wake up every morning with a headache. I swear it's not a hangover! What could be going on? This just started a few months ago.*

A A lot of things could cause this problem, and you should see your doctor to get an accurate diagnosis. One possibility is a sleep-related breathing disorder. If you have trouble drawing in enough air when you're sleeping, you raise the carbon dioxide level in your blood; this increases the blood flow and raises the pressure in your brain. Before you go to the doctor, ask your husband or partner whether you make any gasping noises when you sleep. It could be an indication of sleep apnea. (For more on sleep-related breathing disorders, see Chapter 4.)

MOUTH PROBLEMS

BURNING MOUTH SYNDROME

Q *I've got this dry, burning feeling in my mouth and on my tongue, and food doesn't taste the same to me. Could this be related to menopause?*

A What you're describing is burning mouth syndrome. According to a report in the journal *American Family*

Physician, 10 to 40 percent of women seeking treatment for menopausal symptoms experience some variation of this problem, compared with less than 3 percent of the general population, but its direct link to menopause is unknown. Women usually get a burning feeling on the tongue and along the lips and sides of the mouth. It tends to get worse as the day goes on. Some women say it's especially bad late at night, when it keeps them awake; if they do get to sleep, the discomfort goes away. The pain varies from mild to severe (some women compare it to a bad toothache) and is often accompanied by dry mouth. Many foods—especially salty, peppery, and sour things—don't taste the same. There may be a persistent metallic or bitter taste in the mouth and an increased sensitivity to cold and hot foods.

WHO GETS IT. While a burning sensation in the mouth is associated with diabetes and anemia (and can be a side effect of a medication, such as one of the medications for high blood pressure called angiotensin-converting enzyme inhibitors), the classic case of burning mouth syndrome appears out of nowhere, with no obvious cause, and lasts for years. Women who are depressed and anxious tend to experience it more than others, which may explain why doctors once thought it was largely psychosomatic. Now, however, it's more common to assume that the lack of sleep and chronic pain associated with burning mouth syndrome may be the cause of those mood problems rather than the other way around.

WHY IT HAPPENS. There's no consensus about what causes this syndrome or even agreement that all cases have the same cause. Scientists have known for a while that menopausal women lose the ability to detect bitter tastes over time, and some wonder if there's a connection between this tendency and burning mouth syndrome. There's also the intriguing fact that many people who report this problem have recently had some dental work or an upper respiratory infection, either of which could have resulted in nerve damage—another possible cause of the syndrome. Generally, the pain subsides during the process of eating, which could indicate that the nerves busy sending taste signals to the brain don't have the capacity to cause pain.

Burning mouth syndrome has also been associated with a very dry mouth. Some doctors routinely screen all patients with this syndrome for Sjögren's syndrome, an autoimmune disease that often causes dry mouth and eyes (see Chapter 11). Nine out of 10 people with Sjögren's are women who often have their first symptoms when they're in their late 40s.

Burning mouth syndrome could also be linked to candidal (fungal) infections, like those that cause thrush in babies. The University of Connecticut's Taste and Smell Center treats many patients who come with burning mouth syndrome for a candidal infection, even if there's no visible sign of it and their oral cultures come back negative. Patients are asked to dissolve Nystatin vaginal troches in their mouths. (These lozenges are sugar-free; people with dry mouths are more susceptible to developing cavities because of the lack of saliva.) If patients get better after two weeks of four treatments a day, this regimen is continued for another 6 to 10 weeks. If the treatment doesn't work, a brain scan may be recommended to see if a tiny stroke has damaged the part of the brain associated with oral burning.

Because burning mouth syndrome is also associated with nutritional deficiencies, some doctors recommend supplements, including vitamins C and B, iron, and zinc, if lab work indicates that these might ease symptoms.

Although there have been few high-quality studies on the treatment of burning mouth syndrome, many doctors now prescribe a variety of drugs, including benzodiazepines, tricyclic antidepressants, anticonvulsants, and topical capsaicin. Your dentist or doctor may also suggest saliva substitutes. In most cases, the burning goes away over time, but without effective treatment this might mean five or more years. One final note: Although no one has established a direct link between burning mouth syndrome and hormone deficiencies, women who use hormone therapy for their other menopausal symptoms sometimes find that their mouth pain disappears along with their hot flashes. This is another reminder that there's still a lot to learn about menopause.

CHANGING GUMS

Q *When I went to the dentist recently, she took one look at my gums and told me I might be entering perimenopause. How does this hormonal change show up in my mouth?*

A Dentists say they often notice a subtle change in the gums of women in their 40s. The tissue may be more swollen, or perhaps there's unusual bleeding. Gum disease is caused by plaque, a sticky film of bacteria that forms on your teeth. You need to remove that plaque with daily brushing and flossing and visit the dentist regularly to get a good cleaning. Left untreated, plaque irritates and inflames your gums. Eventually, your gums will separate from your teeth and form pockets where more bacteria will thrive. The hormonal fluctuations of perimenopause can make your gums even more sensitive to plaque. That's why good dental care is important as you get older. Your dental X-rays can also offer some clues to the health of your bones. Loose teeth can indicate thinning bones. (For more on this, see Chapter 10.)

THYROID PROBLEMS

The thyroid scenario is a little like Goldilocks and the Three Bears. You don't want too much or too little—or, in this case, a thyroid gland that's too active or not active enough.

Located in the front of your neck, the thyroid gland produces hormones that travel through your bloodstream and help keep your brain, heart, and other organs working properly. An overactive thyroid causes *hyperthyroidism,* a condition characterized mainly by nervousness and heart irregularities. At the other end of the spectrum is *hypothyroidism,*

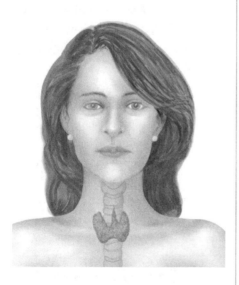

AN IMPORTANT GLAND
The thyroid is a butterfly-shaped gland that makes hormones affecting every part of your body. If it's too active, you're in overdrive. If it's not active enough, you feel tired and sluggish.

Is It True?

Fiction: An underactive thyroid makes you fat.

Fact: Although your metabolism does slow down when your thyroid is low, you don't necessarily gain a huge amount of weight. On average, a person who is hypothyroid could put on up to 10 pounds; more than that would be unusual. When your thyroid is underactive, you're less hungry so you eat less. In any case, the main cause of obesity is too much food and not enough exercise. It's tempting to blame the thyroid, but don't!

caused by an underactive thyroid gland; it is typically evident in a general slowing down of both mental and physical functions.

Both conditions often go undetected because their symptoms, especially in the early stages, are difficult to pinpoint. Of the two, hypothyroidism is more commonly reported.

FEELING RUN-DOWN

Q *I've gained about eight pounds in the last year, and I swear I've hardly touched a peanut, let alone a chocolate-chip cookie. I'm not even very hungry. I'm also incredibly tired, my skin is really dry, and I'm terribly cold all the time. Is it menopause or something else that's making me feel so bad??*

Your symptoms are vague enough that it could be a lot of things, but one possibility is hypothyroidism. When you have too little thyroid hormone, your body starts to slow down. One of the frequent causes of this condition is autoimmune disease, in which your body's immune system mistakenly attacks the thyroid. If enough thyroid cells are destroyed, the gland doesn't make enough hormones. The most common autoimmune form of hypothyroidism is called Hashimoto's thyroiditis.

The incidence of hypothyroidism increases with age, with the peak coming between the ages of 35 and 60. It's estimated that although 10 million Americans are on thyroid medication, 9 million more have untreated hypothyroidism. Thyroid disease is diagnosed by a simple blood test, which measures levels of the thyroid hormones T4 and T3, as well as thyroid-stimulating hormone (TSH) secreted by the pituitary gland. You need all three to get a clear picture of what's going on. You might have normal levels of T4 and T3, but a high TSH at the same time means your body is working extra hard to keep you going. This is known as subclinical hypothyroidism, or mild thyroid failure, and doctors disagree about treating it. In some cases it goes away, but in many others it doesn't, so some doctors wonder why patients should have to wait until they're sick to get help. Others won't begin treatment unless you show both an elevated TSH and symptoms

like dry skin, slow pulse, and diminished reflexes.

The usual treatment for hypothyroidism is to replace the thyroid hormone with a substitute; the most widely prescribed is levothyroxine, sold as a generic or under brand names such as Synthroid, Levoxyl, and Unithroid. Generally, you start with a small dose and get your blood tested periodically until your TSH reaches a normal level. This can take months, but in the meantime you will begin to feel much better. You'll have to take it for the rest of your life.

THE JITTERS

Q I'm feeling jittery and having trouble sleeping. Sometimes my heart feels like it's pounding so fast that it will jump right out of my chest. What's wrong?

A Although these symptoms could signal a number of conditions, hyperthyroidism might be the cause. Only about 2.6 million Americans have hyperthyroidism, while about 9.6 million, most of them women, are afflicted with hypothyroidism.

Hyperthyroidism is often misdiagnosed as heart disease or a mental disorder. But left untreated, it does put you at risk for heart problems (because your heart is working much too hard) and also for osteoporosis. Some other symptoms are heat intolerance, constant hunger, and unexplained weight loss. Some people with Graves' disease, an

What the Tests Mean

Thyroid function tests measure levels of the thyroid-stimulating hormone (TSH) and two thyroid hormones, T3 and T4. Here's how the results stack up:

	TSH	THYROID HORMONES
Overt hyperthyroidism	Low or undetectable	Elevated T4 or T3
Subclinical hyperthyroidism	Low or undetectable	Normal T4 and T3
Overt hypothyroidism	High	Low T4
Subclinical hypothyroidism	High	Normal T4

autoimmune disorder that can cause hyperthyroidism, develop red and bulging eyes with a distinctive stare. In testing, a negligible or low TSH would be a signal of the disease.

Treating hyperthyroidism is more complex than treating low thyroid; consequently, you may be referred to an endocrinologist, a doctor who specializes in hormones. You may be given radioactive iodine to destroy part of the thyroid or drugs that will reduce its function, or you may have surgery to remove the gland altogether. In that case, you would take thyroid hormone for the rest of your life.

WHAT'S A GOITER?

Q I've been feeling tightness in my throat, and my doctor says I have a goiter. How is this related to thyroid disease?

A A goiter is basically an enlargement of the thyroid gland. It can indeed interfere with swallowing and breathing. Until the early 20th century, when iodized salt was introduced in the United States, Americans developed goiters because of a shortage of iodine in their diets, but in your case the cause is most likely a thyroid problem. The treatment depends on the cause. You can get a goiter whether your thyroid hormone levels are high, low, or normal. Some goiters are caused by Graves' disease, when the thyroid is working overtime. Others result from hypothyroidism, when your thyroid is also overstimulated by attempts to produce more hormones. The goiter could come from nodules (usually benign) or, much less commonly, thyroid cancer. Your doctor will put you on an appropriate course of therapy; sometimes your goiter will go away, although often it will not.

A LINK TO ESTROGEN?

Q *It seems that thyroid trouble is more common in women than in men. Does it have something to do with estrogen?*

A Scientists are still learning about the body's immune system, but there is some evidence that estrogen does play a role; in fact, women are five to eight times more likely than men to get thyroid disease. Postpartum thyroiditis, a temporary form of the disease, occurs in 4 to 9 percent of new mothers—often when there is a history of autoimmune disease in the family. The immune system goes from being partially suppressed during pregnancy to being active after childbirth, a switch that can trigger the disease. In most cases, normal thyroid function returns in six to eight months. Changes in estrogen levels also may play into the onset of thyroid disease at menopause.

Gender isn't the only risk factor for thyroid disease. The third U.S. National Health and Nutrition Examination Survey (NHANES) of Americans aged 12 and older found that 14.3 percent of Caucasians had thyroid antibodies compared with 10.9 percent of Mexican Americans and only 5.3 percent of African-Americans. Antibodies are a sign of autoimmune disease. Hashimoto's thyroiditis and other autoimmune diseases run in families, so genetics is another risk factor. Some other autoimmune diseases are type 1 diabetes, Addison's disease, pernicious anemia, rheumatoid arthritis, and vitiligo.

And here's one more finding that might surprise you: prematurely gray hair. It turns out that if your hair turns gray before 30 or if you notice patches of hair loss (a condition called alopecia areata), you're more likely to have thyroid disease.

GENERIC THYROID PILLS

Q *My doctor prescribed Synthroid for my hypothyroidism, but my insurance company will only pay for a generic brand. Should I take the generic?*

A The recommendation of both the American Thyroid Association and the American Academy of Clinical Endocrinologists is to choose a brand-name thyroid medication and stick with it. It's important to keep your thyroid hormone levels stable, and the best way to do that is to maintain exactly the same dose. The trouble with generics is that the pharmacy will probably give you whatever is on hand, and it may not have the same composition as the generic you took the month before. This can screw up your thyroid levels, as indicated by a blood test. The only way to be sure you get the same formula every month is to ask for the same brand name. See if your doctor will explain this to your insurance company. With luck, they'll understand and give you a break on the cost.

Too Little and Too Much	
HYPOTHYROIDISM	**HYPERTHYROIDISM**
Coarse, dry skin and hair	Clammy skin
Feeling chilly	Heat intolerance
Constipation	Increased frequency of bowel movements
Depression	Nervousness and irritability
Diminished sweating	Increased sweating
Fatigue	Fatigue
Tingling or numbness	Muscle weakness
Puffiness around eyes	Blurred or double vision
More frequent periods	Fewer periods
Decreased appetite	Increased appetite
Slow thinking	Distractibility
Slow movement	Tremors
Slow pulse	Rapid heartbeat; heart palpitations
Weight gain	Weight loss
Goiter	Goiter

To Treat or Not to Treat?

Q *My TSH is high, but my thyroid hormone level is normal. My doctor doesn't want to start treatment now; he says he'd rather wait and see if it gets worse. Is that a good plan?*

A It certainly is good that your doctor tested your thyroid levels. Many doctors don't, and that's why thyroid disease often goes undiagnosed. Left untreated, low thyroid increases your risk of cardiovascular disease. Current recommendations are to test women every five years beginning at age 50, when your risk for thyroid disease begins to increase. If there's thyroid disease in your family, you should be tested more often—especially if you're beginning to show symptoms. Your test results show that you have mild (sub-clinical) hypothyroidism. Studies indicate that up to 20 percent of all women fall into this category. Why wouldn't they be treated? It's possible that their disease won't get worse; each year, only 2.6 percent of all people with mild disease progress to full-fledged thyroid disease. It's never a good idea to be on medication if you don't need it.

The risk is higher for people who have thyroid antibodies—an indication of the presence of autoimmune disease. The current recommendation from a 2004 meeting of medical experts on this issue is to test anyone who's at high risk, which means all women over 60. The decision on whether to treat someone with mild thyroid disease is really up to you and your doctor. If a family history or overt symptoms indicate that the patient is likely to get worse, then treatment might be a good idea. Otherwise, you can wait and be retested every six months or so to see how you're doing.

CAN DIET HELP?

Q *Several people in my family have thyroid disease. If I change my diet, can I avoid it?*

A For the most part, thyroid disease isn't affected by diet. The only exception is iodine. Too much or too little can bring on thyroid disease. In this country, iodized salt pretty much takes care of the problem. (It's not in kosher or sea salt, however.) Iodine is also often added to the bread and milk we buy in the supermarket, so most of us get all the iodine we need from our food. Although iodine deficiency isn't a big problem in the industrialized world, it's still a major issue in developing countries—and a major public health issue, affecting a billion people. In children, severe iodine deficiency causes growth and developmental disabilities.

SHOULDER INJURIES

TORN ROTATOR CUFF

Q *I'm a tennis player, and I think of myself as being in great shape. But recently, after a particularly strenuous game, I felt a sharp pain in the top and outer side of my shoulder. Now I even have trouble raising my arm to get dressed. Is this menopause or aging?*

A Shoulder problems like yours keep orthopedists busy. Each year, four million Americans seek medical care for shoulder sprain, strain, dislocation, or other problems. So join the crowd. If you're in pain, you need to see your doctor to get an accurate diagnosis, but it sounds like you might have torn tendons in your rotator cuff, which works with your muscles to keep your shoulder strong and in place. This is a common problem at midlife for men and women . . . because of aging, not menopause. Sports that involve repeated overhead arm motions (tennis, anyone?) make you particularly vulnerable to this injury. It's also a problem for people who have occupations that require lots of heavy lifting. The rotator cuff tendons may be strong but worn down by use and thus susceptible to tearing when they're stressed. In addition to the symptoms you describe, a person with a torn rotator cuff may also hear a click or pop when the shoulder moves.

In a sense, the rotator cuff suffers from what you might consider a design flaw. A third of it has very poor circulation, and this makes it particularly vulnerable to problems, which can develop gradually. One of the main tendons is protected in a tunnel of bone, which weakens as you get older—especially if you're osteopenic or have osteoporosis.

In order to diagnose this problem, your doctor will check to see how much you're able to move your shoulder and where it hurts. You can't always locate the problem during a physical exam, and tests such as X-rays and MRIs have limitations as well. X-rays may appear normal even if there's a tear. MRIs can almost always detect frontal tears and large tears in the rear, but small rear tears can be hard to see. Your doctor might suggest an arthrogram. In this test, a contrast fluid is injected into the shoulder joint and then studied on an X-ray.

The fluid might leak into an area where it doesn't belong (indicating a tear) or be blocked from entering. This helps your doctor pinpoint the location and full extent of the injury. If all your tests come back negative and you still feel pain, be persistent. Return to your doctor and say you need further testing.

Generally, the initial treatment is to rest the shoulder with heat or cold packs to relieve pain. Painkilling medication also helps. You may need to wear a sling for a few days. In more serious cases, you might get a cortisone injection near the inflamed area. Your doctor will probably also suggest exercises to help restore function to your shoulder. If all those alternatives fail, surgery is an option.

FROZEN SHOULDER

Q I was in a bike accident and fell on my side. Now I'm having trouble moving my shoulder. My doctor says it's frozen. What does that mean?

A As we get older, our joints have more trouble rebounding from unusual stress—like falling off a bike. "Frozen shoulder," a popular name for adhesive capsulitis, means your shoulder mobility is severely restricted. If an injury makes it too painful to use your shoulder, it gets inflamed after a while and abnormal bands of tissue called adhesions grow between the joint surfaces. Eventually, the joint becomes so tight and stiff that it's hard to raise your arm. The stiffness and pain often get worse at night. People with diabetes, stroke, lung disease, rheumatoid arthritis, and heart disease are at high risk for frozen shoulder.

Frozen shoulder progresses in three stages. The first stage, the actual "freezing," persists for about three weeks. It's the best time to get treatment. You feel pain even when you're resting and have limited shoulder mobility. In the second stage, you generally have pain only when you're moving, but this doesn't mean you've improved; it's a sign that some of your shoulder muscles have begun to atrophy. (You can actually see this in a mirror; the damaged shoulder will look different from the other one.) The "thawing" stage is when you start to feel better, usually after physical therapy.

Treatment typically begins with anti-inflammatory medication and heat, followed by gentle stretching exercises. Your doctor will probably send you to a physical therapist for these. Physical therapy can break up adhesions. (Sometimes you can hear them pop during a therapeutic workout.) If this doesn't work, a doctor can manipulate your arm under anesthesia to break them up.

BREAST PAIN

Breast tenderness is a common occurrence during perimenopause. It's usually a little less than what you feel right before your period or when you're pregnant, but it can be a little more—and in some cases a lot more. Perimenopausal symptoms vary mightily from person to person, and breast pain (mastalgia) is a good example. Your breasts may feel tender and sore, like a pulled muscle or a bruise. Sometimes the pain starts in the breast, typically the upper outside corner, then radiates to the underarm or the shoulder or back. Some women feel pain in both breasts; others feel it in only one. Usually, this tenderness comes and goes, but it can be persistent. Keep track of the pain so you can determine if there's a pattern. Once you reach menopause and your hormone levels aren't so erratic, the pain usually diminishes or goes away completely. But there are always a few exceptions to the rule; some women experience an occasional twinge into their 70s.

BLAME IT ON ESTROGEN

Q *I've always felt some tenderness in my breasts at certain times of the month. Are hormonal fluctuations the issue now as well?*

A Breast tenderness during perimenopause is usually associated with a hormone imbalance, specifically elevated levels of estrogen. As you know, your hormone levels fluctuate a lot during perimenopause, especially as you near the end of the transition. Your brain is battling with your ovaries over how much estrogen to produce. Your brain says your body wants more, and your ovaries are not responding the way they used to. Sometimes your brain's demands are so intense that your ovaries overreact and produce a lot more estrogen than usual. This estrogen is "unopposed" because your ovaries aren't also making progesterone. One of the telltale signs of high levels of estrogen in your body is breast tissue that's swollen and sore.

PILLS AND SORENESS

Q *My breast soreness began when I started taking oral contraceptives to help regulate my crazy periods. What should I do?*

A Oral contraceptives or hormone therapy can cause breasts to feel extra sensitive. Tell your doctor that your current dose is causing this reaction.

COULD IT BE CANCER?

Q *Of course, my first thought when my breasts became sore was that I've got breast cancer. Your response?*

A What woman doesn't worry about cancer when there's something going on with her breasts? But remember this: Although it's possible that a tumor could hurt, it's not likely. Most of the time, breast cancer reveals its presence by producing small, hard lumps, not pain. Still, it's a good idea to mention this problem to your doctor. After age 40, you should have a mammogram every year or two and a breast exam with every physical. If you're over-

due for either of these, put down this book and make an appointment now. If it's been less than a year since your last mammogram or physical, ask your doctor if you should schedule another appointment earlier than normal or if you should have an ultrasound, which can show cysts that can't be felt but could be causing pain. Cysts can enlarge in response to hormonal changes. If possible, try to schedule your mammogram or ultrasound at a time during the month when your breasts are not tender. If you've been keeping track with a diary, you may be able to predict when that's likely to be.

PAIN RELIEF

Q *The pain in my breasts is keeping me from sleeping, and I'm getting grouchy. What can I do before I get to the doctor?*

A First, try wearing a good support bra, which can help protect tender breast tissue. But since the top of an underwire often hits right about where the pain is, you may want to stick to a bra with no underwire on days when you're uncomfortable. Heating pads and hot water bottles can help reduce the swelling and pain. Some doctors recommend cutting back on caffeine and salt, but there's not much evidence that this helps. In European countries, evening primrose oil is often recommended to relieve breast pain, but studies of its effectiveness have shown mixed results.

You might want to try alternative pain relief techniques like meditation and visualization. Nonsteroidal anti-inflammatory drugs (NSAIDs) such as Advil or Motrin (ibuprofen) are also effective. Besides the pills available over the counter, some women like the cream versions, which have been proven to work in two randomized, blind placebo-controlled studies. (Progesterone creams rubbed into breast tissue are not recommended.) If pain persists, talk to your doctor about prescription pain drugs like danazol and bromocriptine. Be aware, however, that these drugs can have significant side effects, including decreased libido and weight gain.

If pain at night is your biggest problem, talk to your doctor about whether you can use an 8- or 12-hour pain reliever to get you through the night. Nondrug ideas include wearing a supportive bra to bed; the extra protection it provides may be enough to keep you sleeping. You might also want to try taking a hot water bottle to bed with you.

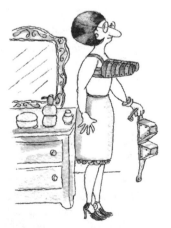

JOINTS AND OTHER CONNECTIONS

Do you wake up in the morning feeling stiff and creaky? This could be a sign of osteoarthritis. Scientists used to think this disease was the result of wear and tear on the joints, but new research indicates that it's the result of a series of events involving various *parts* of joints. That process is probably exacerbated by some combination of aging and others factors: overweight, joint injury, or stresses on the joints from certain jobs or athletic activities. It affects each person differently. Some people never get past early morning creakiness. Others get worse quickly.

Although the most common sites are the hands, knees, hips, and spine, osteoarthritis can hit any joint. The cartilage on the joint surfaces begins to wear away. Spurs form on the bones and the fluid between the bones increases, making the joint swollen and sore. If you're only mildly affected, one of the best treatments is exercise. Avoid anything that increases pounding on your knees, like running on pavement. Target the parts of your body that seem to need help. For example, strengthening the thigh muscle (quadriceps) can ease pain in the knees and prevent more damage. If you're overweight, lose some pounds. Some women find that they can ease the pain with relaxation techniques or biofeedback. Warm towels or cold packs can also relieve pain. Wearing insoles or

Joints 101

Without joints, your body would be a jumble of parts. Your joints enable you to move smoothly; they also absorb the shock of repetitive movements. The five main components of joints are:

◆ **Cartilage.** This hard, slippery coating on the end of each bone breaks down and wears away in osteoarthritis.

◆ **Joint capsule.** A tough membrane sac that holds bones and other parts of the joint together.

◆ **Synovium.** A thin membrane inside the joint capsule.

◆ **Synovial fluid.** The fluid that lubricates the joint and keeps cartilage smooth and healthy.

◆ **Ligaments, tendons, and muscles.** Tissues involved in keeping bones stable and regulating changes in position.

cushioned shoes minimizes joint stress. If your problem is mostly in the morning, try taking a steaming shower to loosen up your joints. Your doctor may also recommend over-the-counter medications like acetaminophen or nonsteroidal anti-inflammatory drugs (NSAIDs), depending on your medical history.

STRAIGHTEN ME OUT

Q *I keep hearing about osteoarthritis and osteoporosis. What's the difference between these two diseases?*

A Both involve bones (that's why they start with *osteo-*, a prefix based on the Greek word for "bone"). Osteoporosis is a loss of bone tissue that leaves bones fragile and vulnerable to fracture; it's a major health threat for postmenopausal women and can cause severe pain and impair your ability to walk. Fortunately, there are a lot of things you can do to prevent damage to your bones. (For more detail, see Chapter 10.) Osteoarthritis is the most common form of arthritis, a disorder of the joints and surrounding tissue *between* your bones. It may develop after repeated overuse of a joint or because of the stress of obesity.

SCARY DRUGS

Q *I've read about problems with drugs for arthritis. What's safe and what's not safe?*

A Vioxx and Bextra, two popular painkillers that belong to a class of drugs called COX-2 inhibitors, were pulled off the market in 2004 and 2005 because of reports of an increased risk of heart attack and stroke. Millions of people had taken these drugs and now need some other sources of relief. The right medication for you depends on your particular needs and risk factors. For example, if you're under 60, have no stomach or intestinal bleeding problems, and aren't taking a blood thinner or oral steroid, you could try an NSAID like Advil or Motrin (ibuprofen) or Aleve or Naprosyn

AREAS AFFECTED BY OSTEOARTHRITIS

A HEALTHY JOINT

A JOINT AFFECTED BY OSTEOARTHRITIS

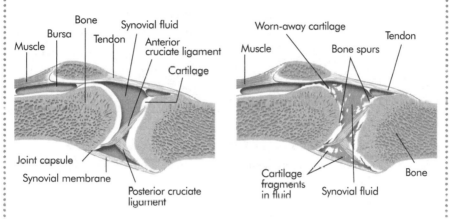

A HEALTHY JOINT labels: Muscle, Bursa, Bone, Tendon, Synovial fluid, Anterior cruciate ligament, Cartilage, Joint capsule, Synovial membrane, Posterior cruciate ligament

A JOINT AFFECTED BY OSTEOARTHRITIS labels: Worn-away cartilage, Muscle, Bone spurs, Tendon, Cartilage fragments in fluid, Synovial fluid, Bone

As you get older, the cartilage at the end of each bone can wear down, causing painful bone spurs.

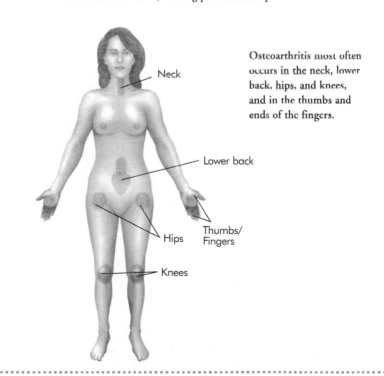

Osteoarthritis most often occurs in the neck, lower back, hips, and knees, and in the thumbs and ends of the fingers.

Labels: Neck, Lower back, Hips, Thumbs/Fingers, Knees

(naproxen). Tylenol (acetaminophen) might also work. Older people might take an NSAID with another drug to protect their stomach. You and your doctor have to work out the correct choice for you.

Why Us?

Q *I know several women who have osteoarthritis, but I've never met a man who has it. Is it strictly a female problem?*

A Both men and women get this disease, although it's more common in women after age 45. Researchers think there's some connection to estrogen. Some studies have found that women on hormone therapy have a lower risk of osteoarthritis, but other studies have shown the opposite. This is a particular problem for women who are taking anti-breast cancer drugs called aromatase inhibitors, which reduce the amount of estrogen in the body. In a 2005 study, patients taking these drugs reported a higher level of pain than did women on a placebo or those who were taking tamoxifen. The pain went away when they stopped taking the drugs.

Stomach Problems

Q *Why do I have to watch out for my stomach when I take medication for osteoarthritis?*

A NSAIDs are a common and effective treatment for osteoarthritis, but there's a downside. They can cause stomach upset and bleeding ulcers. Another approach is to take an NSAID and an acid-blocking drug like Tagamet (cimetidine) or Zantac (ranitidine hydrochloride). Medications called proton pump inhibitors are also helpful; they include Prevacid (lansoprazole) and Prilosec (omeprazole). In addition, your doctor may suggest the following:

Don't drink alcohol. It can increase the risk of gastric bleeding if you're taking an NSAID.

Take your pills with food and water. A little bit in your stomach helps—unless your doctor or the product label says otherwise.

Keep track of medications. Make sure your doctor and your pharmacist know everything you're taking so they can guard against drug interactions that could increase the risk of bleeding.

Chopstick Stress

Q *I have a Chinese friend who claims that her grandmother developed arthritis in the hand she uses to hold chopsticks. Could that really be true?*

A Any repetitive stress can aggravate joints, and that's apparently even true of using chopsticks. In a 2004 study, researchers from Boston University looked at hand X-rays of approximately 2,500 Beijing residents aged 60 or older and found that chopsticks did indeed put stress on certain joints, especially the thumb and second and third fingers of the hand that holds them. Women had more problems than men, which could simply reflect the higher rate of osteoarthritis in women. In any case, that isn't a reason to avoid using chopsticks occasionally—and certainly not Chinese food. Many of the subjects of the study reported feeling no pain in their hands even when the X-rays showed joint damage.

EXERCISE WOES

Q *I know you're supposed to keep moving if you have osteoarthritis, but how can I do that when my joints hurt so much?*

A It does seem like a contradiction, but exercise can actually reduce the pain. You might start by asking your doctor to refer you to a physical therapist who can teach you some gentle stretches that you can do on your own. Once you've got that down, you could progress to yoga, Pilates, or tai chi—all of which will help improve your range of motion, flexibility, and muscle strength. Doing these exercises when you get up in the morning can help you start your day without too much stiffness. Aerobic exercise is important for people with osteoarthritis. Swimming is an excellent choice. You might also think about enrolling in a water aerobics class. You can do almost anything in the water—without the pain. If you're uncomfortable being seen in a bathing suit, remember that you'll be underwater (and out of view). Whatever you choose, try to work on the parts of your body that are most affected. Strengthening the muscles around your knee or back, for example, can help ease the pain.

Rheumatoid Arthritis

Unlike osteoarthritis, rheumatoid arthritis affects both sides of the body at the same time in a symmetrical pattern. In severe cases, it can also affect the eyes, lungs, heart, nerves, or blood vessels. Fatigue and fever are common, and the lymph nodes may swell. It's estimated that about 2.1 million Americans have rheumatoid arthritis, but some recent studies have suggested that the number of new cases may be declining. No one yet knows why that is. It afflicts about two to three times as many women as men, and although it often shows up in midlife, children and young adults can develop it as well.

Rheumatoid arthritis is an unpredictable disease. Symptoms can be mild and then disappear or get worse over a lifetime. There's increasing evidence that a virus or bacteria triggers the disease in people who are genetically susceptible. Because it tends to go away during pregnancy, researchers think estrogen may also play a role.

Early treatment, including medication and exercise, can help stop the damage. But because the disease is so variable, doctors take different approaches in beginning treatment. Some are conservative, starting with small doses and adding medication gradually. Others treat the

SIGNS OF RHEUMATOID ARTHRITIS

◆ Tender, swollen joints that feel warm

◆ Symmetrical pattern of affected joints

◆ Inflammation of the wrist and finger joints closest to the hand

◆ Inflammation of other joints, including the neck, shoulders, elbows, hips, knees, ankles, and feet

◆ Fatigue, occasional fever, a sense of not feeling well

◆ Pain and stiffness lasting more than 30 minutes in the morning or after a long rest

◆ Symptoms lasting for many years

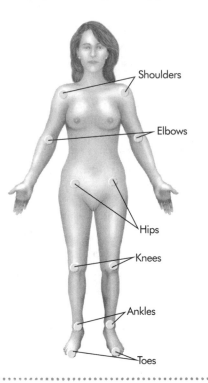

JOINTS THAT MAY BE AFFECTED BY RHEUMATOID ARTHRITIS

Rheumatoid arthritis affects joints symmetrically. The symptoms can fade for years and then reappear.

disease with aggressive drugs from the start. Two types of drugs are used: those that relieve symptoms and others that may alter the course of the disease. Drugs that can relieve symptoms include NSAIDs and aspirin, Tylenol (acetaminophen), and corticosteroids such as cortisone and prednisone. Medications that may alter the process of the disease include Trexall and Rheumatrex (methotrexate), Arava (leflunomide), and

Humira (adalimumab). Research in this area is ongoing, so individual treatment is best decided between patient and doctor.

FAMILY HISTORY

Q *One of my aunts had rheumatoid arthritis. She was in a wheelchair by the time she was 60. How does that affect my vulnerability to the disease?*

Rheumatoid arthritis is an auto-immune disorder, which means that the body's own immune system attacks the tissues of the joints. And autoimmune diseases do seem to run in families. Still, that doesn't mean you will suffer like your aunt. Many factors appear to be involved in the onset of rheumatoid arthritis: genes, environment, hormonal changes during pregnancy. Even if you do get rheumatoid arthritis, the disease's progress is so variable that you might live a long and active life with few physical limitations. However, it's good to know your family history and be familiar with the signs of rheumatoid arthritis so you can be on the watch for them and get treatment early if any show up.

TINGLING HANDS

Q *I don't know if this is arthritis or I'm just nuts. I wake up at night when my hands feel like they've fallen asleep. It's that pins and needles thing. What could cause it?*

A Your sleeping position might be putting pressure on the nerves that go from your spinal cord to your hands. If shaking or rubbing your hands fixes the problem, don't worry. Try changing your sleeping position to relieve the pressure. But if this keeps happening, you should check with your doctor. It's possible that rheumatoid arthritis or hypothyroidism could be behind this; tingling in the hands can be a sign of both conditions. If you're also noticing some tingling when you're at the computer, this could be a symptom of carpal tunnel syndrome. Your doctor might recommend a splint to protect your wrists or an anti-inflammatory drug. Seeing an orthopedist or a neurologist can speed up the diagnostic process.

URINARY PROBLEMS

Why do so many women have trouble with bladder control during the menopause transition? Many scientists believe that loss of estrogen, which normally helps to keep the lining of the bladder and urethra plump and healthy, weakens the bladder muscle. Pressure from exercise, coughing, sneezing, or lifting heavy objects then pushes urine through the weakened muscle, causing *stress incontinence.* This is the kind of incontinence that is most common in younger and middle-aged women.

A second kind of incontinence is called *urge incontinence.* This happens when the bladder muscle squeezes at the wrong time or all the time. You feel a constant need to urinate and may not make it to the toilet in time, resulting in urine leakage. Urge incontinence is more common as women get older and is often found in those who have diabetes, stroke, dementia, Parkinson's disease, or multiple sclerosis. It can also be a sign of bladder cancer.

In the condition called *overflow incontinence,* small amounts of urine leak from a bladder that is always full. Diabetes and spinal cord injury may cause this; in men, it may mean that an enlarged prostate is blocking the urethra.

Functional incontinence afflicts older people who have normal bladder control but can't make it to the toilet in time simply because of limited mobility.

Mixed incontinence involves more than one type of incontinence, usually stress and urge.

A LITTLE LEAKY

Q *Every time I laugh, I seem to leak a little urine. It's gotten so bad that I've started wearing light sanitary napkins every day. I'm really humiliated by this.*

A Before you start investing in cartons of Depends, talk to your doctor. Incontinence can be the result of

Bladder muscle
Pelvic floor muscles
Sphincter muscle
Urine
Urethra

HOW THE BLADDER WORKS
Your bladder holds about 400 to 500 ccs of urine, a little less than a 20-ounce bottle of soda. Strengthening your pelvic floor muscles can help fight leaking.

infection, recent surgery, or illness. Your doctor can give you tests to see what's causing the problem. These might include blood and urine analysis and possibly an ultrasound or other imaging test to see how your urinary tract is functioning.

You can ease your discomfort with some simple changes. Many women do use the light sanitary napkins you've already tried, although pads made especially for incontinence provide better protection and may be less irritating. You might also restrict liquids that can irritate your bladder. These include coffee, tea, alcohol, and acidic juices. Kegel exercises (see pages 118–19) will strengthen your pelvic floor muscles and can reduce or even cure stress incontinence. Losing weight also helps. Many women find that even a relatively small weight loss dramatically reduces stress incontinence. Emptying your bladder more frequently, every two to three hours, will reduce the bladder volume and decrease leakage during coughing, sneezing, or laughing. For urge incontinence, you might also ask your doctor about anticholinergic medications that can help relax your bladder and cut in half the number of times you need to urinate each day.

HOW TO TALK TO THE DOCTOR

Q *I've been leaking a lot lately, but I'm too embarrassed to bring this up to my doctor. Any advice on what I should say?*

A Sample Bladder Diary

Keeping a diary like this one will help you and your doctor pinpoint your daytime problems.

	DRINKS		URINE		ACCIDENTAL LEAKS	Accidents	
						DID YOU FEEL A STRONG URGE TO GO?	WHAT WERE YOU DOING AT THE TIME?
TIME	What kind?	How much?	How many times?	How much? (S, M, L)	How much? (S, M, L)	(Circle one.)	Sneezing, exercising, having sex, lifting, etc.
Sample	coffee	2 cups	✓✓	M	S	(Yes) No	running
6–7 A.M.						Yes No	
7–8 A.M.						Yes No	
8–9 A.M.						Yes No	
9–10 A.M.						Yes No	
10–11 A.M.						Yes No	
11–noon						Yes No	
12–1 P.M.						Yes No	
1–2 P.M.						Yes No	
2–3 P.M.						Yes No	
3–4 P.M.						Yes No	
4–5 P.M.						Yes No	
5–6 P.M.						Yes No	
6–7 P.M.						Yes No	

A Write down your symptoms and your questions, and bring them with you. Okay, we know: Many people find it difficult to talk about intimate bodily functions like urinating. If you're worried that you're someone who might clam up at the last minute, try keeping a "voiding diary" for a week or two before your visit. We've included a sample diary above, but you can use any form that works for you. It's a helpful tool because you may detect a pattern to the problem that may give your doctor an idea of what to look for and how to treat you.

Knowledge is power, and the more you can tell your doctor about your symptoms, the better he or she will be at treating them. At your appointment, you might just say that you've been having a problem and then hand over the diary. You might also list all the medications you're taking, including over-the-counter drugs, because some can make incontinence worse. Your doctor will take over from there. Don't be afraid—doctors have heard it all.

In the Past

Ancient Egyptians believed that the pesky uterus was the source of most of a woman's health problems. The 4,000-year-old Kahun Medical Papyrus, a gynecological text, gives physicians specific instructions for dealing with this willful organ. If a woman's legs and calves hurt after walking, the doctor is told to identify the problem as "discharges of the womb"; the remedy is massaging the legs with mud. If her teeth and ears hurt, the diagnosis is "terrors of the womb" and the doctor is advised to remove detritus from her uterus. If her eyes hurt and she's having trouble with her vision, the doctor should tell her there is material in her eyes from her overflowing uterus. (No word on what they would tell a man with the same problem!) The solution: exposing her vulva to the vapors of frankincense and fresh oil and exposing her eyes to the vapor of oriole thighs. After that, the woman should eat fresh donkey liver. For burning urine—caused again by "discharges of the womb"—the doctor is instructed to treat the woman with a mixture of beans and other plants boiled in a jar of beer. The patient drinks it four mornings in a row after fasting.

In her book *The Wandering Womb,* author Lana Thompson says the Egyptians believed that the womb was "an entity unto itself capable of 'wandering' throughout the body if sexually unfulfilled, crowding the other organs and causing tissue damage, suffocation, and a variety of illnesses." Even Plato supported this idea; in *Timaeus,* he described the uterus as "an animal, which longs to generate children. When it remains barren too long after puberty, it is distressed and sorely disturbed, and straying about in the body . . . and provokes all manner of diseases." Hippocrates, the ancient Greek physician, argued that wombs didn't start to wander until women were older: "In such situations, the uterus dries up and loses weight and in its search for moisture, rises toward the hypochondrium" where "it causes convulsions similar to those of epilepsy."

The second-century physician Aretaeus told his female patients that only by taking a lover would they get their uteruses to behave. These ideas persisted well into the 16th century, when physician Ambroise Paré wrote a book on obstetrics in which he described the womb as capable of expressing a wide range of emotions and insisted that he had personally seen serpents and other fantastic creatures residing inside women's uteruses.

WHY US?

Q *I know urinary tract infections are more common in women than in men. Is this because of estrogen? Or is it something else?*

A In this case, it's a structural issue. We'll try to explain it delicately. In women, the urethral opening is closer to the anus than it is in men. Also, the female urethra is shorter, which means germs have a quicker trip into the bladder. The vast majority of urinary tract infections are caused by *Escherichia coli* (usually called *E. coli*), one of the most common organisms in fecal matter. That's why it's important to wipe from front to back.

PAINFUL URINATION

Q *I feel a burning sensation when I urinate, and I've also noticed drops of blood in my urine. What could this be?*

A Blood in your urine is a major warning sign; you need to see a doctor right away. One possibility is a urinary tract infection. A healthy bladder is generally free of bacteria, but the germs on your skin—especially in your vaginal and rectal areas—can travel up your urethra into your bladder. Most of the time, your bladder gets rid of these nasty intruders naturally, but if they're not evicted they can cause an infection. Be sure to wipe from the urethra back toward the rectum to prevent spreading

of fecal bacteria to the urinary system. When you have a urinary tract infection, the lining of the bladder and urethra becomes red and irritated. You may feel pain in your pelvic area and may need to go the bathroom much more often. Sometimes, when you urinate, you'll produce only a few drops and feel burning as the urine comes out. You may also find that your urine is cloudy or smells unusually bad.

It's important to treat a bladder infection promptly because it can spread to your kidneys. The signs of a kidney infection are pain under the lower ribs, fever, and chills. Immediate treatment with antibiotics should get everything under control.

THE ROLE OF HORMONES

Q *I had a problem with leaking when I was pregnant, and now I have it again as I'm entering menopause. That makes me think estrogen plays a part in all this.*

A Stress incontinence is common during pregnancy and after childbirth, particularly in women who've had vaginal deliveries. While many doctors say that's because the pelvic floor muscles are often stretched out and weakened during pregnancy, recent research indicates that women who haven't given birth have almost the same rate of stress incontinence as women who have had children. In any case, incontinence associated with pregnancy can be temporary,

TREATMENTS FOR INCONTINENCE

Treatment depends on the type of bladder control problem you have and how severe it is. Here's a quick rundown:

Things you can do yourself. Kegel exercises strengthen the muscles near the urethra and take only a few minutes a day. Next time you urinate, stop your stream right in the middle. The muscles you use to do that are the same ones you strengthen with Kegels. You should do them for the rest of your life.

Don't try to "hold it in" for as long as possible. Urinating regularly will decrease the amount of leaking with coughing or sneezing. If you're overweight, losing a few pounds almost always helps. In any case, you should watch what you eat and drink—certain foods make it harder to control your bladder. This is especially true of caffeine drinks (coffee, tea, or cola), which have a diuretic effect.

Electrical therapy. Your doctor may use brief doses of electrical stimulation to exercise the muscles around your urethra, making them stronger and tighter. Electrical stimulation can also stabilize overactive bladder muscles. Biofeedback helps to make sure you're exercising the right muscles when you're doing Kegels. A physical therapist places a patch over the muscles and a wire connects the patch to a TV screen, which you can watch to see if the right muscles are moving when you squeeze.

Medications. Drugs can attack different types of incontinence. Some inhibit the contractions of an overactive bladder. Others relax muscles, enabling you to empty your bladder more completely. Still others tighten muscles at the bladder neck and urethra to prevent leakage.

Pessaries. A pessary is a stiff ring inserted by a doctor or nurse into the vagina that pushes against the vaginal wall and the nearby urethra. That pressure helps reposition the urethra, reducing leakage. It can be a good choice if your incontinence is the result of a dropped (prolapsed) bladder or uterus. One drawback: a possible increase in vaginal and urinary tract infections.

Surgery. A very common procedure to help support the urethra, surgery works by providing a backboard for the urethra to close against. Various types of surgery can be effective. f your bladder or uterus has slipped out of position, a surgeon can reposition it. In women, the most common and popular treatment for stress incontinence is the sling, a strip of abdominal tissue or synthetic material that prevents leaks by forming a kind of hammock for the urethra.

---

lasting just a few months after delivery. Kegel exercises (pages 118–19) and losing pregnancy weight help a lot.

Since loss of estrogen has been linked to incontinence during the menopause transition, you would think that hormone therapy might do the trick. In fact, doctors used to prescribe hormones for this purpose. However, recent research indicates that estrogen may exacerbate the condition. A clinical trial of low-dose estrogen patches also showed no effect on incontinence. These new studies have sent researchers back to the lab to try and figure out exactly how estrogen or the lack of it affects the female urinary tract. Until we know more, the best advice would be to avoid hormone therapy to treat incontinence alone.

BERRY GOOD FOR YOU

Q *I've heard that cranberry juice can help to ward off urinary tract infections. Is this just a folktale? Do I have to actually drink it? Would cranberry pills work just as well?*

A This falls into the category of things that can't hurt and might help. Cranberry juice is quite an old remedy for urinary tract infections; it was used by Native Americans to treat bladder and kidney ailments. In more recent times, scientists have tried to figure out if it works and, if so, how. Although studies are mixed, there is reasonably good evidence to suggest that cranberries may indeed help prevent infections in some women but won't cure an infection that's already there. The current theory is that chemicals in cranberries prevent *E. coli* from sticking to the bladder; instead, the germs get washed out in urine. Cranberry pills seem to work just as well as cranberry juice. If you want to try this out yourself, the American Academy of Family Physicians recommends eight ounces of unsweetened juice three times a day or one tablet (300 to 400 milligrams) twice a day. Despite this, the best way to prevent infection is to drink lots of fluid in order to decrease the bacteria load. After intercourse, urinate immediately to help wash away bacteria, and be sure to use adequate lubrication during sex if you're a little dry.

AFTER MENOPAUSE

Q *What happens after menopause to make us more vulnerable to urinary tract infections?*

A After menopause, the entire vaginal area becomes more fragile. Tissues in the vagina, urethra, and base of the bladder become thinner and more susceptible to infection. Although scientists have identified estrogen receptors throughout this area, it's still not clear whether adding estrogen helps to reduce the chances of infection. Estrogen administered locally to the vagina through tablets, creams, or a ring appears to ease symptoms like burning and irritation, but the effect on recurrent infection is unclear. Oral estrogen may even slightly increase the risk of infection. Despite this uneven evidence, many doctors continue to believe that topical estrogen helps women who get repeated urinary tract infections. If your doctor is one of them, ask about alternatives. Make sure you understand the pros and cons of estrogen if you decide to give it a try.

KILLER HEELS

Pointy shoes with stiletto heels may look great, but they can do some real damage to your feet as you get older. Squeezing your toes into triangular prisons exacerbates deformities like bunions (enlargement of the joint at the base of the big toe) and hammertoes (contraction of the toe that makes it look like an upside-down V). If your toenails are turning a yucky color, you could have a nail fungus aggravated by too-tight shoes. The higher the heel, the more pressure on your foot and the possibility of a neuroma, a pinched nerve that causes pain in the ball of your foot and a tingling in your toes. Your soles suffer as well. The fat pads under your toes begin to thin as you age, and wearing high heels accelerates that process, which means you'll feel more pain when you're walking or even just standing. Longtime high-heel wearers are at higher risk for bursitis, capsulitis, and arthritis, all of which cause painful swelling around joints.

High heels also strain tendons, which can lead to inflammation. Some women find it hard to wear sneakers after years of wearing heels. That's because their Achilles tendons have contracted so much that they can no longer get their feet flat down on the ground. Bone spurs aggravated by the wrong shoes can also form at the back of the heel, causing a "Haglund deformity" or "pump bump."

All of these problems get worse as women age. One study found that older women who need knee surgery are more likely to have worn heels all their lives because their knees have become shock absorbers. That's supposed to be the foot's job; if you're walking on your toes all the time, your foot is basically out of commission and the shock travels up your leg.

To make sure the shoes you buy actually fit, ask to have your feet measured while you're standing. The size you wore 10 years ago is irrelevant—your feet get bigger as you get older because of wear and tear on your joints and a general loss of elasticity. Always buy shoes late in the day, when your feet are at their most swollen; if they fit snugly in the morning,

SORE FEET

CHRONIC FOOT PAIN

Q Soon after I get up in the morning and start walking around, I get a nagging pain near my heel. It disappears after an hour or so. My mom told me that a lot of women in their 40s and 50s get this pain. Is it menopause-related?

A A lot of midlife women get this pain, but so do a lot of midlife men. This condition is known as plantar fasciitis (FASH-EE-EYE-TIS), and it's often related to degeneration (a nice word for aging) or overuse and abuse of the feet. It can also be brought on by a variety of muscle problems; for example, women with flat feet or very high arches are particularly vulnerable. The fact that it often crops up during menopause is strictly a coincidence. And despite its

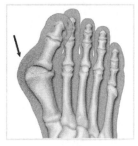

Bunion

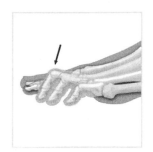

Hammertoes

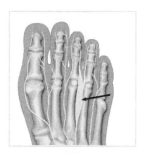

Neuroma (between third and fourth toes)

you might have blisters by evening. One foot is usually bigger than the other, so you should buy shoes that fit the larger one; try on both shoes and walk around the store. Stick to heels that are no more than an inch and a half high. Look for a more rounded or square toe box. Shoes that fit well should have wiggle room for your toes. Give your feet a break by wearing more comfortable flats to and from work. Carry higher heels in a tote bag and wait until you're in the office to slip them on. Reserve the stilettos for really special occasions, treating your feet kindly before and after by wearing supportive flats. Padded inserts in the front of

the shoe help to reduce pressure on the ball of the foot. If you're on the heavy side, you need to be extra cautious when wearing higher heels. The more you weigh, the more problems you'll have, and the negative effects are cumulative.

If you love Mary Janes, go for it. Shoes with a strap at mid-foot mean you don't have to grip so hard to keep them on your feet. If you're gripping, you're more likely to get blisters, arch pain, and foot fatigue. Avoid backless slides. They can easily slip off if you're not constantly tensing your feet to keep them on. The same goes for flip-flops. Save them for the beach.

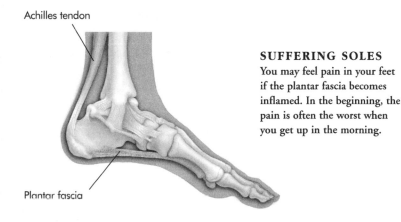

Achilles tendon

Plantar fascia

SUFFERING SOLES

You may feel pain in your feet if the plantar fascia becomes inflamed. In the beginning, the pain is often the worst when you get up in the morning.

old nickname "gonorrheal heel," it has nothing to do with sexually transmitted diseases. (People used to think venereal disease caused heel pain.)

The plantar fascia is the flat ligament that runs along the bottom of your foot, parallel to the arch. It stretches (and takes on all your weight) every time you flex your foot or take a step. It's also your foot's shock absorber. When you take a long run on an uneven surface in old athletic shoes, it takes a pounding. When you misstep and awkwardly twist your foot, this is the ligament that strains. When you spend all day on your feet, this is the part of your foot that gets stressed. Young feet generally rebound from these insults quickly. Over time, however, everyday wear can tear at the plantar fascia (especially where it's anchored to the heel) and cause swelling and pain. Typically, the pain is dull and intermittent at first, becoming sharp and constant as time goes on. Many people feel the ache soon after they get out of bed, but in the most severe cases it's worse at day's end. Doing weight-bearing exercises and running are good for a lot of reasons, but they can make you particularly vulnerable to this kind of inflammation. On the other hand, so can

obesity . . . so don't think you've finally found a good excuse not to exercise! People with flat feet and tight Achilles tendons are more likely to develop this problem—as are those who wear too-small shoes.

To treat plantar fasciitis, many doctors recommend starting with the most conservative interventions and moving on to more aggressive treatments only if the pain doesn't lessen. That means rest, stretching, strengthening, and icing your foot (especially after stretching and strengthening). Buy a new pair of running shoes; your old ones may have lost their ability to absorb pounding. You might also want to put some extra padding in your other shoes. Some other treatments: taping your arch, using arch supports or orthotics (individually cast supports), taking anti-inflammatories, or using night splints to stretch the ligament while you sleep. Finally, there's surgery to release the ligament. Some doctors are also trying laser, ultrasound, and shock wave therapies. All these methods work for some people, but there doesn't seem to be one cure-all for everyone. If you start treatment early, you have a better chance of success. But it still takes a long time to fix—6 to 18 months is typical.

CHAPTER 8

Moods and Emotions

*A*re you singing the midlife blues? You're usually a pretty upbeat person, but lately you're shifting from neutral to super cranky in less than five seconds and barking at everyone who comes within earshot. You know you're being unreasonable, but you can't seem to help yourself no matter how hard you try. Maybe you're not crazy about all the changes that are starting to come your way. Or maybe you've been depressed or anxious in the past and worry that menopause will prompt a relapse.

Be reassured that menopause doesn't cause a major mood problem in most women. While all of us can be irritable at times (okay, bitchy), most of us will navigate our way through midlife just fine. In fact, the majority of women between 45 and 55 describe the menopause years as the best of their lives.

But there's no denying that some of us are in for a bumpy ride,

even clinical depression, maybe for the first time. Some women's moods are highly sensitive to hormonal changes. It probably comes as no surprise that hot flashes and insomnia have been known to leave more than a few women moody and depressed. Side effects of medications or an undiagnosed thyroid problem could also be responsible. Or maybe the stresses that many

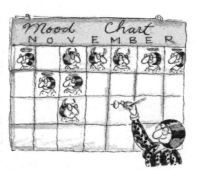

of us deal with at midlife—trying to juggle too many balls, coping with teenagers, caring for elderly parents, sometimes all at once—are just too much. Whatever has put you on this emotional roller coaster, this chapter has ideas that will help you cope.

WHAT YOU NEED TO KNOW ABOUT DEPRESSION

Despite what many people believe, you can't will yourself out of depression. Just like cancer or diabetes, depression is a genuine disease that can have a huge impact on your body. And women are roughly twice as likely as men to develop it. Genetics is probably also a determinant, since depression runs in families. Traumatic life experiences, especially in childhood, may raise your risk. And the painful events of midlife—the death of a parent, for example—can leave your body's stress response in overdrive. Long-term heightened anxiety, usually reserved for the rare reaction to an imminent threat, can also sow the seeds of depression.

Hormones and Mood

How do sex hormones affect this potentially combustible mix? Unclear, but another risk factor for depression is being one of a small subset of women whose moods change in response to fluctuating levels of estrogen and progesterone. That's about 10 percent of all women experiencing midlife depression. In these women, hormonal fluctuations may make it harder for parts of the brain involved in controlling emotion to communicate with one another. When this happens, it may be easier for basic emotions like irritability and anxiety to slip past the regulators in your brain that normally modulate them, making you more vulnerable to depression.

Estrogen (specifically, estradiol) may act as one of nature's antidepressants. In lab studies, it seems to help some of the brain's signaling and regulation systems work more efficiently. It performs some of the same services that make chemical

What Can Happen

◆ If you've never had a serious mood disorder, there's no reason to assume that you're going to have one now. Although many women experience some moodiness during the menopause transition, most don't develop full-blown depression or anxiety.

◆ If you do have a history of depression or anxiety, you may be at higher risk for recurrence at any time. Make sure you know the symptoms to watch for and get help if you need it.

◆ If you've had significant mood problems during times of hormonal disruption (before your period, after a pregnancy, during infertility treatments, while taking oral contraceptives), you may be at higher risk for mood fluctuations, particularly during perimenopause.

antidepressants so effective in treating depression. It may also be involved in protecting against the kind of cell death brought on by stress and aging, which is believed to indirectly affect depression.

Several studies have shown that estrogen has short-term antidepressant effects on some depressed perimenopausal women. (Similar results have not been seen in postmenopausal women.) While most doctors try traditional antidepressants first, estrogen may be prescribed as an alternative or additional treatment for perimenopausal women when other antidepressants prove ineffective or only partially effective. If you're suffering from moderate to severe hot flashes and if your mood problems are relatively mild, your doctor may suggest that you try hormone therapy before adding antidepressants.

Because of the health risks associated with long-term use of hormone therapy, many questions remain about which mood problems might benefit from it. Scientists at the National Institute of Mental Health think estrogen may have potential to treat some forms of depression within three to six weeks with no

A Boost for Your Brain

In the last few years, a lot has been learned about how to treat depression. Some of the most effective new medications affect levels of neurotransmitters in your brain that allow signals to travel from neuron to neuron. The best-known neurotransmitter is serotonin, whose levels typically fluctuate more in women than in men. Although scientists don't know exactly how serotonin works, they think it's an important regulator of sleep, mood, depression, and anxiety. Other important neurotransmitters include dopamine (associated with emotion and pleasure; increases with stimulants and sex), norepinephrine (associated with drive and motivation), and acetylcholine (may be critical for sleep, attention, and memory).

When you have the right levels of serotonin and these other neurotransmitters in your brain, you're more likely to feel emotionally balanced and in control of your feelings and behavior. When levels drop, you can feel unusually apathetic or hopeless and have trouble sleeping—symptoms of clinical depression. Low serotonin levels can even generate suicidal tendencies.

In some women, this very delicate balance can be thrown off during the perimenopause years because of the connection between estrogen and the way your body manufactures serotonin. Nerve cells create serotonin using a stored amino acid called tryptophan. Estrogen seems to increase tryptophan availability in your brain. One group of antidepressants is called SSRIs (selective serotonin reuptake inhibitors). You've probably heard the brand names of some of them—Prozac, Paxil, Lexapro, Celexa, and Zoloft—because they're among the most commonly prescribed medications. SSRIs prevent your brain from quickly metabolizing (or inhibiting reuptake of) serotonin; the result is that these natural chemicals are available to the brain for longer periods.

When to See the Doctor

If mood problems last longer than two weeks and interfere with your ability to function at home or at work, you should get help. These problems might include:

❖ MORE THAN ONE PANIC ATTACK

❖ A GENERAL SENSE OF UNHAPPINESS OR A PERSISTENT NEGATIVE MOOD

❖ INABILITY TO EXPERIENCE PLEASURE OR TO ENJOY THINGS YOU USED TO DO

❖ CONSTANT OR RUMINATIVE WORRYING

❖ CHRONIC ANXIETY

❖ OBSESSIVE THOUGHTS OR COMPULSIVE ACTIONS THAT YOU CAN'T CONTROL

❖ PARANOIA (AN INESCAPABLE FEELING THAT OTHERS MEAN TO HARM YOU)

❖ SYMPTOMS OF PSYCHOSIS, SUCH AS HEARING VOICES OR OTHER HALLUCINATIONS

❖ SUICIDAL THOUGHTS OR RECURRING THOUGHTS OF DEATH

need for supplemental long-term use of other antidepressants. This research is in its very early stages, and it will take more study to determine whether these preliminary results hold up.

SCREENING FOR SYMPTOMS

Q *Does every perimenopausal woman get depressed? My doctor just screened me for depression and said he routinely does this for women headed toward menopause.*

A Midlife is not a time of increased risk of depression for the majority of women. In fact, you're more likely to be diagnosed with major depressive disorder before the age of 44 than when you're older. But some of the warning signs of depression are common during the menopause years. You may find that you're a little more irritable than usual, or that you have trouble sleeping or making decisions. Maybe you can't concentrate or enjoy your usual activities. You may have headaches, dizziness, and appetite changes. These symptoms don't quite reach the level of a full-blown

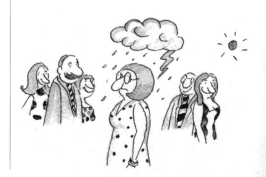

mood disorder, but they can cause significant distress if they persist. There's also an association between hot flashes, insomnia, and depression. Your doctor will want to not only help you move through this transition but also catch true depression early, since it's often overlooked and underdiagnosed.

Even if you're not clinically depressed, your doctor may recommend medication or other therapy to relieve some of your symptoms. Proper treatment now can improve your long-term health.

Depressive symptoms put you at higher risk for many problems, including cardiovascular disease, dementia, stroke, and osteoporosis. If you're suffering from depression and another health problem, your overall prognosis worsens.

Treatment may mean medication, talk therapy, or some combination of the two. Nonpharmaceutical alternatives are also available. Your mental health might benefit from regular exercise and a healthier diet. Your doctor can help figure out what will work best for you.

TYPES OF DEPRESSION

Seasonal affective disorder: a cyclical disorder that worsens at a particular time of the year, typically when daylight hours are shorter and there's less sunlight.

Complete remission occurs at another time of year, usually in the spring, when daylight hours lengthen. The pattern must persist for at least two years for diagnosis.

Major or clinical depression: chronic feelings of sadness, apathy, or hopelessness that are out of kilter with whatever's going on in your life.

A diagnosis depends on the presence of five or more specific symptoms (see page 202) that have persisted for at least two weeks and interfere with your ability to live your life.

Minor or mild depression: similar to major depression, but with fewer symptoms; can occur in those with serial bipolar disease.

This needs to be taken seriously, especially if it's recurrent and makes it difficult to function normally.

Moderate depression: a significant number of symptoms impact your ability to participate in most activities.

Severe depression: functioning restricted with all or almost all symptoms present.

Dysthymic disorder: a less well-known form of chronic depression that persists for long periods at a lower intensity; diagnosed when there are more bad days than good days for at least two years (one year in adolescents and children) and when accompanied by at least two other symptoms of major depression.

Patients with dysthymic disorder may have periods of major depression as well. It usually begins in childhood or adolescence, but may not get diagnosed until adulthood.

TESTING FOR DEPRESSION

Q *Is there something like a blood test for diagnosing depression?*

A Not yet, but researchers are trying to determine if biological markers for depression can be detected in blood tests or with brain imaging. The hope is that eventually doctors will be able to identify a variety of depression "profiles" and know which treatments work best to prevent or treat each type.

AN OUNCE OF PREVENTION

Q *I'm big on stopping problems before they start. Is there something I can do to reduce or avoid feelings of moodiness or irritability during the menopause transition?*

A Fortunately, you can be extremely proactive about your mental health. You've probably heard most of these suggestions before, but now is the time to stop ignoring them. If you're using illegal drugs or drinking too much alcohol, stop. Both can trigger episodes of depression. Are you getting enough exercise? Physical activity improves just about everyone's mental outlook. It can also help you reduce your weight and improve your cardiovascular health, two additional boosters for good mental health. And since a regular dose of natural light may keep your mood sunnier, do some of that exercise outside (protected by sunscreen or in a shaded area). Make a conscious effort to put a smile on your face, and give yourself opportunities to laugh. Smiling and laughing release endorphins, natural chemicals in your brain that are associated with a good mood.

Try to reduce stress, which can bring on depression. Find healthy ways to relax: a yoga class, a massage, a manicure and pedicure. Improve your self-image and your overall fitness by losing some weight. Eating right can help you achieve that goal. Make sure your diet includes adequate levels of calcium and iron. Don't forget to schedule your annual physical. While you're there, make sure your cholesterol levels and blood pressure are checked. Take on a new career challenge, and emphasize your maturity and experience as prime assets. Go back to school to increase your skills or get a degree that will make you more marketable. Get involved in some meaningful volunteer work. Even if you've tried some of these things before without much success, use the motivation of wanting to feel good, look

Is It True?

Fiction: Depression isn't a real disease.

Fact: Although scientists still don't fully understand the causes of depression, they know that it's linked to physical changes in your brain and can increase your risk for other health problems, such as heart attack, dementia, and osteoporosis.

What to Tell Your Daughter

If she's a teenager, your daughter is on the other end of the same hormonal seesaw you're riding during perimenopause. Your experiences can help her understand what she's going through. But know this: The average adolescent navigates these years with only a few bumpy spots. Don't assume that excessive moodiness is normal. Your daughter (or son, for that matter) may be suffering from depression if she's persistently morose and alienated, sleeping too much or too little, disinterested in school or activities she used to enjoy, and pushing old friends away. Studies indicate that one in five teens considers suicide. Teens who abuse alcohol or drugs may actually be making a misguided attempt at self-treatment. (Research suggests that it may happen the other way around as well. Substance abuse may cause teens to become depressed.) Effective early treatment will not only help depressed teens feel better, but will also help prevent recurrence in the future.

better, and age well to stick to a new routine more faithfully.

Menopause is a major life transition. Expect it to inspire some introspection and reevaluation; this kind of deep thinking can trigger painful feelings of regret and sadness. But if it's transitory, it doesn't constitute depression. It may be that you need to get a second wind or make overdue changes. Many women find it helpful to talk to a therapist or social worker as they rethink their priorities and goals during this time.

PMS AND PERIMENOPAUSE

Q *My doctor asked me a lot of questions about PMS and about my emotional state while I was taking fertility drugs and after my children's births. What connection does this have to my mood at menopause?*

A Women who have a history of severe mood problems during times of normal hormonal change (after giving birth, before a period) may be particularly vulnerable to depression and anxiety during perimenopause, when hormone levels are most likely to be bouncing around. It's not the actual hormone level but a sensitivity to changing levels that appears to trigger distress.

The best evidence comes from research on women suffering from severe premenstrual syndrome (PMS) or premenstrual dysphoric disorder (PMDD). A National Institute of Mental Health study identified a subset of women whose moods improved and then worsened in response to suppression and supplementation of their ovarian secretions. Their reactions were markedly different from those of the women in the control group, whose moods were unaffected by the same experiences. A few other studies have demonstrated a link between mood problems during perimenopause and similar problems after the birth of a child or while using oral contraceptives. According to the data provided by these studies, women with a history of mood disruption during times of hormonal flux may be particularly susceptible to emotional problems at perimenopause. But no strict cause and effect has been identified. Not every woman who has a history of severe PMS or postpartum depression will experience a return of mood problems at perimenopause.

The hormonally sensitive group is estimated to be pretty small, representing about 10 percent of the depression seen in women at midlife. It does not include everyone who ever got a little cranky or out of sorts the day before her period or a little weepy the week after giving birth. While many women feel exhausted and somewhat blue after childbirth, only 10 percent have the severe symptoms associated with postpartum depression. About 50 to 80 percent of women have had some experience with premenstrual symptoms sometime in their life, but only 3 to 7 percent of all women qualify for a diagnosis of PMDD. If your experience is more typical, there's no reason to anticipate mood problems directly related to hormone shifts during perimenopause.

Newly Cursed by PMS

Q *I've never had PMS, but now, at age 40, it has come on with a vengeance. What's going on?*

A Sometimes severe PMS or PMDD comes on just as you describe. These disorders are characterized by a wide range of emotional and physical symptoms that include irritability, mood swings, weepiness, bloating, headaches, breast tenderness, sleeplessness, fatigue, food cravings, stomach and intestinal distress, joint pain, anxiety, depression, memory problems, and trouble concentrating. Even if you never had any problem with PMS when you were younger, it can become an issue in your 30s or 40s. It's not clear why this happens. It could be aging or the effects of stress. You could also be experiencing the beginning of perimenopause. It's hard to tell exactly what's happening without a little detective work. Start by charting your symptoms daily for a few months. If you find that you're only uncomfortable during the week before your period (the luteal phase of your menstrual cycle, when your uterine lining is being built up), PMS or PMDD is the likely issue.

There are some indications that certain low-dose antidepressants can help. Another promising treatment is light therapy (see pages 210–11), especially if you're interested in a nondrug solution.

From the Past

enopause and mood have been intertwined for centuries. The renowned second-century doctor and philosopher Galen proposed that menopause was the result of a hardening of women's blood vessels. This condition, he wrote, could prompt rising levels of blood to flood a woman's brain and cause her to go insane. The way to treat such a "plethora" was with periodic bleedings. This approach was based on the mistaken belief that the body was a closed system and that without a monthly bleed, a woman could be harmed by having too much blood raging through her veins.

For many, many centuries, it was thought that the workings of a woman's womb and her brain were closely related. That helps to explain the evolution of the word *hysterical*. (*Hystera* is Greek for "uterus"—think hysterectomy.) In *On the Preservation of the Health of Women at the Critical Periods of Life* (1851), Dr. Edward John Tilt listed these symptoms of "menopausal insanity": uncontrollable peevishness, melancholia, perversion of moral instincts, impulse to deceive, delirium, mania, suicidal tendencies, uncontrollable impulses, dipsomania, "demonomania," and "erotomania." An influential gynecologist and president of the Obstetrical Society of London, Tilt backed up this claim by disclosing that about a third of the 1,320

women admitted to a local hospital for the insane were between 40 and 45 years old. Besides bloodletting, surgeries such as hysterectomies and "ovariotomies" were seen as possible treatments for psychiatric problems. Alternative treatments included Lydia Pinkham's Vegetable Compound (composed of black cohosh root extract, a popular herbal treatment even today, and 19 percent alcohol) and "water cures," a regimen that required drinking a lot of water, eating lightly, and taking many baths. Even as late as 1888, the *Surgeon General's Index Catalogue* told readers looking for information on menopause to "See also: Insanity in Women."

In the Victorian era, when illness was proof of gentility, the notion that menopause left a woman mentally vulnerable seemed to resonate. In *Psychiatrie* (1909), German psychiatrist E. Kraepelin wrote about the onset of "involutional melancholia" during menopause—a diagnosis that persisted into the 20th century and was included in the first and second editions (1952, 1968) of the American Psychiatric Association's *Diagnostic and Statistical Manual of Mental Disorders*. Not until the third edition (1980) was it removed for lack of evidence. Despite that, the idea that menopause predisposes all women to erratic behavior lingers on.

Symptoms of Major and Minor Depression

To be diagnosed with major depressive disorder, you must have five or more of the symptoms listed below (including one of the first two). These symptoms must persist most of the time for two weeks, must represent a change from your previous state of mind, and must prevent you from functioning normally. After conducting a comprehensive interview and physical exam to rule out other possible causes of a mood disorder, your doctor will categorize the severity of your depression. Major depression usually appears for the first time in the late 20s, but it can occur anytime. Minor depression is diagnosed when at least three of these symptoms in the list below interfere with your ability to function well.

◆ Persistent sad mood

◆ Loss of interest or pleasure in things you once enjoyed

◆ Changes in appetite and body weight

◆ Sleep changes, such as difficulty sleeping as well as oversleeping

◆ Physical displays of agitation or, at the other extreme, listlessness

◆ Loss of energy; exhaustion

◆ Sense of worthlessness and futility or inappropriate guilt

◆ Difficulty making decisions, concentrating, and thinking clearly

◆ Recurrent thoughts of death or suicide

BAD TIMES IN THE PAST

Q *I'm generally healthy and usually in pretty good spirits. However, I did go through a bad patch a few years ago. Eventually I felt better, so I didn't go to my doctor for help. Could I be at risk for depression at menopause?*

A If you've suffered from depression in the past, even if it wasn't formally diagnosed, you're more likely to have a recurrence than someone who has never been depressed. Women who have had one episode of depression have a 50 percent chance of a second. Those who have experienced two episodes have a 70 percent chance of recurrence. Those who have had three or more episodes have a 90 percent chance of experiencing another. Women with a genetic predisposition to depression coupled with a difficult life (periods of social isolation, trauma, or childhood deprivation may permanently alter brain function and possibly brain structure) are especially susceptible.

Women who have a history of depression during hormonally sensitive periods (like postpartum depression) also may be particularly vulnerable, but more study is needed to establish this link.

SWEATS, SLEEP, AND MOOD

Q *Hot flashes at night are not only ruining my sleep, they're also having a terrible effect on my mood. Is it possible that all this is connected to depression?*

A It makes common sense that hot flashes at night would disturb your sleep and make you cranky in the morning. But you're obviously talking about more than irritability here. Research indicates that a lot of perimenopausal women get hit with hot flashes, sleep problems, *and* depression all at the same time. A study conducted by Massachusetts General Hospital in Boston found that perimenopausal women with hot flashes are more than four times as likely to become depressed as those who never flash. Interestingly, this seems to hold true only while you're perimenopausal. The researchers did not find the same link among premenopausal or postmenopausal women who experience hot flashes. What's the connection? During perimenopause, estrogen levels are at their most erratic, and these zigzagging levels reduce the availability of neurotransmitters such as serotonin. We know that serotonin levels have an effect on mood, but some researchers theorize that they may also affect the body's ability to regulate temperature. This may explain why antidepressants like Prozac and Paxil, which have an effect on serotonin, have been shown in randomized studies to be effective treatments for both hot flashes and depression. Another antidepressant, Effexor, is also used to treat both problems. Using antidepressants to reduce the frequency and number of hot flashes is an "off-label" use—they haven't been FDA-approved for this purpose—but this is a common practice and is not necessarily

unsafe. Some doctors may want their patients to try oral contraceptives first if they're perimenopausal or hormone therapy if they're postmenopausal; both can reduce hot flashes and may have an effect on mood as well. If you're interested in trying either hormones or an antidepressant for your situation, talk to your doctor about the potential side effects, benefits, and risks for someone like you. If your mood problems are mild, be sure to consider the nondrug alternatives as well.

SHADES OF BLUE

Q *Are hormones always involved when you experience mood problems at midlife?*

A Not always. Mood disorders at any time of life can be a side effect of medications such as oral contraceptives, tranquilizers, some types of heart drugs, and diet pills. Symptoms of depression are also associated with an underactive thyroid, many serious illnesses, and poor overall health. Personal traumas and losses, stress at home or in the office, cultural attitudes toward aging, or a combination of all these things may affect your mood.

Sleeplessness can have a huge impact on mood, and sleep disorders such as obstructive sleep apnea become more common in women at midlife. Unfortunately, many doctors overlook lack of sleep because they have no training in sleep science. Look through Chapter 4 for symptoms and solutions.

<hr>

━━━ STRESS AT MIDLIFE ━━━

The menopause years are a time of many changes beyond the end of fertility. Here are some of the other reasons that women at midlife might be vulnerable to stress-induced depression:

◆ Marriage and relationship problems

◆ Involuntary childlessness

◆ Raising young children or teens, or both

◆ Empty nest

◆ Returning adult children

◆ Personal or family medical problems

◆ Body changes associated with aging

◆ Divorce

◆ Widowhood

◆ Aging parents

◆ Career and work issues

<hr>

STRESS AND MORE STRESS

Q *What kinds of stress can increase your chances of having mood problems now?*

A Stress is a major factor for everyone dealing with depression, but it seems to have a greater impact on women. Research funded by the National Institute of Mental Health indicates that stressful incidents are more likely to provoke a recurrence of depression in women than in men.

Relationships, career, health, family —almost any source of stress—can have a big impact on your emotional health. One reason: Stress increases levels of the hormone cortisol, which is associated with depression. Stress that develops into a mood disorder might result from one major challenge (a bout with breast cancer, for example), or it could be the cumulative result of everything in your life. Imagine that we're all walking around with our own personal mental health bucket. As the amount of stress in our lives rises, so does the level in the bucket. Because of your genes or biochemistry or experiences (like childhood abuse or traumatic loss) or chronic disease or a combination of these things, the level in your bucket might be higher to start with. Over the course of our lives, it's not surprising that our levels rise and at some point may spill over, resulting in depression and anxiety. When that happens, it doesn't mean there's anything wrong with your bucket; it's just too full. One way of thinking about depression, the kindling theory, suggests that if you have recurrent bouts of depression, it takes progressively smaller levels of stress to precipitate the next episode.

At this time of life, your stress level may rise because of something directly related to menopause, such as sadness about the end of your fertility or distress about aging. Abusive and otherwise toxic marriages have a particularly profound effect. Many women are struggling to juggle multiple demands. Maybe you're the main breadwinner for your family as well as the main caretaker at home. The age of your children plays a major role, and we're not just talking about teenagers, who have certainly been known to increase tension in the home. Having children under the age of five is most closely associated with depression, and more perimenopausal women have young children today than ever before. You may also be actively involved in the care of aging parents. Meeting both of these responsibilities at the same time makes you a member of the "sandwich" generation, a common marker for stress.

TOXIC MARRIAGES

Q *I have a miserable marriage that I would call abusive. I'm taking medication for depression, but I don't feel much better. How do I know how much of my distress is related to my mental state vs. my relationship with my husband?*

A Because your living situation may be interfering with your ability to get better, depression coupled with a toxic marriage is challenging to treat. And just taking medication is unlikely to lead to real relief. As one psychiatrist we know put it, "Antidepressants are not anesthetics." If you're not receiving any talk therapy, now is a good time to ask for a referral. Keep in mind that living for long periods of time in a debilitating relationship takes a toll not only on your mental state, but on your physical health as well. Don't put this off.

IS IT JUST US?

Q *Do women who live in cultures where aging is celebrated experience fewer mood problems?*

A The little research done in this area seems to indicate that they do. For example, anthropologists have found that Mayan women look forward to menopause partly because their culture puts more value on older women than on younger ones. In the United States, we celebrate youth above almost everything else. One study of American women found that 80 percent of those surveyed associated an increased risk of depression with menopause. Some feminist psychologists theorize that the overemphasis on youth is responsible for a lot of the mood problems American women experience at midlife.

WILL IT GET WORSE?

Q *I'm just starting to get irregular periods and already I'm feeling moody! Will this get worse over time?*

A Most women find that their moodiness hits its zenith at the end of the menopause transition, around the time of their last period. Since you only identify your last period retrospectively, it's hard to know when that moment has come. Interestingly, surveys have found that many women in their early 50s describe these years as the happiest in their lives. So even if it feels like tough going right now, you can be optimistic about the future.

LOW THYROID

Q *I went to the doctor because I felt depressed. After running some tests, he told me that I had a problem with my thyroid and gave me medication to treat it. I feel better, but I'm still depressed. Does it make sense to raise this issue again?*

A Yes. As part of the process of diagnosing depression, doctors look for alternative causes. A malfunctioning thyroid can bring on depressive moods, and mood problems sometimes disappear as your thyroid function improves. If they don't, it's a sign that something else may be going on. For instance, you could have hypothyroidism *and* depression. Your doctor needs to hear that the mood symptoms are still bothering you so he can determine what to do next.

DEPRESSED INTO MENOPAUSE?

Q *I'm in my late 30s and my ob-gyn thinks I'm perimenopausal. She said it might be related to my years of struggling with depression.*

A Harvard researchers discovered that women with a history of major depression were 20 percent more

likely to experience early natural menopause. Women with severe symptoms had double that risk. The subgroup of women with severe symptoms who were also using antidepressants were almost three times as likely to transition into perimenopause early. It's not clear why this happens, but it might be related to the fact that depressed women have elevated levels of the stress hormone cortisol for extended periods.

However, other research suggests that many women who experience premature ovarian failure become depressed *after* they're diagnosed. This has raised speculation that perhaps the same thing that sends some women into early menopause may also cause them to develop depression. More research is clearly needed.

CANCER SIDE EFFECTS

Q *My breast cancer treatments have sent me into early menopause and an emotional spin. How do I know whether I'm just upset about being sick or suffering from depression?*

A When you have a serious or chronic illness, it's very common for depression to join the mix. About 10 to 15 percent of all cases of depression occur in people dealing with serious medical problems (like cancer, heart disease, thyroid problems, or neurological conditions). It's unclear to researchers whether depression occurs because of an emotional reaction to the illness or is somehow part of the illness itself. In your case, the abruptness of your transition to menopause could be a contributing factor.

It's not surprising that people dealing with serious illness feel sad some of the time. But if such emotions last for two weeks or more and you have other symptoms of depression, you should seek treatment. The exhaustion and apathy that come with depression could hinder your ability to follow through on the treatments prescribed for your cancer. Untreated depression can also put you at higher risk for a variety of other health problems. You may need to be your own advocate on this, since many doctors miss depression symptoms while focusing on a more immediate medical problem.

IS IT TESTOSTERONE?

Q *Does testosterone affect mood? I have a friend who self-treats her mood problems with DHEA.*

A Androgens like testosterone may indeed play a role in mood regulation, although it's not clear how or why. Depressed perimenopausal women appear to have lower levels of the androgen steroids DHEA and DHEA-S in the morning than nondepressed women do. However, testosterone levels drop earlier than estrogen levels during the natural menopause transition. By the time you're 40, you have only about half the testosterone you had in your 20s, which is why

testosterone usually isn't associated with midlife mood problems. But here's the exception: Taking supplemental estrogen during the menopause transition can lead to lower levels of free testosterone, which in turn may lead to low libido. If a diminished sex drive is your issue, talk to your doctor about your options. Just remember, it's generally a bad idea to self-treat with hormones, even over-the-counter products like DHEA. There's also some question whether the kind of DHEA found in many health food stores (created in labs from wild yams) converts to DHEA in the body.

THE NEXT STEP

Q *A lot of the symptoms of depression seem to match the way I'm feeling. Should I make an appointment with my physician or with a psychologist or psychiatrist?*

A Some people like to start this process by getting a complete physical from their regular doctor to rule out medical conditions with symptoms that mimic depression. However, if you have to wait a long time for an appointment, don't. Depression is a serious illness that needs prompt attention. Since psychiatrists are medical doctors, they can diagnose depression as well as other conditions that could be causing or contributing to your symptoms. Many people also see a psychologist to get the psychotherapy that's usually recommended as part of a treatment program.

THE SECRET TO HAPPINESS

Can you make yourself happy? It appears that you can. In recent years, researchers have become increasingly intrigued with "positive psychology," the science of happiness. Happy people not only enjoy life more; they also live longer and are less vulnerable to mental and physical ailments. Surprisingly, however, the road to happiness isn't reached through wealth or fame or an endless stream of lovers. Those things afford you moments of pleasure, but that's a lot different from the kind of "authentic happiness" that leads to life satisfaction. According to University of Pennsylvania psychologist Martin Seligman (the "father" of positive psychology), increasing life satisfaction begins with identifying your personal strengths, spending more time doing things that you're good at and that truly engage you, and using your talents to create a life that has meaning. To help you get started, go to Seligman's website (www.authentichappiness.sas.upenn.edu), which offers 18 scientifically validated questionnaires to help you identify your strengths as well as areas that need work.

Here are some other research-based ways to boost your happiness:

◆ Work on fostering close relationships with your family and friends. Invest time and energy to become a valued member of a community. You're much more likely to feel true happiness if you connect in healthy, vibrant ways to people you care about. If you think you don't have good social skills, there are therapists who specialize in developing them.

◆ Take the time—and make the time—to notice and savor the good things in your life, whether it's something simple (a hot shower) or sublime (reading poetry).

◆ Be proactively grateful. You might want to start out by keeping a "gratitude journal" (once a week, make a written list of three things you're thankful for) or keeping track of your blessings (once a day, write down three things that went well and why they happened). Or go out of your way to express gratitude to someone who has made a significant difference

WHAT WORKS?

A number of nondrug treatment methods have been proven effective, either on their own or as part of a multitiered approach, especially if you have a mild or moderate case of depression, or if your depression has stabilized and you're trying to prevent a recurrence. But be sure to discuss your mental health history and preferences with your doctor before you decide what course to take.

PSYCHOTHERAPY. Effective talk therapy can literally change the way your brain functions by teaching it new ways of reacting to stressors that may be generating a depressive response. Cognitive-behavior therapy, which shows patients

in your life (parent, teacher, mentor), preferably in person. These types of positive exercises give you an instant lift and can reduce depression, boost your energy level, and even lower your perception of pain.

◆ Be kind to others. Not only will this make you feel good about yourself, but such efforts often trigger gratitude from others, which in turn will make you feel more connected to and valued by your community.

◆ Forgive someone. No matter how justified your resentment and anger might be, you will continue to pay a personal price (constant ruminations, desire for revenge) for refusing to let go of these negative emotions.

◆ Develop your spiritual side. Science shows that people with religious faith feel more supported when going through hard times (although it's hard to

tease out how much of this is due to religious fervor vs. being part of a caring community).

◆ Exercise helps everything, including your disposition. People who get regular exercise feel better and have more energy. Spend enough time on the track and you'll experience a runner's high, thanks to increased levels of endorphins.

◆ Look for opportunities to laugh and smile. Doing so is an instant mood-lifter.

◆ Find activities that make you feel creative and totally engaged. Psychologist Mihaly Csikszentmihalyi describes this uplifting state as "flow" in a book by the same name.

◆ Get older. Studies indicate that older people as a group are more satisfied with their lives than twentysomethings and spend fewer days (2.3 vs. 3.4) each month feeling sad.

how to recognize and alter the negative reactions and behavior that can accompany depression, is often very helpful, but it can be difficult to find a therapist trained in this technique. Interpersonal therapy can be a good option for women dealing with reactive depression, which is brought on by personal trauma, crisis, or transition (think divorce, retirement, empty nest). It works by helping you sort

through the troubled relationships that may be contributing to your depression. Some of the best programs for women at midlife are those that focus on changing family or societal roles. In some cases, marital or family therapy should be part of the mix. For mild cases of depression, psychotherapy alone may work well. In moderate to severe cases, the most effective programs combine psychotherapy with medication. A National Institute of Mental Health study found that patients treated with a combination of psychotherapy and medication had fewer recurrences over a three-year period than those who just got one or the other.

MINDFULNESS MEDITATION. A derivative of Buddhism, mindfulness encourages people to live in the moment. By learning to recognize and acknowledge painful emotions as they occur and accepting that they will pass, those skilled in mindfulness diminish the likelihood that depressive symptoms will return. Research indicates that mastery of mindfulness helps make cognitive behavior therapy more effective; as a result, some specialists offer eight-week courses that teach both therapies.

EXERCISE. Another reason to go to the gym. Exercise can reduce and manage depression and may even prevent it. Why this is so is still under debate, but there are plenty of theories. Exercise typically produces a small but significant improvement in self-esteem, which can distract your attention from negative thoughts. It also boosts the levels of neurotransmitters such as serotonin and dopamine, which are linked to mood, as well as the feel-good endorphins that create the euphoria commonly known as runner's high.

At the same time, exercise seems to reduce your body's levels of cortisol, the so-called stress hormone. Movement helps to release tension from your muscles and improves sleep quality. And all this comes fairly easily. Depending on your current fitness level, you may benefit from something as simple as a 10-minute walk. In any case, don't push yourself to the point where the exercise itself becomes stressful. And recognize that the more depressed you are, the less motivated you may be to get moving. That's why some doctors start people on psychotherapy or medication first and encourage exercise as a second or alternative therapy once they start feeling better.

LIGHT THERAPY (PHOTOTHERAPY). Bright light has long been accepted as an effective treatment for seasonal affective disorder (SAD), which is associated with the darker months of the year. Many SAD patients get significant relief by sitting in front of specially made "light boxes" first thing in the morning for specific amounts of time, usually from 15 minutes to an hour. To the brain, exposure to a 10,000-lux light (a lux is the scientific unit of light intensity) is the equivalent of a dose of bright sunshine without the risk of the ultraviolet rays associated with skin cancer. It's significantly more than what you'd get sitting inside a house with normal lights on. Most indoor settings have lighting that ranges from about 50 to 500 lux; sitting outside in the shade is about 2,000 to 3,000 lux. Some pilot studies indicate that exposure to bright light may also be effective in treating some cases of major depression and bipolar disorder, usually as an adjunct therapy combined with medication. Many patients feel better in a week or two. It's not clear yet why light therapy works, but some think it may be especially effective for dealing with depression that occurs in the winter. Since depression is a disorder of deregulation, it could be that an effective brain regulator like light helps to balance things out.

In any case, make sure you talk to your doctor before starting light therapy. You need a specific prescription about how close you should sit to the box, when to use it, and for what length of time. Too much time under a light box could make it harder for you to fall asleep at night; too little won't be effective. A prescription may help you get insurance reimbursement (the light usually costs at least $200). There have been some reports of side effects, including headaches, eye irritation, and nausea. In rare cases, light therapy can trigger bipolar episodes, although it's more likely to help alleviate them. In some situations, time spent in bright daylight sun can be substituted for the light box.

OMEGA-3 FATTY ACIDS. Both clinical and epidemiological evidence suggests that increasing the amount of EPA, one of the long-chain fatty acids, can help you bounce back from depression. (Depression can be associated with notably low blood levels of EPA.) This supplement seems to help even those who aren't adequately responding to antidepressants. Many doctors recommend that their depressed patients take a supplement that contains about 1 gram of EPA or more per day. EPA has also been proven effective in treating bipolar disorder.

SLEEP DEPRIVATION. It seems counterintuitive, but losing sleep can make some severely depressed and bipolar patients feel better. Brain scans of depressed patients before and after periods of sleep deprivation reveal that those who benefited experienced a drop in activity in the area of the brain associated with regulating emotion. Sustaining that improvement can be a challenge, however. Some patients feel worse after they get some sleep; this type of therapy can trigger depression in bipolar patients. Patients who were taking antidepressants or using light therapy as part of their treatment plan seemed best able to prevent relapse after recovery sleep.

In any case, sleep deprivation remains largely experimental and should be attempted only under medical supervision. It is typically reserved for giving a quick lift to severely depressed or suicidal patients before their medications can reach therapeutic levels.

ELECTROCONVULSIVE THERAPY (ECT).
Formerly known as shock therapy, this treatment is now used only when other treatments fail. Patients are placed under general anesthesia before electrodes are placed on their scalp. Electricity stimulates the brain and prompts it to go into a seizure. About 80 to 90 percent of those who undergo these treatments experience substantial improvement, making it one of the most effective treatments for acute depression. However, patients often experience some cognitive problems and memory loss immediately after treatment. These problems usually dissipate quickly, but not always; in some rare cases, they never go away. ECT is also not a permanent solution. Several rounds are typically required in order to effect maximal improvement, and even then, many patients eventually relapse.

VAGUS NERVE STIMULATION (VNS).
Electrical impulses generated by a pacemaker-like device surgically attached to the left vagus nerve in the neck stimulate the mood centers of the brain to reduce depression in medication-resistant patients. Originally developed for use in patients with drug-resistant epilepsy, VNS improved their moods as well, which led to its use for depression. Placebo-controlled trials did not show any benefit, but in open trials about one-third of the patients experienced a 50 percent decrease in their depression. Among the downsides: It can take up to a year to work, and antidepressants may need to be continued as well. It is

BOTOX DEPRESSION AWAY?

Can Botox be used to get rid of the blues and wrinkles at the same time? A Maryland cosmetic surgeon did one small study (reported in the journal *Dermatologic Surgery*) in which he injected muscle-paralyzing Botox into the foreheads of 10 depressed women, effectively preventing them from frowning. The treatment eliminated depression in 9 of the 10 women; the mood of the 10th woman improved. While some have suggested that the women's moods brightened because their looks improved, the cosmetic surgeon who did the study says some of the younger women had no furrows for the Botox to erase and their moods improved anyway. The study is intriguing because there is extensive research suggesting that you can boost your mood by smiling and laughing, even if you're faking it. Could the same be true if you're frowning less? Is it possible that one shot could make you look younger *and* feel better? Too bad that this little study is far from definitive. There was no control group; the participants were not randomized into treatment groups, and they all knew exactly what they were getting (so it was not blind). Plus, there were only 10 women participating. Altogether, this means that the results should be considered with caution. But you can bet there will be continued interest and research in the near future.

approved for use in the United States (where it is being monitored closely), Canada, and Europe.

TRANSCRANIAL MAGNETIC STIMULATION (TMS). Since a handheld coil with an electromagnetic discharge stimulates areas of the brain involved in mood regulation, TMS has been compared to electroconvulsive therapy. But the differences are huge. TMS does not prompt seizures, it isn't painful, and it doesn't cause cognition problems. Efficacy studies show mixed results; some patients do better than others. In some comparative trials, TMS did no better than placebo. Still considered experimental in the United States, it has been approved in Canada and Israel. This treatment is generally used for drug-resistant cases of depression.

ACUPUNCTURE. This Chinese import is one of the rare alternative treatments that show potential as a sole source of therapy for single episodes of depression. Talk to your doctor about finding an experienced and certified acupuncturist in your area.

LOW-CARB DIET

Q *I've heard that eating a low-carb diet can aggravate symptoms of depression. Is there any connection between food and mood?*

A There may be a link between carbohydrates and the availability of serotonin in the brain. Some women who suffer from premenstrual syndrome find that boosting their carbs during the second half of their cycle (when hormone levels are starting to drop) reduces their symptoms. There are only a few studies on this, but you've got nothing to lose by adding more whole-grain foods, vegetables, and fruits to your diet. But don't fool yourself—a few extra Twinkies are not going to help you feel better.

ALCOHOL AND DEPRESSION

Q *My doctor doesn't want me to drink alcohol while I'm taking antidepressants. Why?*

A Alcohol reduces serotonin levels, which can increase your chances of experiencing depression. The result is that it makes antidepressants less effective. The combination can also reduce your body's ability to efficiently metabolize alcohol, which means you may get drunk more easily.

GET A JOB

Q *Someone suggested that I get a job to help overcome my depression. Why would that make a difference?*

A There's not a lot of research on this, but some studies indicate that women who work are slightly less likely to develop depression than are women who stay home. The assumption is that working women have more social contacts, better support systems, and more dependable income. Clearly, this isn't true of everyone. Some working women are exposed to a lot more stress and get fewer opportunities to exercise, sleep, and eat right. Some women who stay home are well plugged into social networks and have very active, healthy lives. If working reduces your sense of isolation and gets you involved in something that lifts your spirits, it could be therapeutic.

Prescription Help

About 80 percent of depression responds to a treatment plan that includes some type of prescription medication. For many women, these drugs have been lifesavers. The frustration is that many people have to try a couple of different medications or combinations before they find one that's right for them. A study published in the *New England Journal of Medicine* found that about one in every three or four people who do not find relief after trying SSRIs (see below) eventually are helped by changing to another prescription or using a combination of drugs. This process can take months. Typically, you have to give each drug a chance to have an effect—at least two to six weeks of use—before you move on to another and perhaps yet another. In any case, drugs seem especially effective when there is a family history of depression, severe symptoms, or repeated episodes. Most antidepressants are believed to work by influencing the availability of neurotransmitters in the brain, primarily serotonin and norepinephrine. And like any class of drugs, antidepressants have both benefits and risks. Some affect your sleep; some boost your libido, while others dampen it. If you have problems with insomnia or your sex drive, make sure you mention them to your doctor before you get your first prescription. In some cases, doctors prescribe more than one antidepressant at a time to get a more effective response, but there's little research on this strategy. Because of possible drug interactions, be sure to tell your doctor about any other medications (prescription and over-the-counter) or botanicals you're taking before you start using any antidepressants. Below is a primer on the different types that are most commonly prescribed:

Selective serotonin reuptake inhibitors (SSRIs) are among the newest and most widely used antidepressants. By helping the brain maintain adequate levels of serotonin, SSRIs help stabilize your mood within a few weeks. Some studies indicate that these antidepressants are especially effective in women. They don't cause as many side effects as some of the older medications, but about half of the patients who take them report being bothered by side effects during the first four to six weeks of use. These often disappear over time. Common side effects include dry mouth, nervousness, nausea, dizziness, sleeplessness, constipation, skin rashes, fatigue, and weight gain or loss. Sexual problems can also occur; about a third of the women who use SSRIs have difficulty reaching orgasm.

Ask about the specific side effects associated with your prescription. SSRIs include Celexa (citalopram), Lexapro (escitalopram), and Zoloft (sertraline). Celexa and Lexapro seem to cause fewer interactions with a range of other medications; Lexapro is particularly fast-acting. Check the labels for specific drug information. Two other SSRIs, Prozac (fluoxetine) and Paxil (paroxetine), have been shown to reduce hot flashes. In other cases, however, they have caused hot flashes in women who never had the problem before.

SSRIs also affect platelet stickiness in your blood, so ask your doctor about discontinuing them if you're scheduled for surgery.

Serotonin and norepinephrine reuptake inhibitors (SNRIs) boost the availability of norepinephrine and serotonin in the brain. They are often tried on women who don't respond to SSRIs. The best known of this class is Effexor (venlafaxine), which can also reduce hot flashes. Side effects of SNRIs include sleepiness, dizziness, constipation, and sexual dysfunction. At high doses, they are also associated with increased blood pressure and cholesterol levels. Cymbalta (duloxetine) has been shown to reduce diabetic peripheral neuropathic pain and seems to be a particularly good choice for women dealing with both depression and diabetes.

Tricyclic antidepressants (TCAs) aim to increase levels of serotonin, dopamine, and norepinephrine. They also seem to work on other chemicals in the body, which may explain why they tend to have more side effects than the SSRIs and SNRIs. TCAs include Elavil (amitriptyline), Norpramin (desipramine), Tofranil (imipramine), and Aventyl and Pamelor (both nortriptyline). Among the common side effects include impaired thinking, blurred vision, difficulty urinating, constipation, fatigue, worsened glaucoma, and orthostatic hypotension (low blood pressure when standing up). Some types affect heart rate and blood sugar levels.

Monoamine oxidase inhibitors (MAOIs) were discovered by accident in the 1950s when researchers were looking for new treatments for tuberculosis. Common monoamine oxidase inhibitors include Nardil (phenelzine) and Parnate (tranylcypromine). Like TCAs, MAOIs attempt to increase the functioning of both serotonin and norepinephrine. Although they're very effective for some patients, strict dietary and alcohol restrictions, drug interactions, and side effects have made oral MAOIs a less popular choice. For example, users are prohibited from ingesting any aged foods, including red wine, soy sauce, and certain cheeses. Dietary restrictions don't apply to the new lowest-dose MAOI patch (transdermal selegiline); check with your doctor about the restrictions associated with your dosage.

HORMONES AFTER MENOPAUSE

Q *Can hormones be used to treat depression after menopause?*

A The answer seems to be no. Once the hormone fluctuation stops, estrogen appears to have no effect on depression.

HOW LONG DOES IT TAKE?

Q *I'm on antidepressants now, but I don't like the idea of chemicals in my body. What's a realistic time frame? When can I get off them?*

A The answer varies from person to person, and the ultimate decision should be made by you and your doctor. If this is your first episode of depression, the shortest amount of time you can expect to be on medication is six to nine months. The general rule is one year. If you want to get off (and stay off) faster, take your doctor's advice about seeing a psychotherapist, getting more exercise, or using light as an adjunct therapy. The more you can do to eliminate factors that add to your vulnerability, the better off you'll be. Concern about relapse prompts doctors to keep patients on antidepressants even after symptoms wane. Usually, each recurrence means staying on medication longer. Three or more episodes would probably mean being asked to stay on medication for the foreseeable future.

ANTIDEPRESSANTS AND SEX

Q *I've been treating my depression with Prozac. I feel better most of the time, but I rarely feel sexually aroused anymore. Could Prozac be the problem?*

A Sexual problems are a common side effect of some antidepressants. Nobody knows why, but medications like Prozac reduce the amount of dopamine in your brain and this affects your perception of pleasure. But arousal problems could be related to lower levels of another neurotransmitter, norepinephrine. The drugs' effects on serotonin (also one of those neurotransmitters) could be the culprit for orgasm troubles. A University of Virginia study of 6,300 people with antidepressant-related sexual dysfunction found notable gender differences. Two-thirds of the men complained about desire and orgasm problems (often delayed ejaculation), while the women were much more likely to have trouble with arousal. Although there has been more attention to this problem with the increased use of SSRIs, older antidepressants also cause sexual problems.

Doctors take these complaints seriously because they worry that people will stop taking their medication in order to improve their sex lives, and stopping without supervision could have long-term health consequences. Although you may be hesitant to discuss your sex life with anyone (even your doctor), force yourself to bring it up anyway. If your medication is the problem, your doctor can give you an array of choices. One option is to wait it out, since sex problems often decline after you've been on a drug for a while and have built up tolerance. You may also try another antidepressant to see if it has fewer sexual side effects. Some doctors suggest substituting or adding Wellbutrin. Others suggest Cymbalta. Both tend to cause fewer sexual problems and even enhance some patients' sex lives. Serzone, an antidepressant that is not an SSRI, SNRI, TCA, or MAOI, is also associated with fewer sexual problems. Finding a solution to both depression and sexual dysfunction can be complicated, so you might consider asking for a consultation with a psychiatrist or psychopharmacologist who has expertise in this area.

ESTROGEN AND MOOD

Q *I'm considering hormone therapy to treat my hot flashes. Will it have any effect on depression?*

A Estrogen not only reduces the number and intensity of hot flashes, but also seems to reduce some women's vulnerability to depression. Even without that benefit, estrogen may boost mood, but more research is needed in this area.

In the meantime, most doctors prefer to start with a traditional antidepressant. You might be asked to take hormone therapy in addition to an antidepressant if the latter hasn't worked or has worked only partially; estrogen could make the crucial difference. It might also be helpful if your moods seem to be hormonally sensitive. But remember, hormone therapy has risks. (See Chapter 2 for more details.)

ESTROGEN ALONE

Q *Can estrogen alone treat depression?*

A It's controversial, but some good-quality research indicates that estrogen (estradiol) alone might be an effective short-term treatment for mood problems in some perimenopausal women and that follow-up with traditional antidepressants might not be necessary. But the research is still in its early stages, and it remains unclear who might benefit from this strategy.

If you have other menopausal symptoms and are interested in using hormone therapy to treat them, your doctor may be willing to see what effect hormones have on your mild to moderate depression symptoms before prescribing anything else. However, if hormones aren't doing the job within three weeks, don't be surprised if a traditional antidepressant is added to your drug mix.

HELP FOR HOT FLASHES

Q *I'm struggling with depression and hot flashes. Should I try hormones or an antidepressant?*

A So far, no high-quality studies have directly compared one treatment with the other. If your depression is severe and your hot flashes are not, your doctor will probably recommend antidepressants first. If your hot flashes are really bad but your mood symptoms are mild, he'll probably suggest trying hormones (either an estrogen-progestogen combination if you have a uterus, or estrogen alone if you don't). If you're concerned about the health risks of hormones or if you try hormones and your mood problems get worse, an antidepressant may be recommended. Only a few antidepressants are known to alleviate hot flashes: Effexor, Paxil, and Prozac. Even those three aren't as effective as hormones in reducing their intensity and frequency. While antidepressants often take about six weeks to work on depression, you'll know within a week if they're making any headway against hot flashes.

If it tutns out that neither hormones nor antidepressants work for you, your doctor may want you to try using both at the same time, as well as nonpharmaceutical solutions like exercise, light therapy, and psychotherapy.

It's Getting Worse

Q *I'm perimenopausal and recently started a low-dose combination hormone therapy to help me with the hot flashes and night sweats. But instead of feeling better, I actually feel more out of control—more moody and irritable. My energy is low, and I'm not sleeping any better. Is it possible that my real problem is depression? I've had trouble with it in the past.*

A A couple of different things may be happening. If you have a history of depression, you're at higher risk for renewed symptoms. If you have a history of mood problems at hormonally sensitive times, you might even be at higher risk during perimenopause. You should let your doctor make the call as to whether your depression has returned and whether you're better off treating your symptoms with hormones, an antidepressant, or a combination of the two.

Because your mood got worse after you started the combination therapy, another thing your doctor is likely to consider is whether the progestogen in your combined hormone therapy is the culprit behind your mood problems. You may be advised to try a different progestogen, a different dose, or a different schedule. You might even be asked to take estrogen alone for a few months to see if you feel better. If that works, you and your doctor will need to discuss how you will be monitored so that you don't increase your risk of endometrial cancer. (Keep in mind that there are no high-quality data indicating that taking a progestogen less often than monthly will give you all the protection you need against the increased risk of endometrial cancer.) You will also have to be scrupulous about reporting any irregular bleeding to your doctor. That's often the first warning sign of gynecological cancer.

ON TAKING PROGESTERONE

Q *I still have my uterus, so if I use estrogen to treat my hot flashes and mood problems, my doctor wants me to take progesterone, too. Won't that make my moods worse?*

A Progestogens (the group of hormones that includes progesterone) have long had a reputation for ruining mood, but they don't have this effect on everyone. It's also not clear if progestogens have a negative effect on mood all by themselves or whether they neutralize the beneficial effect of estrogen in some women. The main purpose of the progesterone your body makes is to help your uterus prepare for a possible pregnancy each month. It does this by prompting the walls of your uterus to thicken. When progesterone (and estrogen) levels drop at the end of your cycle, they signal your body to shed the uterine lining and your period begins. Progesterone's levels peak the week between ovulation and the start of your period, during what's known as the luteal phase. This is the time when PMS typically occurs. Some women seem particularly sensitive to rises and falls in their progesterone levels.

A few small studies indicate that certain progestogens (micronized progesterone, for example), as well as ultra-low doses, may cause fewer mood problems when combined with estrogen. Talk to your doctor about what might work best for you.

Another option is to take estrogen alone. However, if you still have your uterus, your doctor will want to monitor the thickness of its lining. Depending on your specific medical history, it might be possible to take estrogen alone if you're extremely rigorous about getting an annual biopsy or ultrasound of your uterus. This is serious business. The number one cause of endometrial cancer is taking estrogen without a progestogen.

END POINT?

Q *I'm taking hormone therapy for both my mood and hot flashes, but I don't want to stay on it too long. How soon can I stop and be confident that neither problem will recur?*

A Unfortunately, we can't give you a good answer, because there are no clinical recommendations about how long you need to stay on hormone therapy to maintain a stable mood. The standard advice on hormones and hot flashes is to take the lowest effective dose for the shortest amount of time possible, but no one really knows what that means for any individual woman. Most women's hot flashes begin and end fairly quickly; many last about five years, and others go on and on. Research indicates that some women may simply be delaying the resolution of their hot flashes by taking hormones. Right now, there's no good way to determine which group you're in. That's one reason why getting off hormone therapy can be so tricky. Because you're concerned about long-term use of hormone therapy, be sure to raise the issue with your doctor every six months. Together, you can see if the time is right to wean yourself. You may need to experiment with slowly dialing down your dose as opposed to going cold turkey to see which method works best for you. There are no good studies to advise you on this, either. (For more detail on these issues, see Chapter 2.)

ANTIDEPRESSANTS ALONE

Q *Will antidepressants help my hot flashes even if I don't have any mood problems? I'm scared to take hormones, but I'd like to find relief!*

A They may. The original studies on antidepressants and hot flashes were part of an effort to find something that would reduce hot flashes in women who were recovering from breast cancer. Because of the link between estrogen and some breast tumors, hormone therapy is not an option in many such cases. Since the antidepressants Prozac, Paxil, and Effexor did prove helpful for these women, doctors assume that the same is true for women who have not had breast cancer.

Like many other drugs, antidepressants can have unpleasant side effects, so you'll have to decide if the benefits are worth it for you. You might also want to consider nondrug alternatives. We offer lots of ideas in Chapter 3.

FLASHES AND BIPOLAR DISORDER

Q *I have a history of bipolar disorder. Can I use hormone therapy for my severe hot flashes?*

A Combination hormone therapy (estrogen and a progestogen) can make bipolar symptoms harder to control. Estrogen can also induce mania. Talk to your doctor about your specific risks.

WHAT ABOUT TIBOLONE?

Q *Some of my European friends use a drug called tibolone that's supposed to be good for mood, hot flashes, and bones. Can I buy it in the United States?*

A The manufacturer of tibolone has not yet sought approval from the FDA for sale in this country, but it does appear to be a promising treatment. It seems to share some of the properties of estrogen, progesterone, and testosterone and may help with mood and bone health. It may also reduce hot flashes and boost sex drive. It's not a perfect drug, however. Early indications are that it lowers HDL (the good cholesterol), and there is concern about its effect on heart disease. In the British Million Women's Study, it also appeared to increase the risk of breast cancer. More research into its effectiveness and safety are currently under way, but it's not clear when the manufacturer will seek permission to sell it here. It's available in Canada and in many places in Europe.

TYPES OF BIPOLAR DISORDER

Once known as manic-depressive illness, bipolar disorders are characterized primarily by cycles of major depression and mania (abnormal bursts of energy and activity). Type I is characterized by at least one manic episode, with or without depression. The manic behavior can seem more like extreme irritability than euphoria. Impulsive and reckless behavior is common. Symptoms worsen with use of antidepressants. At least three of these symptoms must be present for a diagnosis of Type I:

◆ Inflated sense of self

◆ Little need for sleep

◆ Extreme talkativeness

◆ Racing thoughts

◆ Increased distractibility

◆ Physical agitation

◆ Obsessive focusing on a goal

◆ Reckless behavior

Type II is characterized by a milder form of mania (called hypomania) and at least one episode of depression. This is the most common type, although it's harder to diagnose; it's also closely associated with increased suicide risk. Symptoms worsen with use of antidepressants.

Cyclothymic disorder is a less severe but more chronic version of Type II; it may be a precursor to Type I or Type II.

While all three may be part of the same disorder spectrum, some believe that each type may be a totally separate disorder with distinct biologic and environmental causes.

OTHER MENTAL HEALTH ISSUES

It's more than normal worrying. Your heart starts pounding, you feel like you can't breathe, and you begin to sweat all over. You have a sense of something terrible happening—even though everything is actually pretty normal.

What's going on? These are symptoms of an anxiety disorder, probably caused by a biochemical imbalance that set off a "fight or flight" response.

GENERALIZED ANXIETY DISORDER. You have persistent feelings of anxiety that aren't prompted by a specific event or concern. These can be intense as well as moderate and sometimes include panic attacks.

PANIC ATTACKS. These acute and overwhelming episodes of anxiety seem to come out of nowhere and include physical symptoms like rapid heartbeat, shortness of breath, dizziness, and trembling. They may be triggered by stressful situations and too much caffeine or other stimulants.

PANIC DISORDER. Often referred to as a fear of fear, panic disorder is diagnosed if you suffer recurrent and unexpected panic attacks and have at least one of these three experiences: 1) you spend at least a month being extremely fearful of suffering another panic attack; 2) you worry about the implications of having panic attacks, or 3) you change your behavior to avoid certain places or activities for fear they'll bring on a panic attack.

SOCIAL ANXIETY DISORDER. You avoid social situations because of a deep fear of embarrassment or humiliation.

PHOBIAS. Specific, chronic, and irrational fears seriously impair your ability to do certain things, like board an airplane or go into the snake house at the zoo.

OBSESSIVE-COMPULSIVE DISORDER (OCD). This involves repetitive actions (compulsions) and/or thoughts (obsessions) that are difficult to resist, even though you're aware that they don't make any sense. OCD vulnerability is associated with rising levels of estrogen; the likelihood of an episode increases with pregnancy.

POST-TRAUMATIC STRESS DISORDER (PTSD). This can occur after a trauma such as sexual abuse, time in a war zone, or an automobile accident. Emotions may alternate between terrifying rage and feelings of vulnerability and may involve flashbacks and nightmares. PTSD increases your vulnerability to developing depression.

NEW ANXIETY

Q *I'm a pretty calm person and used to working under stress, but in the last few months I've begun to feel extreme anxiety in new situations. Is this part of the craziness of menopause?*

A Anxiety affects twice as many women as men. If you first develop this problem at midlife, it's possible that the menopause transition has something to do with it. But there's a big difference between feeling anxious (a short-term emotion you might experience when faced with a worrisome problem like being laid off) and developing an anxiety disorder (an involuntary and exaggerated response that seems out of whack with the situation or challenge you're facing). In the latter case, areas of the brain that monitor and react to danger, along with the adrenal system, go into overdrive. Why this happens isn't thoroughly understood, but genetics and life experiences are thought to play a role. Your disorder might be triggered by bereavement, repressed feelings about a past trauma, or some ongoing stress.

Menopause might be the source of that stress if you're upset that your fertility is ending or if you're struggling with the idea that you're getting older. Erratic hormone levels may also play an indirect role. We know from studies of younger women who have panic attacks that the frequency of their episodes increases just before they get their monthly period. This seems to indicate that hormonal fluctuations may make some women more vulnerable to developing the imbalance. If you've experienced anxiety or depression in the past, especially during hormonally sensitive periods like menstruation and pregnancies, you may be at higher risk for a return, increase, or initiation of anxiety symptoms as you move through perimenopause. A pounding or racing heart, a jittery feeling, lack of concentration, nausea, and exhaustion may intrude into your life only occasionally. But in the most extreme situations, these interfere with your ability to work, plan, and take care of everyday needs. More than one form of anxiety disorder may appear at the same time, or the anxiety may crop up with depression.

Effective treatments are available. Cognitive-behavior therapy can help you learn to manage your anxiety and increase your sense of control. Medications, including antidepressants such as SSRIs and tricyclics, can also be helpful in some cases. Consistent and regular exercise (every day or at least five days a week) can reduce anxiety attacks, elevate your mood, and reduce your stress level.

Some medications and physical conditions (including thyroid problems and chronically low blood sugar) can be responsible for similar feelings. So can too much caffeine and other stimulants. Both anxiety and panic attacks are also symptoms of mitral valve prolapse, a heart abnormality.

PANIC ATTACKS

Q *There's a tunnel that goes under a bay near my house, and I've driven through it many times without a second thought. But the other day I panicked at the entrance. My heart was pounding like crazy, and I had to force myself to keep driving. It took about 10 minutes to calm myself down. I figure it was a panic attack. Is this somehow associated with menopause?*

A Although it's long been known that panic attacks are twice as common in women as in men, they've had the reputation of being a young person's problem because they usually crop up for the first time in adolescence or early adulthood. But there's evidence that they also occur regularly among midlife women. In a study of 3,369 postmenopausal women aged 50 to 79 enrolled in an arm of the Women's Health Initiative, about 10 percent of the participants reported having had a full-blown panic attack over the previous six months and another 8 percent said they had experienced something close to it—what researchers characterized as a "limited symptom attack." Both numbers were much higher than the researchers expected to find. (Previous estimates had put the national rate for experience with panic attacks at about 1.6 percent.) Interestingly, women at the younger end of the spectrum reported having more attacks than the older women. After adjusting for age, race, and ethnicity, the researchers found that the women most likely to report the attacks had a history of migraines, emphysema, cardiovascular disease, and symptoms of depression. They were also associated with a trauma or major stressor in the previous year.

While recent research indicates that panic attacks involve an overreaction by the amygdala (a part of the brain that monitors and reacts to danger), it's not clear how menopause plays a role. It could have something to do with the availability of neurotransmitters or a heightened sensitivity to the secretions of the adrenal glands as estrogen levels fall. Genetics may play a role as well. Because panic attacks can also be caused by an overactive thyroid (hyperthyroidism) or a heart problem, you need to mention this incident to your doctor.

Panic attacks, which usually peak within 10 minutes but may last 20 to 30 minutes, can be one-time incidents or can recur. If you experience recurrent attacks and develop a fear of feeling afraid or worry about the implications of these attacks or change your behavior (like avoiding tunnels), you've developed panic disorder. A third of the people who have panic disorder go on to experience an intense fear of leaving the house or going to new places; this particular fear is known as agoraphobia. You may feel increased anxiety between attacks. Depression can also become part of the mix.

When the first attack occurs, some doctors would encourage you to face your fear and force yourself to duplicate the action that set off the attack (i.e., get back in your car and drive through the tunnel again). This can help you disassociate the action from the fear before it becomes a phobia. If you experience a series of panic attacks, talk to your doctor about the range of medications (including antidepressants, anti-anxiety medications, and anticonvulsants) and behavior modification treatments that have been proven to help. Improvement is often seen within two months. In the meantime, more exercise and relaxation can decrease symptoms. Don't ignore the problem if it doesn't go away on its own. Not only can panic attacks add to your stress levels and hamper your ability to live a normal life, but they've also been associated with increased risk of cardiovascular problems.

HOT AND BOTHERED

Q *If I suffer from an anxiety disorder, am I more likely to have a lot of hot flashes?*

A It appears that you are. In a six-year study at the University of Pennsylvania, researchers monitored the moods and menopausal symptoms of more than 400 randomly selected women between the ages of 35 and 47. The women whose tests revealed a moderate level of anxiety were three times more likely to get hot flashes than were those with anxiety levels in the normal range. Subjects with high levels of anxiety were almost five times more likely to get hot flashes than the group with normal-range scores. Using early scores on anxiety tests, the researchers were also able to predict which premenopausal women would go on to experience severe and frequent hot flashes as they moved closer to menopause.

TROUBLING SYMPTOMS

Q *I'm a perimenopausal woman dealing with depression, but I'm wondering if it's possible that I have obsessive-compulsive disorder as well. Some of my symptoms aren't on the depression chart.*

A It's relatively common for depression to show up accompanied by another mood abnormality: anxiety, post-traumatic stress disorder, a social phobia, panic disorder, or obsessive-compulsive disorder. This is particularly true in the case of post-traumatic stress disorder, which can surface days, weeks, or even months after a frightening or disturbing incident. About 40 percent of patients suffering from post-traumatic stress are also diagnosed with depression. Be sure to share all your symptoms with your doctor, because you'll need to be diagnosed and treated for each problem. This is particularly true if you're experiencing panic attacks; research indicates that the combination of panic disorder and depression puts people at higher risk for attempted suicide.

ONSET OF SCHIZOPHRENIA

Q *Can menopause bring on schizophrenia in someone who has never had it before?*

A There is a very, very small chance that this can occur. The timing of schizophrenia (the most severe of mental illnesses, often involving delusions and hallucinations) differs between men and women. Men tend to exhibit the initial symptoms earlier and are diagnosed on average between the ages of 20 and 24. Schizophrenia shows itself later in women, typically between ages 25 and 29. However, after age 44, there is another, smaller peak in first-time schizophrenia diagnoses in women that does not occur in men. The presumption is that this blip in late-onset schizophrenia occurs because a very small percentage of women are biologically predisposed to develop these symptoms in response to the drops in estrogen levels during perimenopause or after the ovaries are removed. In some cases, symptoms of both schizophrenia and depression can appear simultaneously. You need a good diagnostician to determine whether you're suffering from depression with psychotic episodes or schizophrenia with depressive episodes. In any case, these are all rare events.

Does Estrogen Play a Role?

Q *If I've been diagnosed with schizophrenia, am I likely to have a harder time during menopause?*

A   That depends on how closely you're being monitored by your doctor and on your own personal history. While there's still a lot that's unknown about the relationship between estrogen and schizophrenia, the hormone may help protect against the disease. We know that some women's symptoms get worse as their estrogen levels fall during each menstrual cycle. (As a result, some doctors put women patients on a cyclic dosage schedule to correspond to their estrogen levels.) Younger symptomatic women tend to need less antipsychotic medication than men do, but they may need higher dosages during the menopause transition and afterwards. Research also shows that pairing antipsychotic drugs and hormone therapy tends to relieve symptoms faster in symptomatic women.

Raise the issue with your doctor when you first start noticing signs of perimenopause or hit your mid-40s, whichever comes first. If you're considering adding hormone therapy to your regimen, make sure you review all the risks associated with it and carefully consider the pros and cons in your particular case.

Take some comfort in the fact that, as a general rule, schizophrenics tend to have fewer psychotic episodes as they age.

CHAPTER 9

Thinking and Memory

*Y*ou struggle to retrieve the right word. Your ability with names (never great) is worse. Your mind feels as if it's working at half speed, and you have more trouble paying attention. Maybe you find yourself reading the same passage over and over, or perhaps you're wondering if you're a little dyslexic. Your first instinct is to blame menopause, and it's true that women who have had their ovaries removed or who have gone through cancer treatments complain the most about a general sense of fogginess. But stress, depression, sleeplessness, medications, and a host of other things can also be responsible for what you're feeling.

Fuzzy thinking isn't inevitable, however. While all of us have our "senior moments," they're usually brief: enough to get your attention, maybe enough to annoy or embarrass you, but not proof that you're not as smart as you used to be. And that fogginess is almost never a sign of early dementia. Still, the health and lifestyle choices you make at midlife can have a big effect on your mind 30 years from now.

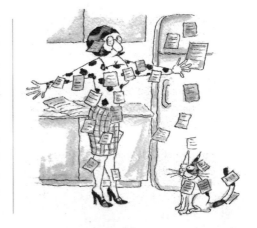

YOUR MIDLIFE BRAIN

Infant brains may get all the press, but there's a lot more going on in your midlife brain than scientists once thought. They used to believe that brain

What Can Happen

✣ Practically nothing. Many women experience few problems with memory or thinking.

✣ Difficulties with verbal memory, word retrieval, and articulation are the most common cognitive glitches associated with menopause. While not indicative of impending dementia, these may be particularly noticeable if you undergo a surgical or chemical menopause.

✣ You may notice more memory lapses (you forget someone's name or why you came into a room). This is very common and probably has nothing to do with menopause. Like a lot of modern women, you may be just too busy or too stressed.

✣ Lower estrogen levels may affect your reading fluency, although vision changes associated with aging eyes may also affect your ability to read easily.

✣ Some women (and men) experience occasional problems with concentration, attention, and thinking clearly during midlife, but a direct link to hormonal changes remains unclear.

development was pretty much over by the time you went to kindergarten. That was because the shape, size, and proportion of the brain appeared to be largely set by then. They also thought that nerve cells died off as you aged, never to be replaced. The fact that older brains physically shrink and become shallower and wider over time seemed to be further proof of an inevitable downward slide.

But it turns out that those ideas were wrong. Your brain is growing, developing, and adapting all through your life. You even continue to produce new nerve cells. Scientists now have evidence that younger and older minds recruit different regions of the brain to perform certain tasks—a fact that not only challenges the idea that each part of the brain performs very specific tasks forever, but may prove that the brain remains more "plastic" than we previously thought.

This doesn't just happen, however. It appears that the more challenges you give your brain, the more nerve proliferation you earn. Neuropsychologist Elkhonon Goldberg, author of *The Wisdom Paradox: How Your Mind Can Grow Stronger as Your Brain Grows Older,* says there's now strong evidence that new mental challenges may be the key to keeping your brain agile. He stresses that it's not enough to do the hard things you've always done; you need to push yourself out of your mental comfort zone. So, for instance, it's not enough for a tax lawyer to keep up with IRS rulings. That lawyer needs to do something

TYPES OF MEMORY

Not all types of memory are affected by hormone fluctuations. While you may find yourself struggling to remember a word, you're probably not having any trouble remembering how to walk (procedural memory) or conjuring up that cozy feeling you got as a child when your grandmother hugged you (emotional memory). Take a quick look at the breakdown below. You'll find it reassuring that most parts of your memory are probably working just fine.

DURATION

◆ *Immediate memory*—retained for only a few seconds. Ex.: the type of car that just passed you on the road

◆ *Short-term memory*—lasts a few minutes. Ex.: the phone number the operator just gave you

◆ *Long-term memory*—held on to for a long time. Ex.: your street address or your wedding day

CLASSIFICATION
Explicit memory

◆ *Semantic*—general knowledge. Ex.: the names of the continents (involves the cerebral cortex)

◆ *Episodic*—Recent and remote events in your life. Ex.: your graduation day or what happened yesterday (involves the hippocampus, cerebral cortex)

Implicit memory

◆ *Procedural memory*—retrieval is so automatic that you don't even think about it. Ex.: walking without consciously remembering how to do it (stored in basal ganglia)

◆ *Classical conditioning*

  *Visceral   automatic linking of one thought with another, like Pavlov's dog salivating upon hearing the bell (stored in cerebellum)

  *Emotional—automatically linking a memory with an emotion. Ex.: feeling panic at the sound of a gunshot (stored in amygdala)

Direction

◆ *Retrospective memory*—remembering something that happened in the past

◆ *Prospective memory*—remembering to remember to do something

really challenging to jump-start her brain, like learning Italian . . . especially if she's not very good at languages. That's why a number of researchers are developing cognitive exercise programs (see page 250) to help us maintain our brains. Another example of midlife brain vitality involves myelination, the process of insulating nerve fibers with a fatty,

high-cholesterol coating that helps speed messages around the brain more efficiently. You can literally see this happening when a flailing infant with almost no control over his limbs becomes a preschooler who can pick up tiny beads with his pincer grasp. For a long time, it was thought that myelination took place only when we were very young.

WHAT IS NORMAL FORGETFULNESS?

◆ Forgetting where you left something, like your keys or cell phone

◆ Forgetting to buy something at the store, including what you went to buy

◆ Forgetting someone's name

WHAT IS ABNORMAL FORGETFULNESS?

◆ General confusion

◆ Disorientation, or forgetting the way to a familiar place

◆ Not being able to remember a very recent event like a phone call or visit

Recently, however, a Harvard researcher investigating the origins of schizophrenia accidentally discovered an extra large stash of myelin in the medial temporal lobe, the part of the brain that integrates memory and emotion. After carefully inspecting 162 brains of different ages, she was able to show that myelin production doubles during the teen years before plateauing. It then revs up again in the 40s and 50s, generating about 50 percent more insulation before leveling off. This discovery has made scientists rethink our notion of wisdom that comes with age. Maybe it's actually a combination of biology (the highly efficient midlife brain, made possible by this increased level of myelin) and hard-earned life experience.

This may not be all good news, however. Researchers at UCLA point out that myelin contains a lot of cholesterol. They wonder if, at some point in some people, all that increased cholesterol in the brain triggers the creation of a toxic protein that degrades myelin, disrupts brain operations, and eventually leads to the plaques and tangles characteristic of

Alzheimer's disease (see pages 232–33). They also speculate that it may be possible that healthy living (a low-fat diet, lots of physical exercise and mental challenges) help mitigate the negative effects of the increased cholesterol in the brain.

SPACIER AT MENOPAUSE?

Q *Does menopause cause problems with memory and learning? I feel spacier than I used to.*

A Lots of women complain of this problem at midlife. In the ongoing Study of Women's Health Across the Nation (SWAN), almost 40 percent of the more than 12,000 women aged 40 to 55 interviewed on this issue said they had experienced problems with forgetfulness in the past two weeks. Premenopausal women were less likely to say they had trouble remembering things than women in perimenopause or postmenopause.

These findings made sense to the researchers. After all, high estrogen levels are associated with the availability of brain chemicals that can be transformed into neurotransmitters (the chemical messengers that help move information from one nerve cell to another). For your memory to be in good working order, you need to have adequate levels of a variety of neurotransmitters. So it wouldn't be surprising if a drop in estrogen temporarily affected your memory or thinking.

But other research indicates that menopause doesn't affect all women's brains the same way or to the same degree. Memory and thinking skills seem to be much more affected by the steep drop in hormones following surgical or chemical menopause than by the more gradual decline associated with the natural menopause transition. For example, when the SWAN researchers repeatedly tested a randomly selected and diverse group of 803 women aged 40 to 55 who were in various stages of the natural menopause transition, they found no evidence that menopause was accompanied by a decline in working memory or perceptual speed. In fact, over the course of the six years of testing, many of the women's scores went up. Similar results came out of the Melbourne Women's Midlife Health Project, in which 326 naturally menopausal women were tested on their ability to recall word lists; no substantial differences were found on the basis of premenopausal, perimenopausal, or postmenopausal status.

Does this mean that naturally menopausal women are mistaken when they complain of memory and thinking problems? Many researchers aren't will-

---

Is It True?

Fiction: Dementia is an inevitable part of aging.

Fact: Most people in their 50s, 60s, and 70s report little decline in mental sharpness as they get older. More typical are problems with working memory, like the ability to keep a new phone number in your head. You may also need more time and effort to learn new things. However, your ability to retain information should remain nearly as good as that of someone decades younger. Some skills even improve; for example, your vocabulary will probably continue to expand as you get older.

---

ing to go that far. It just may be a difficult area to study. Maybe those memory lapses are so transient that they don't show up as functional impairments on periodic tests. Or maybe the kind of testing done so far isn't sensitive enough for true quantification.

So while there's no strong evidence that natural menopause directly causes significant and ongoing problems with thinking or memory, some scientists still suspect that hormonal fluctuation may be a contributing factor for *some* women *some* of the time. Keep in mind that sleep deprivation brought on by bothersome hot flashes, stress, mood problems, and a variety of midlife medical issues can also affect your memory and ability to stay sharp.

WHAT IS ALZHEIMER'S DISEASE?

The most common type of dementia, Alzheimer's disease is characterized by slow, progressive memory loss. Rather than occasionally forgetting a neighbor's name, Alzheimer's patients might find it difficult to remember how to drive to the homes of close friends, how to unlock the front door, or whether they ate breakfast that day. The disease rarely appears before the age of 65.

Those with Alzheimer's often become increasingly uninterested in doing things they once enjoyed and may sit for hours just looking out a window. It's not unusual for them to exhibit significant changes in mood, behavior, and even per-

A NORMAL BRAIN

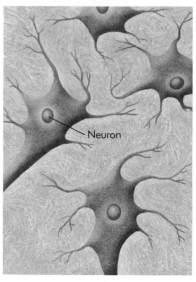

A DISEASED BRAIN

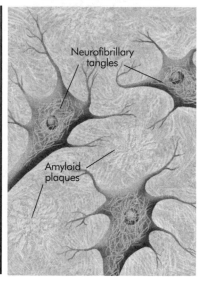

HOW TO DIAGNOSE ALZHEIMER'S DISEASE

The quantity and location of amyloid plaques and neurofibrillary tangles in the brain seen on autopsy determine that a diagnosis of Alzheimer's is accurate.

ON THE TIP OF MY TONGUE

Q *I seem to be struggling for the right word much more often than I used to. Can this be related to menopause?*

A Verbal memory appears to be particularly affected by estrogen levels. You may not have realized it, but this has been true for most of your life. We tend to perform better on verbal tests when our estrogen levels are higher than

sonality. People with this disorder can have many different combinations of symptoms. That's one reason researchers suspect that we may eventually identify multiple types of Alzheimer's—just as we did many years ago with cancer.

When Alzheimer's is suspected, your doctor will order a detailed medical history, a physical exam, a series of mental tests, lab work, and perhaps brain scans. A tentative diagnosis will be made on the basis of a combination of symptoms and the elimination of other possible causes. But amazing as it seems, no test or scan can definitively identify this disorder in a living person. Doctors can't really be sure that someone truly has Alzheimer's until after the patient dies and an autopsy of the brain reveals lots of the neurofibrillary tangles (inside diseased brain cells) and amyloid plaques (between cells) that characterize the disease. Alzheimer's hits many women with a double whammy. Not only are we twice as likely to get it, we're also much more likely to be caretakers to those with Alzheimer's. About 80 percent of the people who provide care for those with the disease are women.

In the chart below, it's important to note that only a minority of those with Alzheimer's have the severe form of the disease at any one time; the numbers indicate individuals who have some symptoms of the disease.

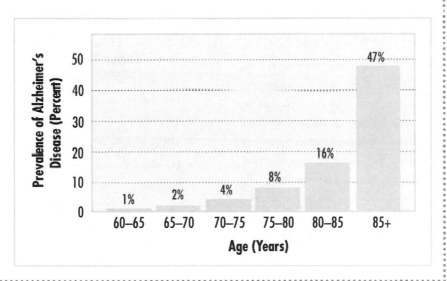

around the time of our periods, when our estrogen levels are low.

One way that the brain stores verbal information is by letter-sound combinations called phonemes. For example, the word *cat* is composed of three phonemes: "k," short "a," and "t." Research at Yale suggests that estrogen's relationship to memory and language may be closely tied to its effect on the brain's storage and processing of phonemes. Think about the times you struggle to remember a word; often, you can remember only the sound of the first letter. It's possible that if your hormone levels weren't bouncing around so much, you might be able to remember the word more quickly. This estrogen-phoneme connection may also explain why some women find that their reading ability suffers during the transition.

AM I BLUE?

Q *When I mentioned to my doctor that I was having problems concentrating and remembering things, he started asking about my mood rather than menopause. Is there a connection between midlife depression and memory loss?*

A Doctors suspect that many of the memory and concentration complaints they hear from women moving toward natural menopause may be related to untreated or undiagnosed anxiety or depression. The fact that you're experiencing these symptoms now may be a coincidence and have nothing to do with menopause; memory and concentration problems are common complaints among depressives at any time of life. The good news is that these types of memory issues can usually be eliminated with effective treatment of the mood problem.

You should be motivated to seek treatment for another reason as well. In the long term, depression seems to be associated with an increased risk of late-onset dementia. This is a relatively new area of research, so not a lot is known about this correlation. Some scientists suspect that since depression puts you at greater risk for heart disease, perhaps there's a vascular connection between depression and dementia. Another theory is that persistent depression keeps stress hormones high for inordinate amounts of time, which may in turn have toxic effects on the brain that increase your vulnerability to dementia. Right now, it isn't clear whether depression causes dementia, or dementia causes depression, or if treating depression significantly reduces your future risk of developing dementia. Until we know more, think of this as another incentive to monitor and manage your depression effectively.

COMMON CAUSES OF MEMORY LOSS

◆ Inactive thyroid

◆ Depression

◆ Sleep problems

◆ Hormonal fluctuations

◆ Stress

◆ Genetic vulnerability to dementia (such as early Alzheimer's)

◆ Head injuries

◆ High blood pressure

◆ Medication side effects

◆ Neurological diseases of the brain (such as Parkinson's, stroke, brain tumor)

◆ Chemotherapy

◆ Alcoholism

A SAD LINK

Q *After my mother died, my father became depressed. Three years later, he was diagnosed with dementia. Could these things be linked?*

A Yes. For a person who has an episode of depression after age 70, the risk of developing dementia in the next three to five years increases by an estimated 50 percent. Let us repeat ourselves: Take depression symptoms seriously.

TROUBLE FOCUSING

Q *My ability to concentrate is really hampered these days. Could this be related to my hot flashes?*

A The fluctuating hormone levels that predispose some women to hot flashes also have an effect on the availability of neurotransmitters in your brain, which can affect your ability to concentrate. So it would make sense that the two might be related, except that studies done to date have not shown a direct link. It could be that your hot flashes are keeping you from getting enough deep sleep and that this is affecting your ability to focus. Try some of the suggestions in Chapters 3 and 4 directed at helping you get a better night's sleep. They couldn't hurt . . . and they might help.

What to Tell Your Daughter

A lot of us grow up thinking we'll go to school while we're young and then be done. But that's not a good idea. Be your child's role model for lifelong learning by taking courses, studying a new language, or learning a new skill. While there are no guaranteed ways to stave off dementia, challenging your mind might offer some protection. Two other ideas: Read to your children when they're young, and encourage them to read on their own. These activities help to develop rich vocabularies and strong reading comprehension skills, both of which are associated later on in life with brains better able to fight off Alzheimer's.

ADD AT 50?

Q *I have a kid who has ADD, and lately he's been teasing me that I seem to have the same problems he has. Is it possible that menopause could do that?*

A It's true that some women complain about their inability to pay attention and concentrate during perimenopause (when hormone levels are fluctuating the most) or after surgical menopause; however, the relationship between hormone fluctuations and concentration isn't clear. Luckily, most of the time it's a short-lived problem. In any case, it doesn't result in a chronic condition like attention deficit disorder. ADD, by definition, must begin during childhood. It continues into adolescence and adulthood in many people, but the symptoms usually become more subtle. Rather than the external symptoms that characterize childhood ADD (like nonstop hyper levels of activity), ADD in adults is characterized by "internal" symptoms like disorganization, impulsivity, and inability to stay focused.

However, it's possible that you've had attention issues all your life, and the additional problems you're experiencing now will prompt you to seek professional help. This diagnosis is overlooked in many kids, especially girls, if they're not causing any disruption in the classroom. Many women discover that they have this disorder only after their own children are diagnosed.

From the Past

*D*oes menopause make women stupid? Early medical books often implied that it did. The 1869 edition of *The Physical Life of Woman: Advice to the Maiden, Wife and Mother* by Dr. George Napheys explains that menopause is "sometimes accompanied by a sense of fullness in the head, a giddiness, and a dullness of the brain . . . a slowness of comprehension." One popular marriage guide of the era warned women "to avoid all intense mental application" or their menopausal symptoms would get worse. And in his 1901 *Text-book of Gynecology,* Dr. C.A.L. Reed wrote that "sometimes a curious mental exaltation would occur early in menopause, and a woman would meddle with business affairs that did not concern her."

But some women struck back against the prevailing prejudice. Starting in 1892, Dr. Clelia Duel Mosher conducted a survey of women's health experiences to document their own thoughts on the subject. Here's an excerpt from one woman's story: "About 1909 . . . my menses began to decline and in the course of a year, ceased altogether. . . . During this time, I was doing heavy intellectual labor—published a statistical and sociological book in 1906, another in 1908 and another in 1912; gained some weight (from average 110 to 120) and did my own housework besides lecturing frequently in public. My health has steadily improved during the last 7 years and I am (at 53) much stronger and capable of doing both more physical and mental work every day than any woman of my acquaintance and more than most women of 40. I can walk 15 miles without feeling it and lift my own weight. Although my passionate feeling has declined somewhat and the orgasm does not always occur, intercourse is still agreeable to me."

CHEMO BRAIN

Q *Does chemotherapy affect memory?*

A Talk to women going through chemotherapy, and chances are you'll hear about "chemo brain." Some chemicals are more toxic to the brain than others, but higher doses and longer treatments are also associated with more cognitive problems. Memory loss, which is often subtle, tends to go away a year or so after chemo stops. However, in a few patients, the problem can be durable and disabling, affecting a range of cognitive functions. Perhaps some women are more genetically vulnerable to brain changes as a result of chemotherapy; no one knows. But the risk of memory loss is something your doctor should discuss with you before you start chemotherapy.

SLOWER RECALL

Q *I'm using tamoxifen to prevent a recurrence of breast cancer. Obviously, that matters most, but I read somewhere that it can lead to memory loss. True?*

A It might. A randomized pilot study of about 100 women compared the mental processing speed and immediate verbal memory of women without breast cancer with those of women with breast cancer who were taking either tamoxifen or the aromatase inhibitor anastrozole, or a combination of the two. Both drugs reduce the amount of estrogen in a woman's body. The women who were taking drugs scored worse on both measures than those who weren't taking the drugs. More research needs to be done to verify these results.

SENIOR MOMENTS

Q *The other day, I had another "senior moment"—I couldn't remember where I left my keys. The day before that, I couldn't remember an old friend's last name. These memory lapses seem to be happening more often. Am I right to be worried that they may be early signs of Alzheimer's?*

A At some point, usually starting in her 40s and 50s, just about every woman has this experience—and it rattles all of us. But what you're experiencing isn't close to qualifying as Alzheimer's disease. It's irritating, but it's not seriously interfering with your ability to function.

A diagnosis of Alzheimer's, the most common type of dementia, is rare before age 60. Even among people 65 to 75, it occurs in less than 5 percent of the population. Symptoms become more apparent as we age. Among those 85 and older, as many as 47 percent may have some symptoms. However, Alzheimer's is a progressive disease; many of those diagnoses are at the early or intermediate stage. The initial symptoms—increasing forgetfulness about recent events (not remembering that a loved one called earlier the same day, for instance) or appointments—may become more noticeable when people begin having trouble doing things they've done for years, like solving simple math problems. As the disease progresses to the middle stage, they forget how to do everyday tasks, like how to tie shoelaces and neckties. They may find themselves increasingly confused and have trouble reading, writing, speaking, and paying attention. That's when people around them recognize a problem (they rarely recognize it in themselves) and a diagnosis is sought. Sometimes it turns out that other medical conditions, such as thyroid problems, depression, brain tumors, or diseases of the blood vessels, are responsible for these symptoms. Mental confusion can be a side effect of a medication or be brought on by stress. When the medication is changed or the stress is reduced, the symptoms can disappear.

THE ROLE OF GENDER

Q *Is menopause the main reason that more women than men have Alzheimer's disease?*

A No, that honor belongs to longevity. But hormones may play some role. A recent study of the brains of deceased women found less estrogen in the brains of those who had Alzheimer's than in the brains of those who didn't have dementia. Interestingly, lab mice bred to have both Alzheimer's and low levels of estrogen developed more numerous and more severe brain plaques than other mice. While this is all a long way from proving cause and effect, it's possible that there may be some individual interplay between Alzheimer's and the declining levels of estrogen associated with menopause. But remember that most women show no signs of dementia until decades after menopause, and not all women become demented—even though we all go through menopause.

IN THE GENES?

Q *What role does genetics play in dementia?*

A Okay, first the scary news. For some people, as much as 70 percent of the risk of eventually suffering from dementia may be connected to genetics. And now the good news. You may be able to lower your risk or delay the onset of the disease by the way you live your life.

Nowhere has this been more obvious than in the research of Dr. David Snowdon and his famous Nun Study, which looked at the prevalence of Alzheimer's over several decades in 678 School Sisters of Notre Dame, all of whom were between the ages of 75 and 106. One of the things that made Snowdon's work remarkable was the fact

When to See the Doctor

It's time to make an appointment with your physician if:

✦ MEMORY PROBLEMS ARE MAKING IT HARD FOR YOU TO FUNCTION NORMALLY.

✦ YOU HAVE TROUBLE REMEMBERING HOW TO DO EVERYDAY TASKS, LIKE BUTTONING A SHIRT OR TYING A SHOELACE.

✦ YOU'RE GETTING LOST WHILE ON YOUR WAY TO PLACES YOU KNOW WELL OR FIND YOURSELF UNABLE TO REMEMBER WHAT YOU DID EARLIER IN THE DAY.

✦ YOU'RE EXPERIENCING UNEXPECTED OR PROFOUND DIFFICULTY READING, WRITING, OR SPEAKING.

✦ YOU'RE EXHIBITING SIGNIFICANT PERSONALITY CHANGES OR INCREASES IN AGGRESSION OR INAPPROPRIATE BEHAVIOR.

✦ MENTAL CONFUSION COMES ON SUDDENLY (RATHER THAN AS A RESULT OF A SLOW, PROGRESSIVE DECLINE). THIS MAY BE A SIGN OF DELIRIUM, WHICH CAN BE CAUSED BY A MEDICAL CONDITION (SUCH AS HEART DISEASE), AN INFECTION (SUCH AS AN ACUTE URINARY INFECTION), OR A COMPLICATION RELATED TO A MEDICATION (TAKING THE WRONG MEDICATION OR HAVING A BAD REACTION).

that his team autopsied the brain of every participant upon her death, whether or not she exhibited any symptoms of Alzheimer's. As a result, they made some unexpected and amazing discoveries. Some of the nuns who seemed to have the most severe symptoms of Alzheimer's had very few of the characteristic brain plaques and tangles. Others whose brains contained masses of plaques and tangles had never shown any outward sign of the disease while they were alive. What made the difference? It appears that the health of their vascular system (e.g., normal blood pressure, low cholesterol) gets some of the credit. The other factor: their language skills. The nuns whose writings in their 20s displayed "high idea density" (a lot of ideas packed into one sentence), as well as a rich vocabulary and complex thoughts, were less likely to develop dementia than were those who expressed themselves simply and had a more limited vocabulary.

CHILL OUT

Q *What's the relationship between stress and dementia?*

A Stimulation is good for your brain, but chronic stress, worry, and anxiety are not. The Rush Memory and Aging Project has been following 800 Catholic nuns, priests, and brothers as they age and annually checking them for signs of memory loss. When the study began, the participants, whose average age was 75, were questioned about how they dealt with stress. After the first five years, about 140 of the participants had developed signs of Alzheimer's. Those participants who described themselves as people who become easily tense and worried were twice as likely to develop Alzheimer's as those who said they dealt with stress in a calmer fashion. The results held true no matter what their level of depressive symptoms. Since worrying tends to be part of a lifetime pattern, researchers are trying to determine whether drug treatment, cognitive-behavior therapy, or other coping strategies can further reduce these risks.

BONES AND BRAINS

Q *Is there some link between osteoporosis and dementia?*

A People who experience fractures related to osteoporosis are more likely to get lower-than-average scores on cognitive tests; women with healthy bone mineral density are more likely to score higher than average on those same tests. Furthermore, postmenopausal women with osteoporosis who take a substantial amount of the prescription medication raloxifene (sold as Evista) to prevent bone loss are less likely to have symptoms of mild cognitive impairment than are those who don't take this bone remodeler.

CAN HORMONES HELP?

Doctors used to encourage women to take hormones as a preventive strategy against dementia because observational studies seemed to indicate that those who used hormone therapy were less likely to experience cognitive decline or Alzheimer's disease than were those who didn't. But it was also well known that the women who once used hormone therapy tended to be better educated and had access to higher-quality health care. To settle the question, about 7,500 women aged 65 and older were recruited to participate in the Women's Health Initiative Memory Study (WHIMS) at 39 centers across the country. In the largest randomized, controlled clinical trial ever done in this field, women were given combined estrogen and progesterone (Prempro), estrogen alone (Premarin), or a placebo. Participants stayed on the pills for four or five years.

Analysis of the results revealed that the women taking estrogen alone did *not* experience a drop in dementia and that those who took the combination of hormones appeared to have increased their risk. Researchers had hoped that hormones might protect women from milder forms of dementia (like mild cognitive impairment), but that didn't happen, either. The WHIMS results were right in line with other studies showing that women with naturally high levels of estrogen in their bodies, as well as those with the greatest number of reproductive years (because they started menstruating early, reached menopause later than average, or both), were at higher risk of getting Alzheimer's.

A Window of Opportunity?

Now, what about taking hormones at an earlier stage in life? Some researchers theorize that healthy women who initiate hormone therapy right around menopause might be able to prevent or delay future dementia. This "window of opportunity" theory has been encouraged by animal and observational studies indicating that using hormone therapy around the menopause transition lessens the likelihood of dementia later in life. For example, a large study in Utah found that women who started using hormone therapy around menopause and continued using it for more than 10 years had an 83 percent reduction in their risk of developing Alzheimer's. Interestingly, in that same study, women who started hormone therapy after age 60 saw a 112 percent *increase* in their risk of Alzheimer's—similar to the increase seen in the WHIMS study.

More recently, an intriguing clinical study in Denmark followed 343 women who had been randomized to take hormone therapy or a placebo for two or three years around age 50. Years later, when they were about age 65, they were given a test to identify symptoms of cognitive decline. Those in the group taking hormone therapy were less likely (5 percent vs. 13 percent) to show signs of men-

WHAT IS MILD COGNITIVE IMPAIRMENT?

◆ Deterioration in memory with symptoms falling short of full dementia

◆ Symptoms typically include lapses in short-term memory, such as difficulty keeping up with the flow of conversation

◆ Normal reasoning and thinking skills

◆ No trouble speaking, concentrating, or comprehending

◆ No confusion about identity (who you are) or location (where you are)

◆ Association with an increased risk of dementia (Every year, about 10 percent of patients with MCI go on to develop some form of dementia, compared with 1 percent of those with a normal memory.)

◆ Unclear whether it's a distinct memory disorder on its own, a step on the road to dementia, or both

tal impairment than were those who had never used it. The same held true for the 82 women who had decided to stay on hormone therapy after the prescribed two to three years or who had later initiated hormone use on their own. These results have added fuel to the speculation that we might someday identify a hormonal inoculation against dementia for women. It's possible that hormones might protect against dementia during one stage of life and contribute to it in another; there also might be a lot of individual variation.

HORMONES AS A TREATMENT?

Q *Is there any possibility that hormones could help women who have already been diagnosed with dementia?*

A Until recently, scientists held out a lot of hope that estrogen might be an effective treatment for relieving the symptoms of dementia. Since 1999, five good-quality (but relatively small) randomized, double-blind placebo-controlled studies have examined this question. In three of these studies, estrogen tablets were given to dementia patients who were in their 70s for periods ranging from 12 weeks to 12 months. Researchers found no improvement in those who were taking oral estrogen.

The other two studies used a transdermal estradiol and got mixed results. One study found improvement on one of two verbal memory tests and on one of two attention tests, but the measures of overall dementia severity didn't improve. The other study revealed improvement on one of three attention tests, one of three visual memory tests, one of two verbal memory tests, and a semantic memory test. But the overall functional assessment scores did not increase.

Those mixed results have left the door open for further study in this area, but there's not a lot of optimism that estrogen is a potential breakthrough treatment.

WHAT ABOUT STOPPING?

Q *If the WHIMS study concluded that older women were more likely to develop dementia while on hormone therapy, will their minds improve if they stop taking the hormones?*

A The women who participated in the WHIMS study are still being followed by researchers, who hope to get an answer to that question in the near future.

DYSLEXIA RETURNS

Q *I had a hard time learning to read when I was a kid, but eventually I overcame my dyslexia. Now that I'm going through menopause, I find that I'm again having reading problems.*

A For years, the only hint that what you're describing actually happens came from anecdotes like yours. However, Dr. Sally Shaywitz, a well-known dyslexia researcher at Yale, recently did a randomized double-blind study in which she tested the reading ability and verbal memory of 60 postmenopausal women. (The average age was 51, but ages ranged from 32 to 64; some of the women had gone through surgical menopause, others natural menopause.) All of the study subjects were tested twice. Half got supplemental estrogen for 21 days before their reading ability and verbal memories were tested. The other half took a placebo for the same 21 days. After a 14-day wash-out period without drugs, each group switched pills for another 21 days before being tested again. In the end, it turned out that the women got significantly higher reading and memory scores when taking estrogen than when taking the placebo. Scans revealed brain reorganization in the postmenopausal women taking estrogen. This resulted in more activity in a part of the brain called the inferior parietal lobule, where the letter-sound connection so essential to reading occurs. Problems in this area of the brain help to explain dyslexia. Because it was such a small study, more research is needed to confirm these results. But the data indicate that there may well be a biological reason why reading becomes more difficult for some women around menopause and that supplemental estrogen might help.

READING BOOSTERS

Q *Out of the blue, reading has become a struggle for me. I'm not having hot flashes and don't particularly want to take hormones. What else can I do?*

A Typically, women who experience this problem at menopause have not lost their ability to read accurately; rather, they have trouble reading fluently. Reading may no longer feel automatic. Dr. Sally Shaywitz of Yale University says you'll find the best solution by doing some experimenting. For starters, if you're reading for pleasure, don't be overly concerned about getting every word right. Try skimming instead of focusing on each syllable. In cases where you need to get the exact meaning of a text, use your finger or an index card to mark the line you're reading so you don't lose your place. Do your important reading in the morning or whenever your energy and concentration levels are at their height. You might want to try reading with the help of a clear bar magnifier, which not only increases the size of the type but also helps you keep track of your place on the page. Large-print publications may also be helpful. Some women find it easier to understand things when they read out loud rather than silently. Another alternative is listening to books on tape instead of reading them yourself.

If you're worried about your ability to give a speech or read something in front of a crowd, give yourself a couple of extra rehearsals before the big event. Whenever you find yourself stumbling over a word, underline or highlight it and say it out loud a few times until you feel confident that you've nailed it.

One other thing worth mentioning: Many midlife women experience vision changes that add to their reading problems. Check with your doctor to see whether you need reading glasses, a new prescription, or more direct (or brighter) light on the pages you're reading. (There's lots more on this topic in Chapter 11.)

AFTER A HYSTERECTOMY

Q *I'm 45 and recently had a hysterectomy. I also had my ovaries removed. I'm dealing with hot flashes and night sweats, sleeplessness, an unreliable memory, and what I would call foggy thinking, all of which are making it very hard for me to get through each day and each night. Will estrogen therapy help?*

A If you've experienced light-speed menopause because of a hysterectomy or cancer treatments, you're more likely to notice problems with verbal memory, attention, concentration, and reading ability—probably because your levels of both estrogen and androgen have declined so steeply and abruptly. You're also more likely to experience hot flashes and night sweats that can affect your ability to sleep and feel well rested. You may be more stressed out, too. All these things can affect how clearly you're thinking and how well your memory is working. Individual experiences can vary a lot.

Because of your multiple symptoms and your age, you're in the group of women who seem to be most helped by estrogen therapy. In five small studies (each with about 20 participants), women who had had their uterus and ovaries removed and experienced menopausal symptoms afterwards scored better on at least one cognitive test (usually, immediate verbal recall, motor speed, or attention) after taking estrogen for two to six months. Other studies indicate that hormone therapy is the most effective treatment available for hot flashes and night sweats. With these other symptoms under control, you may also find that you sleep better. For women like you, who are younger than the typical age of menopause (51), the benefits of using hormones are thought to outweigh the risks for most women, since

STRATEGIES FOR IMPROVING MEMORY

◆ Improve your organizational skills. Write yourself notes. Make lists. Keep a calendar or pocket diary.

◆ Create special places to keep track of things. For example, hang a hook by the garage door for your car keys or always put your purse in the same place when you get home.

◆ Reduce stress. When you're juggling too many details, you're more likely to drop a few balls.

◆ Use alarms or timers to help you remember appointments or deadlines.

◆ Try to reduce information to small chunks. For example, it's a lot easier to remember 2007 and 2008 than 20,072,008.

◆ Form associations, like remembering Mrs. Waters' name because she lives near a lake. Translate other things you need to remember into acronyms, rhymes, and songs.

◆ Repeat things to yourself until you've memorized them. Mentally rehearse information.

they would naturally have estrogen in their bodies. This is a theory, however; no long-term clinical studies have tested this premise.

That said, hormone therapy is not for everyone. If you had a hysterectomy because of an estrogen-sensitive cancer (such as breast or endometrial), your doctor may advise against supplemental estrogen, even for a short period of time. In any case, your doctor will consider your age, your general health, and your individual medical history to help you make the decision that's right for you.

If you decide to use estrogen therapy for menopausal symptoms that include memory and cognitive problems, consider a transdermal or injectable estradiol preparation rather than an oral estrone. While the data are a little conflicting, the studies that used estradiol to treat menopausal memory lapses tended to have more positive results. The patch also has the advantage of getting right into your bloodstream without going through your liver.

Remember to revisit your decision regularly (at least once a year) and determine with your doctor's help how long you need to stay on hormones and whether your dose should be lowered over time. Keep in mind that few women need to stay on hormones for years. (Chapter 2 has more details.)

STRUGGLING AT WORK

Q *I'm 51 and recently had my uterus and ovaries removed, sending me into surgical menopause. I decided not to take estrogen because I wasn't having much trouble with hot flashes. My real problem is that I'm not thinking as sharply as I did before the surgery. This has me worried, since I have a very responsible job. Will estrogen help me?*

A There hasn't been a lot of research on your problem, but the one small study that purposely looked at women who never got hot flashes found that they did not get better scores on a battery of cognitive and memory tests after taking estrogen for three months. Anecdotally, women taking hormones sometimes credit estrogen with helping them think more clearly, but their improvement may be due to a placebo effect. Some researchers argue that we might see different results if we did a better job of matching the symptoms experienced by postmenopausal women and the tests used in this type of research project. Others argue that estrogen may help some and not others. Both of these points may be valid, but we don't have the data to prove it one way or the other. The recommendation of groups like the American College of Obstetricians and Gynecologists and the North American Menopause Society is that you should not use hormones primarily to deal with memory or cognitive problems around menopause. If you want to try anyway, talk to your doctor about your particular situation. While it may not work, there are indications from the Women's Health Initiative study that a 50-year-old (with no increased cancer risk) using estrogen-only therapy soon after surgical menopause faces minimal negative side effects for the first seven years. As always, if you decide to try estrogen, opt for the lowest effective dose for the shortest time needed.

There are a few more things you should consider. Some women have night sweats that don't actually wake them up but disturb the quality of their sleep. If there's any chance that this may be happening to you, estrogen might prove helpful and you should confer with your doctor about it. If you think your fuzzy thinking might be related to the fact that you're not sleeping well and it doesn't have anything to do with hot flashes, try some of our suggestions in Chapter 4 for getting better-quality zzz's.

NATURALLY SLOWER?

Q *I'm going through natural menopause and don't feel as sharp mentally as I used to. Should I try hormone therapy?*

A If you're having other menopausal symptoms, you should talk to your doctor about whether you're a good candidate for a short course of hormone

therapy. It's possible that hot flashes, night sweats, or sleeplessness are affecting (directly or indirectly) your ability to think clearly. However, supplemental hormones are generally not recommended for women like you whose only symptom is fuzzy thinking. If your doctor decides that you should give hormones a try anyway, she'll likely recommend a combination of estrogen and progesterone because you still have a uterus and need protection against endometrial cancer. You should know that researchers haven't had as much success alleviating memory and other cognitive problems with this combination as with estrogen alone. It's not clear why.

MAINTAIN YOUR BRAIN

If you're hoping for a magic pill, there isn't one. But researchers are busy trying to identify things you can do to stave off dementia. So far, they have more ideas of things that *might* make a difference and not that much proof that any of them really work. So, for example, scientists know that people who eat more leafy and cruciferous green vegetables (cabbage, Brussels sprouts, broccoli) tend to have less dementia than those who don't, but they don't know whether you'd reduce your chances of dementia if you ate broccoli every morning, noon, and night.

It turns out that much of what's recommended falls into the category of "won't hurt and may help." Generally, says the National Institute of Aging, whatever's good for your heart is probably good for your brain. That's because there's so much overlap between the things that make you vulnerable to heart disease and those that make you vulnerable to dementia.

And here's a news flash: How healthy you are at midlife may be one of the best predictors of whether or not you'll be at increased risk of dementia later on. Researchers at the Karolinska Institute of Sweden followed 1,449 older people for 21 years and found that those who had high blood pressure at *midlife* had double the risk of developing dementia as those who didn't. The same was true for those with high cholesterol and those who were obese, defined as having a BMI above 30. (If you're not sure of yours, the National Institutes of Health has a handy BMI calculator on the web at www.nhlbisupport.com/bmi), or check out the chart on page 381. Researchers found that those risks are cumulative, meaning that if you have two of the three traits, you're likely to have four times the risk of dementia; if you have all three, it's six times the risk. So how do you improve your odds? The best recommendations are listed below.

1. EXERCISE YOUR BODY. Exercise seems to be good for everything—including your brain. Exercise increases blood flow to the brain, helps to maintain an optimal chemical balance, and lowers the levels of stress hormones. It also reduces your chances of developing cardiovascular disease, diabetes, and depression, which are associated with a higher risk of dementia.

Walking is a great way to start. Get a pedometer and start working your way up to 10,000 steps a day. Dancing the night away may be an even better idea. A study published in the *New England Journal of Medicine* in 2003 concluded that dancing provided more protection against dementia than physical activities like swimming or biking. Maybe that's because dancing requires you to multi-task—to keep rhythm, do precise movements, and interact with others all at the same time. Research also indicates that doing at least four distinct activities during the course of your day (gardening, lifting weights, running errands on foot, and attending a yoga class, for example) can cut your risk of dementia in half. Side benefit: This strategy will also make your life more interesting.

Aerobics and strength training are great for your heart and bones, but you might be surprised to learn that they also give your brain's "executive" functions (prioritizing, organizing, multitasking) a boost by literally increasing the volume of gray matter (nerve cell bodies) and white matter (connecting fibers). Marked improvement with these types of exercise was noted in as little as six months. They have also been found to make some of the brain's memory and attention networks operate more efficiently.

VITAMIN POWER

Sometimes, one substance or another appears to have a beneficial effect on the workings of the brain, but when researchers put it to the test, results don't always hold up. However, some vitamins, dietary supplements, and spices do seem to make a difference.

The B vitamins. Which nutrients are in the running for memory superheroes? Folates, which are B vitamins that help fight off heart disease and stroke, and possibly B_6 and B_{12} because of their role in recycling homocysteine, a by-product of protein breakdown that can clog your arteries. The results of a long-term National Institute of Aging study on diet and brain aging indicate that eating at least the daily recommended amount of folates (400 micrograms a day) reduces the risk of Alzheimer's by more than half, probably because they're also essential for making and maintaining new cells.

Several studies also indicate that getting enough folate may improve the memory and verbal abilities of young and midlife women. Found naturally in leafy green vegetables (like spinach and Brussels sprouts), fruit (citrus, strawberries, and bananas), whole wheat bread, lima beans and peas, eggs, milk, liver, kidneys, and yeast, folates can be destroyed by cooking and processing. Because they've also been associated with fewer birth defects, folates have been added to grain products sold in the United States since 1998, so check labels. You can also take folic acid supplements or get them in your multivitamins. The recommended amount of B_6 is 1.3 to 1.6 milligrams per day. Aim for 6 micrograms of B_{12}.

Turmeric. When researchers noticed that the people of India have much lower rates of dementia than Westerners, they started looking for the reason. They soon

2. EXERCISE YOUR MIND. Doing crossword puzzles and playing chess will keep your mind sharp—right? Maybe not. If you do a crossword puzzle every day and you're really good at it, it's probably not the kind of task required to give your mind a workout. As we age, we need to challenge our minds with both new and hard stuff. Learning to play a musical instrument or mastering a new language might qualify, especially if those things don't come easily to you.

People with higher levels of education (specifically those whose written work utilizes a big vocabulary and conveys complex ideas) also seem to get Alzheimer's at lower rates than the general population. Researchers suspect that a well-developed and challenged brain has more "cognitive reserve" and is better able to deal with the assaults that come with age. Scans indicate that less atrophy occurs over time as well.

Does this mean you have to earn a Ph.D. to avoid dementia? No, but anything you can do to keep your brain engaged and challenged is probably a smart move.

focused on the curry spice turmeric and, more specifically, on curcumin, its active ingredient and a potent antioxidant and anti-inflammatory used for thousands of years in Indian medicine. (Epidemiological studies have indicated a correlation between the use of anti-inflammatory drugs and lowered Alzheimer's risk.) To test the turmeric theory, mice were fed diets rich in curcumin, upon autopsy, their brains displayed significantly less of the telltale plaque buildup associated with dementia. The mice also did better on memory tests involving mazes. Researchers at the UCLA Alzheimer's Disease Research Center are now conducting human trials to determine if turmeric stops dementia in humans.

Vitamin E. This one has gotten lots of hype as a "memory wonder drug" because it slows the progression of Alzheimer's (after diagnosis) for about seven months. But it doesn't seem to prevent the disease. In addition, taking a megadose (more than 400 international units a day rather than the 30 IUs found in most multivitamins) has been associated with an increased risk of death, heart disease, stroke, and breast cancer.

Ginkgo biloba. Researchers have had some success treating some Alzheimer's symptoms with ginkgo biloba, but there's no proof that it can prevent dementia or delay its progress.

Antioxidants. Not long ago, antioxidants (beta-carotene and flavonoids) and vitamin C seemed to hold promise for protection against dementia, but many of the studies designed to prove their worth didn't pan out. For example, when researchers retrospectively analyzed the diets of participants in the Honolulu Asian Aging Study, they found that those who ate foods richest in antioxidants were just as likely to have dementia in their senior years as anyone else.

3. BE A SOCIAL BUTTERFLY. Staying social is crucial to your brain health. As you get older, you may be increasingly tempted to take the path of least resistance—the one that leads to the cushy sofa in front of the TV set. Instead, put on your dancing shoes and shimmy on out the door. Being social is not only a good way to protect yourself from dementia; it's also one of the rare things that have been shown to slow its progression. So get connected. Start a book club, sign up for classes, volunteer, throw a party. Get yourself out there.

4. DON'T SMOKE. Longitudinal studies have found that tobacco not only increases the odds that you'll suffer cognitive problems as you age, but also ups your risk of Alzheimer's. One bit of encouragement: Quitting can make a difference in the amount of deterioration you're likely to experience later in life. If you haven't kicked the habit yet, don't give up hope.

5. EAT A HEALTHY DIET. A balanced diet with lots of whole grains, fruits, and vegetables, as well as some low-fat dairy and lean protein, is good for a wide range of things, including heart health, cholesterol levels, and lowering your risk of developing diabetes. By extension, a healthy diet is believed to reduce your risk of dementia. If you find that you have trouble eating well every day, pop a multivitamin with your morning cereal and OJ.

MIND GAMES

If you want stronger arms, you exercise them more. But what if you want a stronger brain? Could specific exercises and games be developed to improve memory, perception, and processing speed in all kinds of people? As evidence mounts that brain plasticity (the capacity of the human brain to change and adapt in response to challenge) continues well into our senior years, researchers suspect that the answer is yes . . . and marketers are jumping on the bandwagon. For instance, Posit Science has put out The Brain Gym, developed by Michael Merzenich of the University of California–San Francisco. Randomized clinical trials indicate that, for some people, eight weeks (one hour a day, five days a week) of Brain Gym training can result in memory and cognitive skills equal to those of someone 10 years younger. More research is under way to determine whether this program is effective for people with mild cognitive impairment as well as those with early-stage Alzheimer's.

Clinical trial results also indicate that MindFit, a range of software promoted by the nonprofit Geron Tech–Israeli Center for Assistive Technology and Aging, can improve memory, attention, and perception. MindFit's manufacturer, Cognifit, also offers a program designed to help older drivers maintain their driving skills; it's called Golden DriveFit, and it recently won Britain's Prince Michael International Award for Road Safety.

Also on the market: Nintendo's Brain Age. A big hit in Japan, it's played on a $130 Nintendo DS handheld game machine. The program was "inspired" by the research of Dr. Ryuta Kawashima, a Japanese neuroscientist. Game reviewers have found Brain Age to be fun and engaging (it claims to assess your brain's "age" and then helps you whittle it down with stimulating games and exercises). However, no clinical trials seem to have been done to verify its effectiveness.

We were also struck that an aging baby boomer who reviewed the program for *The Wall Street Journal* was initially assessed with a brain age 11 years his senior. By the end of the *first day*, he had trained hard enough to be recategorized as thinking as efficiently as a 20-year-old, the youngest age the game can calculate. If only turning back the clock was that simple!

PART III

STAYING HEALTHY FOREVER

CHAPTER 10

Bones

When you hear the word *osteoporosis,* you probably think of Granny hunched over a walker. Not your problem, right? But think about your poor grandmother 30 or 40 years ago. She was just like you, eagerly engaged in the activities of midlife and unaware of the devastation about to be unleashed on her bones. If only she'd known what scientists now know about a woman's changing skeleton during menopause.

Ten million Americans over age 50 already have osteoporosis—a thinning of bones that leaves them vulnerable to fracture—and another 34 million are at risk of developing it. Women are two to three times more likely than men to suffer from osteoporosis because our bones generally start out smaller. And listen to this really scary stat: Half of all women over age 50 will sustain an osteoporosis-related fracture. In fact, more women will die of complications from osteoporosis than of breast cancer.

Now that we have your attention, here's some encouraging news. Osteoporosis is not inevitable. If you get serious and make a few simple changes right now, you can help your bones do their job of keeping you strong, healthy, and upright. Pay attention to your diet to make sure you're getting the right amounts of calcium and vitamin D. And start a regular workout routine with an emphasis on strength- training and weight-bearing exercises, such as walking, jogging, stair-climbing, tennis, and dancing. Believe us, all these efforts will pay big dividends for the rest of your life.

BONING UP
ON BONES

Your skeleton creates the frame for your body, protects your vital organs, and helps you move. Bones are also the body's storehouse of calcium and phosphorus. Because bones are living tissue, they're always changing in ways that have a big impact on your health throughout your life. From infancy through your 20s, your bones grow in length and density, slowly expanding until they create an adult frame. They double in size between birth and age 2, double again by age 10, and double once more before the end of puberty. After age 18, your bone growth continues at a much slower pace, but over the next 10 years your bone masss should increase by an additional 10 percent or so.

What Can Happen

❖ As you age, your body won't absorb as much calcium and vitamin D.

❖ Your bone mineral density will begin to decrease.

❖ Your risk of fracture will increase, especially in your wrists, hips, and spine.

❖ You may gradually lose height.

Your body builds your skeleton through two processes: bone modeling (new construction) and bone remodeling (continual renovation of existing bone). During childhood, both things are going on at once, with bone modeling being the dominant activity. The bone builders, cells called osteoblasts, work with collagen and calcium, among other minerals, to expand bone length and diameter. Resorbing cells called osteoclasts do the nipping and tucking that allow bones to change shape and direction as they grow. (They also make more calcium available to the body when it's running short.) As the osteoclasts resorb (break down and assimilate) areas that have been damaged by wear and tear, osteoblasts tag-team behind to build new bone to replace them. These renovation teams also replace old bone that has lost its resiliency.

While genetics plays a major role in bone formation, the demands you put on your body have an effect as well. Kids who carry heavier loads (like backpacks full of books), exercise more, and generally give their bodies more of a pounding get the skeletons their lifestyle needs. Not surprisingly, those who play high-impact sports like football or competitive rope jumping will have bodies that require—and get—thicker bones than will kids who spend all their time watching television.

If nutrition, exercise, genetics, and hormones have all been working as they should, you hit your peak bone mass

What to Tell Your Daughter

Bones are like bank accounts—the more you put into them when you're younger, the more you'll get out of them when you're older. Genes, environment, and lifestyle all help to determine peak bone mass, generally reached by age 30, but the most critical years are during puberty, when you gain up to 30 percent of adult bone mass. Here's how to help your daughter get off to the right start:

❖ **Encourage physical activity.** When they're little, kids can't sit still. But as they hit those preadolescent years, their activity levels may slow way down. It may be just a phase, but it's one you shouldn't condone. The youngsters who grow up to have strong bones had active play as a part of their lives. This includes not just organized sports, but also hiking, jumping rope, dancing, skating, and even brisk walking as often as possible. Women who were athletic as girls are less likely to develop osteoporosis. Your goal is to give your daughter this edge by aiming for 60 minutes of moderate activity almost every day of the week.

❖ **Make her diet rich in calcium.** For ages 9 to 18, the recommended level is 1,300 milligrams daily; it drops to 1,000 milligrams a day up to age 50.

❖ **Get her outside.** Sunshine is the best source of vitamin D, which plays a critical role in the absorption and utilization of calcium. In most cases, 20 minutes daily with no sunscreen helps people make enough vitamin D. After that brief exposure, sunscreen is a must.

❖ **Help her find her optimum body weight.** This means not too much—or too little. Girls who become anorexic and stop menstruating are at risk for low bone mass and fractures, as well as osteoporosis in later life. Excessive exercising to maintain a low body weight is also bad for bones. Any healthy non-pregnant young woman who stops menstruating should be concerned about her bones.

❖ **Warn her about smoking and drinking.** There are many reasons to avoid tobacco and alcohol during adolescence. Here's another: They make it harder to reach peak bone mass, raising the risk for fractures and early-onset osteoporosis.

around age 30. Your body has created the maximum amount of bone it's capable of producing, but the bone remodelers stay on the job, remaking your skeleton every 10 years.

From about age 35 on, the osteoblasts start struggling to keep up with the osteoclasts as demolition begins to outpace building. Bone mass may start to decrease a little during these years. Then comes the menopause transition and a big drop in estrogen levels. The osteoclasts seize the moment and start working about 20 percent harder, the osteoblast builders can't keep up, and the gap in productivity results in

When to See the Doctor

The symptoms of osteoporosis are hidden. Too many women don't know they have it until they fracture a bone. You should be concerned if you notice a gradual loss of height and a slight curving of your upper back. Some other warning signs:

❖ Sudden severe back pain (a symptom of possible spinal compression fracture)

❖ Bone loss around your teeth and jaw, usually visible on dental x-rays

❖ Difficulty getting up from a chair without using your arms (a sign of muscle weakness that can predispose you to falls)

bone loss. To make matters worse, the decreasing levels of estrogen also signal the intestines to absorb less calcium, the kidneys to excrete more, and vitamin D to be less active. No wonder bone mass shrinks!

During the menopause transition, your hip bones will typically lose density by about 0.5 percent a year for five to seven years. In addition, they'll lose another 5 to 7 percent as a result of estrogen depletion during the two to three years before and the three to four years after menopause. Bone loss in the spine begins about 18 months before you get your last period. Over the next eight years, that thinning will result in a loss of bone density of about 10.5 percent. If you've got genetics and lifestyle working against you, bone loss can be much higher throughout your skeleton, as much as 5 percent a year. Once this rapid menopause-powered deterioration slows, women begin to experience a

steady age-related thinning of the bones at the same rate as men.

In recent years, scientists have begun to recognize the fact that the bone changes taking place during the menopause transition are distinctly different from those experienced later in life. Women who are moving toward menopause will rapidly lose about 5 to 10 percent of hard outer cortical bone and about 20 to 30 percent of trabecular bone, the internal scaffolding of interconnected bony plates and rods. Deterioration of trabecular bone can result in a series of thinned plates and broken rods, some of which no longer connect to anything, and a diagnosis of osteoporosis. The bones that are primarily trabecular—the hip, spine, wrist, and pelvic bones, for example—now become particularly vulnerable to fracture.

Once a woman is four or five years past menopause, the pace of bone loss slows but cortical and trabecular bone

A Quick Rundown of Risk Factors

Anyone can develop osteoporosis, but you're at higher risk if you're a female over age 50 (women can lose as much as 20 percent of their bone mass during the years around menopause). Some other risk factors:

◆ A history of fractures, especially if caused by low-impact trauma

◆ Caucasian or Asian descent

◆ Late onset of puberty

◆ Low bone mass

◆ A history of fractures in a first-degree relative (mother or sister)

◆ A family history of osteoporosis or related bone diseases

◆ Height loss

◆ Being thin or small framed (lighter than 127 pounds or having a BMI under 20)

◆ Low estrogen after premature or surgically induced menopause

◆ Anorexia or bulimia

◆ Temporary discontinuation of menstruation because of excessive exercising

◆ Sedentary lifestyle

◆ Smoking

◆ Excessive use of alcohol

◆ Low calcium intake

◆ Vitamin D deficiency

◆ Use of corticosteroids (such as prednisone and cortisone) or anticonvulsants

◆ Diseases and disorders that are secondary causes of osteoporosis (see Appendix I)

continue to thin. Over the course of the next 30 years, women typically lose an additional 20 to 25 percent of both because of lower levels of hormones, less active lifestyles, and less efficient absorption of calcium and vitamin D. Because of this last problem, the body may eventually detect a significant drop in blood calcium levels. This will prompt the four small parathyroid glands in the neck to release a hormone (PTH) that signals the body to begin pulling more calcium out of the bones, which can further weaken the skeleton. Even fairly small withdrawals of minerals at this time can cause osteoporosis in women who were holding their own.

Nature makes an attempt to balance things out by initiating a partial jump start in the bone-modeling process. New cortical bone is added if too much bone is resorbed from the inside. This helps because bones with a bigger diameter are harder to break than narrower bones. But for many women that assist is not enough.

Some women are particularly vulnerable to bone problems because they never reached their peak bone mass in their youth. Those who spent their adolescence as couch potatoes and junk-food

NORMAL BONE

OSTEOPOROTIC BONE

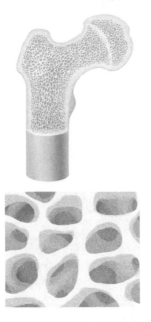
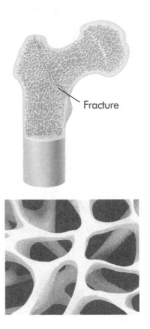

Fracture

HEALTHY BONE VS. POROUS BONE

Inside the hard exterior of your bones is a network of plates and rods called trabecular bone. When you're young and healthy, trabecular bone is sturdy (left). But as you age, this scaffolding can become looser and thinner and weaker (right). When this happens, you're more likely to have a fracture if you fall. A test of your bone mineral density (BMD) will tell you how much internal bone you have lost.

junkies may not have gotten the right combination of exercise, daily calcium, and essential vitamins and nutrients needed to build their bones to the max. Women who suffered from anorexia and bulimia are at high risk, too, as are those who took long-term doses of steroids (like prednisone) or smoked cigarettes. Young women whose periods stopped for long stretches due to excessive exercise or a medical condition may have bones that are less sturdy than they should be. There are also

women who are genetically predisposed to produce thin, slender bones. Whatever the cause, when women who start out with less-than-average bone mass hit the rapid bone-loss years of menopause, their skeletons may soon resemble those of women who are decades older.

The teeth offer other early clues; dentists say they sometimes start seeing bone loss between the teeth of women in their 30s. Also at high risk are women who go through premature or

HOW TO FIND A DOCTOR WHO CAN HELP

Many people are treated for osteoporosis by their primary care physician or gynecologist. Others go to doctors who specialize in muscle or joint problems (orthopedists and rheumatologists) or hormones (endocrinologists). If you want someone who is more of an expert, ask your regular doctor for a referral or call the nearest big hospital or medical school to see if it has a department that focuses on osteoporosis or metabolic bone diseases. A women's health clinic or menopause center may also be able to help.

Before making your appointment, the National Osteoporosis Foundation suggests asking for some background information on the doctor. Has she received any special training in osteoporosis? What proportion of her patients are osteoporotic? Does she have equipment to measure bone mineral density on-site? For additional help, check out the Professional Partners Network directory on the website of the National Osteoporosis Foundation (www.nof.org).

drugs aiming to increase bone formation. If you're concerned about your own risk, talk to your doctor about getting a bone mineral density test. The combination of good nutrition and a smartly planned exercise routine, plus drug therapy in some cases, may go a long way toward reducing your risk of fractures into the future.

A BONE CHECKLIST

Perhaps you have a family history of osteoporosis, or maybe you recently broke a bone and were surprised that a minor fall or accident caused so much damage. Or maybe you're in perimenopause and you know that now is the time to talk bones. In any case, these are some of the topics your doctor should cover during an evaluation of your bone health:

AGE. Around the time of menopause, women begin to lose bone density much more rapidly than men do. That's because they lose the bone-protective benefits of estrogen. Women who experience menopause early are at even greater risk.

HEIGHT. Ideally, your doctor would measure your height with the same scale you've been using for years. No matter what, you should mention any height loss you've noticed. A significant change could be an indication of vertebral compression fractures, a major symptom of osteoporosis.

induced menopause before they reach their 40s.

Growing knowledge about how bones work is leading to more effective therapies and medications. As a result, osteoporosis is increasingly seen as a preventable and treatable disease. The most popular medicines effectively reduce the rate of bone resorption, with the newest

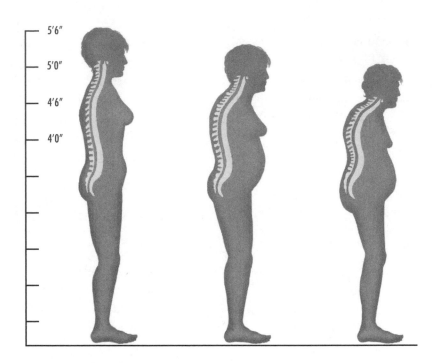

YOUR SPINE THROUGH THE AGES

As you get older, you lose bone in your spine. This process begins about 18 months before your last period. Over the next eight years, your spinal bone density will decrease by more than 10 percent, followed by a slower pace of age-related bone thinning that can go on for the rest of your life. This bone loss can lead to the "dowager's hump" seen in some elderly women.

WEIGHT. Your doctor will want to know not only how much you weigh now, but also your lifelong weight history, dieting history, and whether you've ever had an eating disorder. Inadequate nourishment, especially during the adolescent years, can permanently weaken bones.

FRACTURE HISTORY. Have you broken any bones? What about members of your immediate family? Fractures resulting from low-impact traumas are especially significant. Your doctor will also want to know if osteoporosis or any related bone diseases have occurred in your family.

EXERCISE. How often do you work out? Does your fitness routine include weight-bearing exercises? Do you have a history of excessive exercise that interfered with your monthly period? Significant time without menstruation can make bones more fragile.

MEDICATIONS. Write down everything you take and bring the list with you. Your doctor will also want to know if you've ever taken glucocorticoids, anti-convulsants, thyroid hormone, or a gonadotropin-releasing hormone agonist. All of these medications can affect bone strength.

SMOKING. Whether past or present, it's bad for bones—and everything else.

ALCOHOL USE. A history of excessive alcohol consumption is a red flag for osteoporosis.

NUTRITION. Are you getting enough calcium and vitamin D? Did you get enough in the past? What's your intake of fruit, vegetables, whole grains, sodium, protein, caffeine? Do you take supplements?

REPRODUCTIVE HISTORY. How old were you when you got your first period? How many pregnancies have you had? What was the space between births? Did you breast-feed? Do you have a history of irregular periods? All these questions affect the amount of time that estrogen protected your bones.

MENOPAUSE STATUS. Where are you in the menopause transition? This is particularly noteworthy if your periods stopped earlier than average or if menopause was surgically induced. Are you taking anything for symptoms?

ACHES, PAINS, AND POSTURE. Does your back, hip, or groin area hurt? Did you have scoliosis (a lateral curvature of the spine) as a child? Are there any signs of degenerating posture or an outward curve in your upper spine?

TOOTH LOSS. This could be a sign of bone loss in your jaw.

MEDICAL HISTORY. Red flags include endometriosis, rheumatoid arthritis, an overactive thyroid, parathyroid disease, kidney disease or stones, and malabsorption syndrome.

POOR BALANCE/VISION PROBLEMS. These are important things to track, since they put you at risk for falls.

Depending on the facts learned during this interview, your doctor may request the following:

LAB WORK. This can include a variety of blood tests (complete blood count, erythrocyte sedimentation rate, serum calcium and phosphorus, serum alkaline phosphatase, serum albumin, thyroid stimulating hormone, parathyroid hormone, vitamin D), as well as urine tests (24-hour urinary calcium excretion, calcium, cortisol, pyridinium cross-links, and N-telopeptides). Your doctor may also ask for kidney and liver function tests.

BONE MINERAL DENSITY TESTING. The machine number and name of technician should be noted in your file. Future test data are most reliable when done on the same machine and by the same technician.

DENSITY MEASUREMENTS

If your doctor orders a bone mineral density (BMD) test, there's no reason for anxiety. These tests don't hurt and usually take less then 15 minutes. There are several kinds of measurements. The most reliable is dual-energy X-ray absorptiometry (DEXA) of the spine and hip (and sometimes the wrist). It uses two X-ray beams (hence "dual-energy") to measure bone thickness, which can predict your chances of fracture. A scanning arm scans your body as you're lying down. This test can be used to monitor bone density changes over time and to determine if treatment is working. But it's not for everyone. It doesn't give an accurate measurement of anyone who has had spinal surgery, or who has a spinal deformity or arthritis in the lower spine. DEXA also can't be used on people who have had a hip replacement. Another test is quantitative computed tomography (QCT), which uses computer software to analyze the bone density of your spine and create a three-dimensional image. One of its advantages is that it can give your doctor more information about the quality of your bone than the DEXA scan, but it does expose you to a higher dose of radiation.

If you're over 30, the results are reported as a T score (see opposite), which compares you to a woman at the age of peak bone mass. Z scores, which can even be used for children, compare you to others of your own age. T scores above −1.0 are considered normal. Scores of −1.0 to −2.5 mark you as osteopenic, which means you have a low but potentially stable bone mass. If you have a score of −2.5 or lower, you have osteoporosis. Your risk of fracture doubles for every point below zero. As you get older, your T scores will most likely get worse. And even if your T score doesn't change as you age, your bones will get more brittle

ALL ABOUT CALCIUM

Getting adequate calcium is important throughout your life, but it's particularly critical during the menopause transition, when women rapidly lose bone density. Your body gets calcium in two ways: through your diet and from your bones (which, along with your teeth, store 99 percent of the calcium in your body). The more you take in, the less you'll have to draw from your bones. So what's the best way to get it?

In general, you should start with your diet. People who meet their calcium requirements through food tend to be healthier overall, and there's evidence that your body absorbs calcium from food more efficiently. Start with low-fat or fat-free dairy products and calcium-fortified juice and cereal (the labels will give you the exact amount per serving). (See page 265.)

Try keeping a calcium diary for a few days to see how much you're getting. If it's not the recommended 1,200 milligrams, you probably should consider

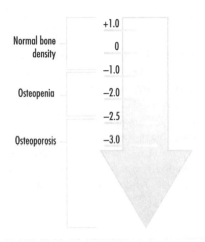

Normal bone density	+1.0
	0
	−1.0
Osteopenia	−2.0
	−2.5
Osteoporosis	−3.0

over time. A 60-year-old woman with a T score of −1.5 has a much lower chance of fracture than the same woman with the same score at age 85. Most women should have their BMD checked every two years, but women who have special risk factors or have already been diagnosed with osteoporosis require more frequent monitoring.

Researchers are trying to find new ways to predict personal fracture risk by using biochemical markers, but there's still much disagreement about what to do with the results of even the most reliable tests. Should everyone below a certain score be treated? That's still a matter of intense debate. Osteopenic women account for half of all fractures in fragile bones. Should they be routinely treated with medications that have potentially serious side effects even if they're only in their 40s or 50s? Many experts say no; some are even opposed to giving drugs to young women with severe bone loss because it's unclear how long patients can safely take them. They argue that everything else should be tried first. The World Health Organization is working to develop a consensus on what to do for these women. In the meantime, if you're under 80 and have evidence of low bone mass, it would be wise to seek the opinion of a bone specialist before starting one of these drugs.

taking a calcium supplement. You won't be alone. Calcium supplements are one of the top-selling nutritional supplements in the United States, accounting for nearly a billion dollars in sales annually. The two main forms are calcium carbonate (which comes from limestone and oyster shells and is used in Tums, Viactiv, and other tablets) and calcium citrate malate (used in juices). Calcium carbonate is more common because it's cheap and easy to take. It's important to remember that neither form is 100 percent calcium.

Calcium carbonate supplements are 40 percent calcium; calcium citrate contains only about 21 percent, but it's slightly better absorbed. The amount of calcium you get from supplements depends on how much total calcium you're taking in at any one time and whether or not you're taking them with food (calcium carbonate works best with food). You absorb the most calcium from supplements when you take in 500 milligrams or less at a time. Don't take calcium with fiber or iron supplements; they

CALCIUM HIGHS AND LOWS

Daily calcium replenishment is essential to strong bones. The specific amount you need to add every day varies with age, but women over 50 should aim for 1,200 milligrams a day. Many doctors think that postmenopausal women who are not on estrogen therapy should get 1,500 milligrams every day.

CALCIUM THIEVES
Unfortunately, certain foods can "steal" calcium from your body. Some of the principal culprits are listed below.

Protein. There's some evidence that large amounts of dietary protein, especially if it's from animals, can leach calcium. More research is needed, but in the meantime pay extra attention to calcium intake if you're on a version of the Atkins diet or if you gulp down a lot of protein powders, drinks, or bars. But don't cut out too much protein; in older people, low protein intake can lead to osteoporosis.

Alcohol. More than seven drinks a week can disrupt calcium balance. Blood levels of calcium are partly regulated by parathyroid hormone (PTH) and vitamin D.

If you drink too much alcohol over a long period of time, you raise your blood levels of PTH, which strains your body's calcium reserves. Alcohol also interferes with the production of liver and kidney enzymes that help activate vitamin D. To make things worse, drinking too much alcohol impairs balance, which makes you more likely to fall. Limit yourself to no more than a drink a day, the government's definition of "moderate" drinking for women.

Salt. This staple increases urinary calcium excretion. The government recommends limiting sodium intake to 2,400 milligrams a day, but many Americans consume more than 6,000 milligrams daily. (This also means that people who are on a low-salt diet may need *less* calcium.)

Oxalates. Foods such as spinach, beans, rhubarb, and sweet potatoes contain oxalates, which reduce calcium absorption. This doesn't mean you shouldn't eat them; just be sure to get your daily allowance of calcium in other foods or in supplements. Even better, try a dish like creamed spinach—some dairy for calcium and all the nutrients of the vegetable.

---

cut down absorption. Some people who use supplements complain of gas, bloating, and constipation. If that happens to you, take the pills with meals, try other brands, or spread out the dosage during the day. Another drawback of supplements is that they can interfere with prescription and over-the-counter medications. Talk to your doctor if you're already taking any of these: digoxin, levothyroxine, tetracycline, anticonvulsants, certain diuretics, glucocorticoids, or fluoroquinolones.

Finally, there is such a thing as taking too much calcium. The Institute of Medicine, a nonprofit scientific advisory

FOODS RICH IN CALCIUM

Dairy products are an excellent source of calcium, but so are numerous fruits, vegetables, grains, and nuts. Another possibility is adding nonfat powdered dry milk (52 milligrams a tablespoon) to recipes. Equivalency tables are usually provided on packages.

	Serving Size	Milligrams of Calcium
DAIRY		
Milk (nonfat)	8 ounces	302
Milk (whole)	8 ounces	291
Yogurt (plain, low-fat)	8 ounces	300
Cottage cheese (1% milk fat)	2 cups	276
Cheddar cheese (shredded)	1½ ounces	306
Vanilla ice cream	½ cup	85
NONDAIRY		
Orange juice (calcium-fortified)	6 ounces	200 to 260
Ready-to-eat cereal (calcium-fortified)	1 cup	100 to 1,000 depending on brand
Sardines (canned in oil, with bones)	3 ounces	324
Salmon (canned)	3 ounces	181
Cornbread	1 piece	162
Almonds (sliced)	1 cup	236
Soybeans (green, boiled)	1 cup	266

group, says you shouldn't ingest more than 2,500 milligrams a day, but some bone doctors urge their patients not to exceed 2,000 milligrams. Too much calcium can also interfere with your body's ability to absorb other minerals, such as iron and magnesium. Don't freak out, though; it's rare to overdose on calcium from food and supplements. A much bigger problem is too little calcium; the average postmenopausal woman consumes only 700 milligrams a day!

MOTHER'S MILK

Q *I breast-fed all three of my children. Does that put me at higher risk for osteoporosis?*

A Pregnancy and breast-feeding may do a number on the rest of your body, but neither one harms your skeleton in the long run. In fact, both may ultimately make your bones stronger. Scientists have spent a considerable amount of time looking into this question, since bone growth in both the developing fetus and the nursing newborn depends on calcium from the mother. There's still a lot to learn, but here's what they've found. When you're pregnant, your body signals your intestines to suck up more calcium than usual. That's why expectant mothers should get extra calcium in their diet, especially during the second and third trimesters. Even if you were really diligent and made sure you had adequate calcium and other nutrients, you will have lost some bone density by the end of your pregnancy. You lose a little more when you breast-feed. But when you wean your baby and start ovulating again, your bone density is restored to pre-pregnancy levels in about a year if you stick to a healthy diet.

So, for the vast majority of women, pregnancy and breast-feeding are not bad for bones. There's even some evidence that women with three or more children may be less likely to sustain hip fractures than women who have never had children. Still, there are a couple of exceptions to this generally reassuring picture: women who go right into menopause after pregnancy or weaning and those diagnosed with weak bones before they get pregnant.

WHEN MILK IS THE PROBLEM

Q *I love dairy products, but they don't love me. I'm lactose-intolerant, and even half a glass of the white stuff sends my stomach into a spasm. Do I have to get all my calcium from supplements? Are there any other ways to make my diet rich in calcium?*

A First of all, your misery has company. Lactose intolerance is surprisingly widespread, affecting more than 30 million Americans. It's caused by insufficient lactase, an enzyme produced in the small intestine that helps to digest lactose, the natural sugar in milk. Without lactase, the lactose in milk turns into a kind of laxative as it travels through the intestine. Before long, you're suffering from abdominal cramping, gas, and diarrhea.

But don't give up. Many foods, including some dairy products, are high in calcium and low in lactose. Yogurt with live active cultures is okay because of its bacterial lactase. You can also eat hard cheeses like Swiss, Cheddar, Parmesan, and Colby; the process of producing these cheeses pulverizes the lactose, leaving only a trace amount behind. Many stores also carry lactose-free or lactose-reduced milk. Calcium-fortified soy milk and orange juice are two other possibilities. Many more foods are now fortified with calcium, including ready-to-eat breakfast cereals and bars and pasta. Check labels for details. Canned sardines (324 milligrams of calcium in three ounces) and canned salmon (181 milligrams) are good sources. Many other foods, including tuna, tofu, beans, and enriched bread, will add to your daily total.

One final note: Studies show that it's possible to build up a tolerance to dairy products. You might try starting with small amounts at meals and then gradually increasing your intake.

A GLASS OF SUNSHINE

Q *I've read that vitamin D may be as important as calcium in protecting bones. But is there really any way to get enough through diet? Aren't supplements the only practical solution?*

A You're right about the growing emphasis on vitamin D. It helps you to maintain normal blood levels of calcium and phosphorus and protects against many bone diseases, including osteoporosis, rickets, and osteomalacia, an abnormal softening of bone. It also plays a role in maintaining muscle strength and may even ward off high blood pressure, depression, and auto-immune disorders like multiple sclerosis, rheumatoid arthritis, and diabetes. In addition, there's tantalizing new evidence that it may prevent or slow cancer and tumor development through its role in cell formation and proliferation.

With all those benefits, it's not surprising that getting too little vitamin D is a serious health concern. Half of post-menopausal women diagnosed with osteoporosis or hospitalized for hip fractures have vitamin D deficiency. A 2003 Mayo Clinic study found that more than 90 percent of patients complaining of nonspecific but chronic musculoskeletal pain were also deficient in vitamin D.

An adult woman 50 or under should get 200 international units (IUs) a day. After age 51, the recommended amount doubles to 400 IUs. At 71, the daily dosage bumps up to 600 IUs. Doctors treating women with osteoporosis often recommend an increase in vitamin D intake to 800 IUs or more, and some researchers are now petitioning the government to raise the recommended daily allowance to 1,000 IUs a day for everyone.

What's the best source? You could start with a glass of milk; it's fortified with about 100 IUs. Not all dairy products are equal, however; the milk used to make most cheeses, ice creams, and yogurts is *not* fortified with vitamin D. On the other hand, some orange juices and ready-to-eat cereals do contain D; check labels to see if your favorite does. Vitamin D is also present in quite a few kinds of fish (herring, mackerel, salmon, tuna, sardines). Cod liver oil is another terrific source, if you can stand the taste; just one tablespoon contains 1,360 IUs.

One of the simplest ways to get enough vitamin D is to just walk around in the sunshine. Ultraviolet rays from the sun trigger the skin to make its own vitamin D. But with our heightened consciousness of the dangers of skin cancer, most of us slather on sunscreen to keep out the rays. So consider a sensible compromise. If you have light skin, get about 5 to 15 minutes of sun exposure to your face, arms, hands, or back at least twice a week (without sunscreen) during warm weather. If you have darker skin, you should add a few more minutes. But don't overdo it. Watch the time, and when you've had enough, slap on sunscreen of at least 15 SPF. And keep in mind that this isn't a year-round solution for everyone. Researchers have found, for example, that between November and February there isn't enough sun in Boston to trigger vitamin D synthesis. Pollution is another factor that cuts down sun exposure. If you live in a colder or rainy climate, you'll need an extra boost. Also, as you age, it's harder to synthesize vitamin D through your skin.

That's where supplements come in. Many health food stores sell vitamin D, but it can be hard to find. Some calcium pills include vitamin D, as do many multivitamins. Check labels to make sure you're getting enough vitamin D for your age and that the supplement contains calciferol, the vitamin's most active form.

EARLY WARNINGS

Q *I recently broke my wrist, and a friend told me this could be an early warning sign of osteoporosis. I'm only 43. Can this be true?*

A Your friend is right. Weak bones can cause trouble at any age, and a broken wrist in your 40s could indeed be the first indication that you're at risk for osteoporosis, especially if the injury resulted from a relatively mild trauma. People who later break a hip or have a spinal fracture often have a broken wrist in their past.

Fortunately, you can improve your odds. Talk to your doctor about how you stack up against the formal guidelines for osteoporosis risk in 40-year-olds. Your doctor will review your medical history to see if you have any of these warning signs: a family history of bone disease, low body weight, a sedentary lifestyle, low calcium intake, loss of height, multiple fractures, or a history of smoking or alcohol abuse, as well as any medication you've taken (current and past) and certain diseases that would put you in a higher risk category. You may be sent for a bone mineral density test along with a blood test to rule out other conditions that can weaken bones, such as hyperparathyroidism (a secondary cause of osteoporosis). If the results show that your bones are thinning, your doctor should explain your options. Ask about how to improve your diet and exercise regimen and whether you should be taking calcium or vitamin D supplements.

A diagnosis of osteoporosis at your age would be scary, but in some ways you could consider yourself lucky for having your problem identified early. In that case, follow your doctor's orders and you can prevent fractures and further bone loss. Your goal is to get yourself reclassified as osteopenic—someone with low but potentially stable bone density.

INCREDIBLE SHRINKING WIFE

Q *I'm in my mid-50s and have already lost a half-inch in height, but my husband still stands as tall as he did on the day we got married. Does being a man protect him from fragile bones?*

A What can we say? Life isn't fair. Osteoporosis is two to three times more common in women than in men, partly because the latter generally start adulthood with larger and stronger bones. Because osteoporosis is primarily a women's disease, there hasn't been as much research on men, but guys who smoke, drink too much alcohol, and don't get enough exercise are generally more vulnerable. Other risk factors include undiagnosed low testosterone levels, a family history of osteoporosis, and long-term use of certain medications, such as steroids or anticonvulsants.

If your husband is a nonsmoking, nondrinking athlete who eats right and gets plenty of sunshine, his odds of beating osteoporosis are even higher than most. Those are good health habits for you, too.

IS IT TOO LATE FOR ME?

Q *I admit it. I've done almost everything on the not-to-do list. My diet isn't particularly good, I smoke, I drink more than I should, and I hate exercise. At 45, is there any hope for me?*

A It's way too early to declare yourself a lost cause. While there are no guarantees that lifestyle changes will prevent you from getting osteoporosis, you could increase your odds substantially by living a healthier life . . . and the sooner, the better. The truth is, because of genetics, some people who do everything right spend decades fighting uphill against the disease. Others, born with bigger bones and inheriting a slower pace of bone loss, will have far more wiggle room—even if they aren't doing everything right. But few people know for sure which category they fall into. Even if you have a bone mineral density test, there's much you still won't know about the overall quality of your bones. The bottom line is that you have nothing to lose and everything to gain by adopting a healthier lifestyle. Even women in their 80s can improve bone health with weight-bearing exercise, calcium supplementation, and osteoporosis medication. And making positive changes will boost not only the density of your bones but your health in general.

Because you have multiple challenges, you should commit yourself now to taking on one goal at a time. A fairly painless way to start is to focus on the 1,200 to 1,500 milligrams of calcium and the 400 international units (IUs) of vitamin D you need each day. Cut back on the junk in your diet, and increase your intake of veggies and fruit, whole grains, and low-fat dairy products. Even if you hate exercising, you can increase your activity level by doing everyday things such as taking the stairs instead of the elevator or walking rather than driving to run quick errands. Keep a set of light weights around the house or at the office and start doing simple lifts. As

you build up strength and start feeling and looking better, you may be surprised to find yourself motivated to experiment with different exercise regimens. Your goal is to do at least 30 minutes of exercise a day. Once you're on a roll, you'll be more likely to find the motivation to cut back on the alcohol and stop smoking. In one study, women in their mid-70s reduced their risk of fracture and increased their bone mass by as much as 15 percent when they started doing the right kinds of exercise, boosted their calcium and vitamin D intake, and improved their diet. If they can do it, so can you.

Too Thin?

Q *I'm short and have always kept a close eye on my weight. I figured that would be a big help in terms of my overall health as I got older. But now I'm hearing that women who weigh less than 127 pounds are at higher risk for osteoporosis. Would I reduce my chances of having bone problems later if I gained weight now?*

A Despite that old adage that you can't be too rich or too thin, the truth is that you can indeed be too thin when it comes to osteoporosis prevention. Slender women are at higher risk for osteoporosis than their bigger-boned sisters. So are women with a history of anorexia and bulimia, extreme dieters, and those who exercise to excess. Even women who are well proportioned but petite in stature can be at high risk because they tend to have smaller bones and less bone mass. (By the way, the 127-pound cutoff comes from one large study of older women, which found that those below this weight were twice as likely to fracture a hip.) Your specific combination of height and weight also matters. Any woman with a body mass index (BMI) of less than 20 is considered at higher risk for bone density problems.

Extra pounds make you more vulnerable to cardiovascular problems and a host of other health problems, but fat does provide some protection against bone loss because it produces estrogen. That means heavier women produce more estrogen (even after menopause), which in turn keeps bones more dense. Heavier women are also loading their bones with more weight, which causes bone density to increase. And if you should fall, extra padding may make the difference between breaking a bone or not, especially as you get older and your bones become more fragile. This doesn't mean the heavier, the better; studies indicate that the hip fracture risk for women of average weight is similar to that of much heavier women.

If your slender frame or BMI puts you in a higher risk category, talk to your doctor about getting a bone mineral density test. Not everyone in the higher risk categories has a problem. Depending on your specific symptoms and history, your doctor might suggest

that you gain a little weight or increase your muscle and bone through weight-bearing exercise. You'll also want to review your diet with your doctor to make sure you're getting enough calcium and vitamin D.

BONES AND RACE

Q *I'm an African-American woman, and I've heard that we're much less likely to get osteoporosis than Caucasian or Asian women. Is this true even if I'm tall and thin?*

A Generally speaking, African-American (and Hispanic) women are less likely than Caucasians or Asians to get osteoporosis. Among women 50 and older, about 20 percent of non-Hispanic Caucasian and Asian women develop osteoporosis, and 52 percent have low bone mass. About 10 percent of Hispanic women have osteoporosis and 49 percent have low bone mass, whereas only 5 percent of African-American women have osteoporosis and 35 percent have low bone mass. Overall, African-American women experience only a third as many fractures as white women do.

But you're smart to zero in on your body type. The main reason that fewer African-American women are diagnosed with osteoporosis is that they tend to have higher bone mass. But this isn't true of all African-American women. Because of the stereotype that osteoporosis is a Caucasian woman's disease, health-care providers are less likely to focus on detection and prevention of bone mineral density problems in minority women. Even after sustaining a fracture, African-American and Hispanic women are less likely than Caucasians and Asians to get referrals for treatment of osteoporosis. So be proactive. If you've checked off more than one or two of the risk factors for osteoporosis on page 257, be sure to bring up the subject with your doctor.

BAD TEETH

Q *My mother-in-law has osteoporosis and blames the disease for the fact that she's losing her teeth. How does this happen?*

A Your mother-in-law is correct in suspecting a link between tooth loss and osteoporosis, but it's more complicated than simple cause and effect. Typically, tooth loss is the culmination of a sequence of events that starts with swollen and bleeding gums. People who are lax about removing all the sticky bacteria that accumulates on their teeth can get irritated gums at any stage of life. That's why you should floss away plaque and brush thoroughly several times a day. During the menopause transition, some women who have had healthy gums start seeing changes because of their fluctuating hormone levels.

(You may have experienced something similar during certain days of your menstrual cycle or during a pregnancy—other times in your life when your hormone levels fluctuated.) Your gums may become more sensitive as well as more vulnerable to bacterial infection. If you have a history of periodontal (gum) disease, your symptoms may get significantly worse.

At the same time, the part of the jaw that includes tooth sockets can be affected by menopausal bone loss and osteoporosis. This may be a second reason for periodontal disease in menopausal women.

In either case, if periodontal disease is not aggressively treated, deep spaces or pockets will develop around your teeth, where the infection will flourish. Over time, the tissue that supports your teeth will weaken, and eventually they'll loosen and fall out. So, to answer your question directly, osteoporosis *can* play a role in tooth loss. But that doesn't mean it's inevitable. To keep your mouth healthy, you'll need to pick up the pace of tooth care in the years before and after menopause. Even if you've been blasé in the past, now's the time to get serious. Consider using one of the newer high-tech toothbrushes for a full two minutes on your teeth and gums. You may also want to dip your brush in 3 percent hydrogen peroxide and treat your gums to a stimulating massage or talk to your dentist about using an antimicrobial mouthwash. Salt water also works well. If you're having a lot of symptoms, consider bumping up to three or four cleanings a year instead of the standard two. Giving your teeth extra attention now may make all the difference in the long run.

And while we're on the topic of your mouth, be sure your dentist knows your menopausal status (especially if you had a hysterectomy or induced menopause at an early age) and ask to be kept informed about any bone loss apparent on dental X-rays or exam. A tip from your dentist may get you on the road to earlier diagnosis and treatment of low bone mass.

WHEN TO TEST

Q *I thought it would be smart to ask for a bone density measurement now, when I'm in my mid-40s, in order to have a baseline that could be used to gauge bone loss later. My doctor is resistant. Why?*

A Doctors agree that all women over 65 need a bone mineral density test, but there's some divergence of opinion within the medical community about which younger women should get measured. In general, however, any woman going through perimenopause with one or more risk factors (see page 257) should qualify for early testing. If you're simply a slender Asian or Caucasian woman, you should be tested to see if you need preventive treatment. The same is true if you've been treated with steroids for a sub-

stantial period of time, have a history of menstrual irregularities, or have recently suffered a low-trauma fracture. After taking your medical history, your doctor can decide whether or not you need further evaluation.

OTHER OPTIONS

Sometimes, bone loss is already so serious that diet and exercise aren't enough. Fortunately, there are other options. Here's a rundown:

HORMONE THERAPY. There was a time in the not-too-distant past when hormone therapy was the darling of the osteoporosis world because research indicated that it not only reduced loss of bone mass but also protected women against heart problems. Postmenopausal therapy with either estrogen alone or a combination of estrogen and a progestin does increase bone density in the first years after menopause, but those benefits must be weighed against the disadvantages, which include increased risk of heart attack, stroke, and blood clots. Combined therapy also increases the risk of breast cancer. The FDA advises women to use hormone therapy only for the relief of menopausal symptoms such as hot flashes and vaginal atrophy—and even then, only at the lowest effective dose and for the shortest possible time. For women younger than 50 who experience early or induced menopause and have significant hot flashes, some doctors may prescribe hormone therapy for longer periods. They tend to agree with the North American Menopause Society's view that "the benefit-risk ratio may be more favorable for younger women who initiate therapy at an early age." But even they acknowledge that the risks associated with this use have not been established through randomized clinical trials and should be implemented with caution.

Low doses of hormone therapy work as well as higher doses for most women when it comes to protecting bones. Your doctor may want to add Fosamax (see below) to the regimen, since one recent study published in the *Journal of the American Medical Association* found that this combination improved bone density in postmenopausal women more than either medication alone.

Hormone therapy is effective for as long as you take it. After you stop, bone loss resumes. The National Osteoporosis Risk Assessment trial found that the risk of hip fracture for former hormone users and women who never used hormones was about the same five years after stopping hormone therapy.

Another option you may hear about is estradiol, the main form of estrogen produced by the ovaries and the body's most active form of estrogen. Estradiol preparations come in patches, pills, or injections and are sold as osteoporosis treatments. There hasn't been much research into their long-term effect, including any potential increase in heart disease or breast cancer, but the assumption is that the risk of using estradiol is the same as for other estrogen formulations.

BISPHOSPHONATES. You've probably seen ads for Fosamax (alendronate), Actonel (risedronate), and Boniva (ibandronate). These bisphosphonates inhibit bone resorption, which increases bone density and lowers fracture risk. Fosamax and Actonel are generally the first choice for treatment. In older women with osteoporosis, Fosamax has been found to reduce the chance of hip and spine fracture by as much as 50 percent and multiple vertebral fractures by 90 percent. In large studies of osteoporotic women, it reduced risk of spinal fracture by 40 percent and hip fracture by 30 percent. The risk of multiple vertebral fractures fell by more than 90 percent. (These are overall numbers; there's no way to predict what would happen to each individual.)

Do these effects last? Unclear. Women just past menopause who used Actonel for only two years lost bone when they stopped taking it; however, women who took it for five years did not lose bone again. Still, Actonel is a fairly new drug, and women have not been followed for very long. In the case of Fosamax, women who took it for 10 years started losing bone a few years after they stopped.

Which of these drugs you take depends on your particular situation. Fosamax may cost you a little more; Actonel tends to cause fewer gastrointestinal upsets (nausea, stomach pain, diarrhea, heartburn, indigestion, and/or peptic ulcers). With both, you must follow a strict routine to ensure better absorption and fewer chances of stomach and esophageal irritations. Bisphosphonates, administered as pills, should be taken with water (not mineral water) before breakfast. You need to wait at least half an hour before eating or drinking anything else, including other medications. During those 30 minutes, you will need to stand, walk, or sit upright. Taking these medications does not reduce your need for adequate calcium, vitamin D, and regular exercise.

Boniva is the most recent bisphosphonate to be approved by the FDA. Like the other bisphosphonates, it reduces bone turnover and increases bone density. It's generally given monthly, which may be a big advantage for some women. Boniva has also been approved for IV administration once every three months.

Another bisphosphonate, Didronel (etidronate), is approved for use against osteoporosis in Canada but not yet in the United States except for Paget's disease, a disorder in which the bones weaken and become more vulnerable to fracture. The trouble is that there's little information on Didronel's long-term safety. It does need to be taken several hours before or after meals, but gastric upsets are rare; that makes the drug attractive to patients whose stomachs simply can't tolerate the other bisphosphonates.

A NOTE OF CAUTION

It's worth emphasizing here that most of the research on bisphosphonates has focused on older women with osteoporosis. The use of these drugs in osteopenic women (and young women with osteoporosis) remains very controversial. While studies continue, some experts are concerned that too many younger women (in their 40s and 50s) are being encouraged to take Fosamax and other bisphosphonates. There isn't much research on its use in these women or its safety and efficacy over several decades of use. The fear is that if women start using these medications too early, the drugs may be useless to them by the time they're in their 80s and 90s. If you fall into this category, carefully review your options with your doctor and consider whether nondrug options (like weight-bearing exercise and a better diet) are worth trying first.

Bisphosphonates that are administered intravenously may also be helpful for patients who can't handle the gastrointestinal upsets caused by Fosamax and Actonel. Research has shown that Boniva, Aredia (pamidronate), and Zometa (zoledronic acid) increase bone density. Aredia and Zometa are not FDA-approved for osteoporosis. Zometa has been found to increase bone mass after one injection. Taking these drugs to treat osteoporosis would be "off-label" use, but it's a common practice.

There have also been rare but troubling cases of osteonecrosis (bone disintegration) of the jaw in some people taking bisphosphonates. While most of them were bone cancer patients taking very high doses, not all were.

CALCITONIN. A hormone that regulates calcium levels in the blood, calcitonin slows bone loss in postmenopausal women and has been shown to increase bone density and strength in the spines and hips of women who have osteoporosis. In women many years past menopause, it reduces the risk of new vertebral fractures by 36 percent. It's not generally the first choice because there's no evidence so far that it reduces fracture risk anywhere but the spine and no evidence that it's effective for women in the first five years after menopause. Sold under the brand names Calcimar and Miacalcin, calcitonin is administered by injection (every day or every other day) or in the form of a nasal spray, the most common delivery method. Possible side effects include nasal inflammation, nausea, loss of smell, and flushing of the face and hands. Synthetic calcitonin comes mainly from salmon; if you're allergic, this drug isn't for you.

RALOXIFENE. Sold under the brand name Evista, raloxifene belongs to a class of drugs called selective estrogen receptor modulators, or SERMs. These drugs mimic estrogen in some parts of the body, such as the bones, and block the effects of estrogen in other places, such as the breasts. Tamoxifen, the first SERM to get FDA approval, is commonly prescribed to prevent recurrence of breast cancer. One of its upsides is that it helps to protect bone in postmenopausal women. But it also slightly increases the risk of endometrial cancer and the likelihood of hot flashes. Raloxifene, the second SERM approved by the FDA, also reduces the risk of breast cancer recurrence and helps to protect bone but does not increase the threat of endometrial cancer. Unlike some of the other drugs, raloxifene doesn't need to be taken at any specific time of day and can be taken with or without food, but its side effects include an increased risk of stroke, leg cramps, blood clots, and hot flashes. More studies are on the way as researchers look at other SERMs that may prevent bone loss while reducing LDL cholesterol levels and preventing menopausal symptoms.

TERIPARATIDE. This genetically engineered parathyroid hormone, sold under the brand name Forteo, boosts the number and productivity of bone-building cells while strengthening interior (trabecular) bone. The result is not only new bone, but stronger bone. In studies, teriparatide increased bone density in the spine by 9 percent and in the hips by 3 percent. After taking the drug for 19 months, postmenopausal women with a history of spinal fractures experienced a 65 percent reduced risk of new vertebral fractures and a 53 percent lower risk of nonvertebral fractures. Long-term safety has not been determined beyond two years, but patients who switch to bisphosphonates at that point are able to maintain their bone gains; however, those who stopped all medication after 18 months quickly lost bone again.

Teriparatide's ability to stimulate bone formation distinguishes it from other medications for osteoporosis, which work primarily by slowing bone loss. Drawbacks: It's expensive and must be administered by daily injection. Some users report feeling dizzy or having heart palpitations the first few times they use it. It's usually prescribed for patients who are at high risk for fracture and cannot take other osteoporosis treatments. In studies required for drug approval, very high doses of teriparatide were given to rats for two years; some developed osteosarcoma, a bone cancer. It is not known whether humans who use Forteo at therapeutic levels are also at risk for bone cancer (no human cases have been reported since the drug was approved in 2002), but it should not be taken by those who have been diagnosed with either bone cancer or other cancers that have spread to the bone and have undergone radiation or by those with Paget's disease. The drug can also cause hypercalcemia, or elevated blood levels of calcium; symptoms of this condition include confusion, muscle or bone pain, vomiting, nausea, and irregular or slowed heartbeat.

TIBOLONE. A synthetic steroid used in more than 50 countries but not in the United States, tibolone (Livial) has intrigued American doctors for years because it seems to do so many things right. It increases bone mass and reduces hot flashes while improving vaginal health and sexual desire. In the body, it can take on qualities of estrogen, progesterone, and androgen but is active only at certain sites; in other words, it behaves something like a SERM. The most recent studies also indicate that tibolone doesn't increase the risk of blood clots or breast density (women with dense breasts tend to have more breast cancer, and dense tissue also makes it harder to spot cancer cells on mammograms). It lowers total cholesterol and increases levels of good cholesterol. It also doesn't appear to cause the uterine walls to thicken the way estrogen alone does.

SUPER STATINS

Q *I have a history of high cholesterol and was told by my doctor that the statins I'm taking could reduce my chance of a heart attack AND build bone. Am I right to assume that I won't need to take any other meds to prevent osteoporosis?*

A Not necessarily. Over the last few years, there were some encouraging results from a variety of animal and human studies indicating that statins might be capable of lowering cholesterol and, as a side benefit, could boost bone growth. But further research paints a less rosy picture. A four-year study following nearly 94,000 postmenopausal women found that there was no difference in rates of hip, wrist, and arm fractures between those who took statins and those who didn't. Even more surprising were results indicating that those taking statins had a slightly higher chance of suffering a spinal fracture. The study also compared the bone mineral density of more than 6,000 of these women and found no difference between the two groups after adjusting for age, race, and weight. More studies are under way. In the meantime, if you're at risk for osteoporosis, go ahead and have your BMD checked, and talk to your doctor about whether other medication should be considered.

CAN TAMOXIFEN HELP?

Q *I am a breast cancer survivor taking tamoxifen. I've heard that this drug also protects bone. Will it protect me from getting osteoporosis?*

A There's some tantalizing evidence that tamoxifen reduces bone turnover and increases bone mineral density, but so far the drug hasn't been approved for prevention or treatment of osteoporosis. As a selective estrogen receptor modulator (SERM), tamoxifen acts like estrogen in some parts of the body but not in others. While looking into tamoxifen's ability to fight breast cancer, researchers were surprised to dis-

cover that it also offered some protection to postmenopausal women against bone loss. One major study involving more than 13,000 women found that those taking tamoxifen had 35 percent fewer vertebral, hip, and wrist fractures than the group taking the placebo. A smaller subgroup was found to have increased their BMD by 2 percent. But in other small clinical trials *premenopausal* women taking tamoxifen lost bone. Still, these studies were aimed at women who had a high risk of breast cancer rather than osteoporosis, so it's unclear if what worked for one group will work for the other. Right now, the only SERM approved for osteoporosis is Evista (raloxifene), which decreases fractures as much as bisphosphonates and has been shown to prevent breast cancer. You may want to ask your doctor about switching to this medication. In any case, you should continue to monitor your BMD to make sure it stays within safe levels. If not, you and your doctor can discuss your options.

SWITCHING MEDS

Q *I've been taking Fosamax to treat my osteoporosis, but I've heard that Evista protects bones and helps to prevent breast cancer. Should I be taking that instead?*

A Generally, if you're taking a bisphosphonate because you have osteoporosis—and are *not* at high risk for breast cancer—your doctor will probably want to keep you on Fosamax because there's more evidence of its safety and efficacy and because Evista has a variety of side effects, including increased risk of hot flashes, stroke, and blood clots. However, if you are at high risk for breast cancer or over 65, it's probably worth having a conversation with your doctor about the comparative merits of the two medications in your particular case.

RADIATION AND BONES

Q *I recently underwent radiation to treat cancer. Did that affect my bones and raise my risk of fracture?*

A It might have. Radiation can kill osteoblasts, the cells that build bone. As a result, women who receive radiation for breast cancer are at higher risk for vertebral fractures, while women who get radiation treatment in the genital or abdominal area may be at higher risk for pelvic or hip fractures. If chemotherapy was also part of your treatment, you're doing a fast-forward through menopause and incurring all the rapid bone loss that goes with it. If you haven't yet had a bone mineral density test, you should talk to your doctor about getting one now.

GOING NATURAL

Q *I've heard that soy helps bones. Is there any research that backs this up? Are there any other alternative therapies that might help?*

A You're probably referring to the flurry of scientific interest in ipriflavone, a synthetic compound similar to the estrogen-like isoflavones found in soy products. Researchers became intrigued with the possibility of a soy-based solution when they noticed significant differences between the hip fracture rate among Caucasian women and women living in Asian countries, where soy is a major part of the national diet. However, closer scrutiny revealed that Japanese women are more likely than Caucasian women to suffer a vertebral fracture, which makes the case for soy less clear. While a number of animal-based studies have indicated that isoflavones encourage bone growth, the results from human studies have been mixed. Some showed little effect; others, none. Critics have complained that many of the studies done to date have been short-term and involved small samples. Longer-term studies are now under way.

Further dampening enthusiasm for ipriflavone is the link between its use and the reduction in the number of circulating lymphocytes, white blood cells that help the body fight infection. There are also mixed data about whether isoflavones increase the risk of breast cancer, the way some hormone therapies do. And like all other botanicals, ipriflavone has earned no FDA assurance that it is safe or effective for the prevention or treatment of osteoporosis.

As of this writing, the National Institutes of Health specifically discourages women from using soy products to prevent bone disease. Some herbalists also suggest wild yam, black cohosh, Asian ginseng, and dong quai because of their estrogen-like tendencies, but there's no scientific confirmation that any of these are effective.

THE MARTINI CURE?

Q *I read somewhere that moderate drinking could be good for bones, but I also know that too much alcohol increases your risk of fracture. What's the real deal?*

A There's good reason for your confusion. The research dealing with alcohol's effect on bones is ongoing, but here's what we know. More than one drink a day, defined as 12 ounces of beer, 5 ounces of wine, or 1.5 ounces of hard liquor, is particularly dangerous for young women who have not yet achieved peak bone mass, because alcohol interferes with the body's ability to build healthy bone. Excessive drinking in adulthood is also bad; it increases the risk of fracture, not only because of the direct effect of alcohol on bones (it's a diuretic and decreases calcium absorption) but also because drinking makes you less steady on your feet and more likely to fall. The effects of moderate drinking on the bones of postmenopausal women are less clear. Some studies have shown that moderate alcohol consumption appears to increase bone mineral density, probably because alcohol raises the level of estrogen in your blood and estrogen has a protective effect on bones, but others have indicated that drinking could increase your risk of breast cancer. So, at this point, it's not likely that your doctor would prescribe a drink a day as a treatment for weak bones without considering your whole medical history. If you like having a drink a day, ask how this might affect your bone health plan. There are better ways to get the same benefits— diet, exercise, and bone-building medication—without the risks.

BONE-BUILDING EXERCISE

You don't have to work the barbells like Arnold Schwarzenegger, but you should try to do 30 to 60 minutes of weight-bearing exercise every day. If you're in good shape, even jumping, hopping, and skipping are great exercises for your bones. No, we're not kidding, and we personally do this in the privacy of our own homes so that no one else can see how ridiculous we look. Aim for 10 minutes a day. Add in a mix of other activities such as progressive weight training (make sure you use all muscle groups), jogging, aerobic dancing, stair-climbing, or active sports like tennis, hiking, and basketball. Also helpful are low-impact weight-bearing exercises like walking (outside and on treadmills), plus elliptical machines and rowing machines.

Remember, you don't have to do all this exercising at one time. You can spread it out, adding 10 minutes here, 10 minutes there. Everyday things like taking the stairs to get from floor to floor at your office and raking leaves in your front yard count toward your exercise total. One word of caution: Never embark on a new exercise regimen without talking to your doctor or healthcare provider.

AN ATHLETE'S DILEMMA

Q *For years, I was a professional athlete in excellent physical shape with very little body fat. Because of that, my periods were really erratic and sometimes didn't come at all for months. Now I'm hearing that I may have inadvertently set myself up for bone problems. Could this be true? I thought exercise was supposed to be good for bones.*

A Exercise *is* good for bones, but you can get too much of it— especially when you're in your teens and early 20s and don't eat right. Those are the years when you're building bone mass (which reaches a peak in most people by the age of 30). When you have so little body fat that you stop menstruating, you also have less estrogen, which protects against bone loss. That may cause irreversible damage. Doctors call this "the female athlete triad," a reference to disordered eating, amenorrhea (no menstruation), and osteoporosis. In several studies, osteoporosis was more common among female runners and ballet dancers. Gymnasts and ice skaters had healthier bones in these studies, even though they may also have had menstrual irregularities. No one knows why that is. You need to talk to your doctor about your medical history and determine whether you're a candidate for a bone mineral density test. So far, there aren't any definitive studies that can tell you what long-term damage you may have done to your bones, but you can get a picture of where things stand now and take action to slow further bone loss.

EVERYBODY OUT OF THE POOL?

Q *I've always been told that swimming is the perfect exercise because it works your whole body and the chance of injury is small. It's kept me in great shape for years, but my doctor is saying I should try something else as well. Why?*

A Swimming is great exercise, but it's not weight-bearing exercise— the kind you need to help build stronger bones as you age. (Ditto indoor cycling, yoga, stretching, and flexibility exercises.) It's not that you have to do any less swimming, but your time in the pool doesn't count toward the 30 to 60 minutes of weight-bearing exercise you should try to get every day. You need a variety of aerobic, load-bearing, strength-training, and balance-enhancing exercises to build up bone and stave off fractures. If you want to stay in the pool, try water aerobics or deepwater walking.

Is Heredity Destiny?

Q My mother and her sister both developed spinal osteoporosis in their late 60s (they have that awful "dowager's hump"). I'm 49 and have been much more careful than they ever were about exercise. I also eat wisely, rarely drink alcohol, and have never smoked. Am I doomed to stoop no matter what I do?

A We wish we could tell you that all will be well because you've been such a good girl—but we can't. There are no guarantees that lifestyle changes will completely prevent osteoporosis if you're genetically predisposed to suffer from fragile bones. It's estimated that as much as 70 percent of a woman's vulnerability to osteoporosis is determined by genetics. But you have greatly improved your odds of staying active for many years by being so conscientious. You're probably at a much lower risk of fracture, which is critical since fractures account for a large percentage of hospitalizations and long-term disability among older people.

At this point, given your family history, you may want to consider even more preventive action. Ask your doctor about a bone mineral density test. If the results show that you've already suffered from bone loss, he may put you on medication to help. Even without medication, there's a lot you can do on your own, including special exercises aimed at strengthening vulnerable points in your body, especially your back (but be sure to get your doctor's okay first). You should be doing weight-bearing exercises every day.

Finally, start thinking about everyday safety. For people with low bone mineral density, certain kinds of movements are dangerous. Avoid heavy lifting, particularly if you have to bend forward at the waist. This sort of movement can lead to a compression fracture in your spine. Think of it as the best excuse you'll ever have to get someone else to do the laundry or the grocery shopping! You should also stay away from twisting movements, which can put extra force on your spine. And do everything you can to make your home a fall-free zone by getting rid of anything you could trip over or slip on. Accidents don't have to happen.

The Osteoporosis
Prevention Exercise Program

Now that we've convinced you that you need to get stronger today in order to be stronger later, you may be wondering exactly what you ought to be doing. The following three-days-a-week program, developed by experts from the Centers for Disease Control and Prevention and Tufts University, is designed for the woman who has done very little exercise in recent years. The idea is to start slowly and move gradually to harder (and more varied) exercises.

Check with your doctor before you start. Then stay with each stage of the program until you're sure you're ready to progress.

PART 1

A Two-Week Plan for Getting Started

For the first two weeks, your focus is on getting stronger and more coordinated. Start each day by walking briskly for five minutes. (If you'd prefer to warm up by riding a bike or using another piece of aerobic equipment, that's fine.)

Exercise 1: Squats

Make sure you don't move too quickly on this one. Also, don't lean your weight too far forward or onto your toes when you're in the standing position.

1. Stand directly in front of a sturdy chair with your feet slightly more than shoulder-width apart. Extend your arms parallel to the ground.

2. Place your weight more on your heels than on the balls of your feet. Bend your knees as you lower your buttocks nearly to the chair in a slow, controlled motion, counting to 4.

3. Pause. Then slowly resume a standing position as you count

to 2. Keep your knees over your ankles and your back straight.

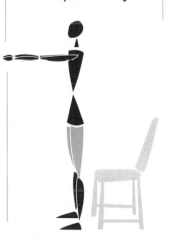
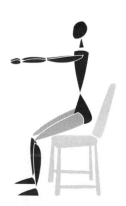

Repeat the squat 10 times. Rest for about 1 minute. Then complete a second set of 10 squats.

Exercise 2: Wall Push-Ups

Keep your hands planted on the wall. Don't round or arch your back.

1. Choose a wall free of any objects such as wall hangings and windows. Stand a little farther than arm's length from the wall. Face the wall, lean your body forward, and place your palms flat against the wall at about shoulder height and shoulder-width apart.

2. Bend your elbows as you lower your upper body toward the wall in a slow, controlled motion as you count to 4. Keep your feet planted.

3. Pause. Then slowly push yourself back until your arms are straight as you count to 4. Make sure you don't lock your elbows.

Repeat the wall push-ups 10 times. Rest for about 1 minute. Then do a second set of 10 wall push-ups.

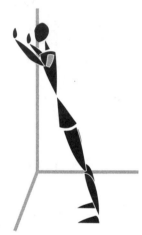

Exercise 3: Toe Stands

Don't forget to breathe regularly when you do this exercise.

1. Stand with your feet shoulder-width apart near a sturdy chair or a counter. Use the chair or counter for balance.

2. Slowly push up as far as you can onto the balls of your feet as you count to 4. Hold this position for 2 to 4 seconds.

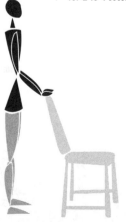

3. Slowly lower your heels back to the floor as you count to 4.

Repeat the toe stands 10 times. Rest for about 1 minute. Then complete a second set of 10 toe stands.

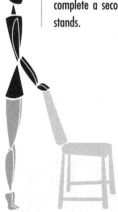

Exercise 4: Finger Marching

Stand or sit forward in a chair with your feet on the floor, shoulder-width apart.

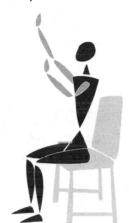

Movement 1: Picture a wall directly in front of you. Slowly walk your fingers up the wall until your arms are above your head. Hold your arms overhead while wiggling your fingers for about 10 seconds. Then slowly walk them back down.

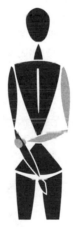

Movement 2: Try to touch your hands behind your back. Reach for the opposite elbow with each hand, getting as close as you can. Hold the position for about 10 seconds, feeling a stretch in your back, arms, and chest. Release your arms.

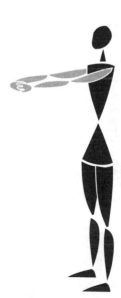

Movement 3: Interlace your fingers in front of your body. Raise your arms parallel to the ground. Rotate your hands so your palms face an imaginary wall. Stand up straight but curl your shoulders forward. You should feel the stretch in your wrists and upper back. Hold the position for about 10 seconds.

Repeat the sequence 3 times.

PART II

Getting Stronger

Continue to do the exercises from Part I of the program, but now add on these strength-building moves. Start out with light weights. Reassess every week, and use heavier weights if an exercise begins to feel too easy. Aim to stay at this level for about four weeks.

Exercise 5: Step-Ups

It's easy to let your back leg do the work, so be sure to press your weight on the heel rather than the ball or toes of your front leg as you lift. When you're ready, try doing this exercise on two stairs rather than one.

1. Stand next to a handrail at the bottom of a staircase. With your feet flat and toes facing forward, put your entire left foot on the first step.

2. Hold the handrail for balance. As you count to 2, place your weight on your left leg and straighten it as you slowly lift your right leg until it reaches the first step. Make sure your left knee stays straight and does not move forward past your ankle as you're lifting yourself up. Let your right foot tap the first step near your left foot.

3. Pause. Then use your left leg to support your weight and slowly lower your right foot to the floor as you count to 4.

Repeat 10 times with the left leg and 10 times with the right leg. Rest for about 1 minute. Then do a second set of 10 repetitions with each leg.

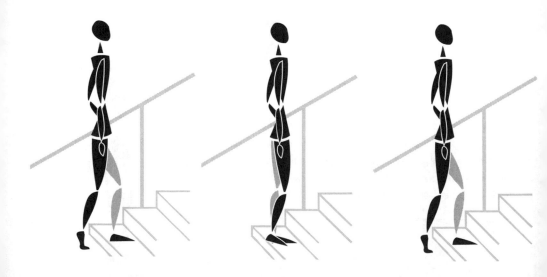

Exercise 6: Biceps Curls

1. Stand or sit in a chair with a dumbbell in each hand. Your feet should be shoulder-width apart with your arms at your sides and your palms facing your thighs.

2. Rotate your wrists and slowly lift the weights as you count to 2. Your palms should be facing in toward your shoulders. Keep your upper arms and elbows close to your sides—as if you had a newspaper tucked under each arm.

3. Pause. Then slowly lower the dumbbells back toward your thighs as you count to 4. Rotate your wrists so that your arms are again at your sides, palms facing your thighs.

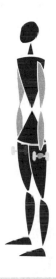
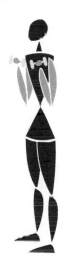

Repeat 10 times. Rest for about 1 minute. Then complete a second set of 10 repetitions.

Exercise 7: Overhead Press

There's a lot to keep track of in this seemingly easy exercise. First off, relax your neck and shoulders. Keep your wrists straight. Don't let the dumbbells move too far in front of or behind your body. And don't forget to breathe!

1. Stand or sit in a chair with your feet shoulder-width apart. Pick up a dumbbell in each hand. With your palms and forearms facing forward, raise your hands until the dumbbells are level with your shoulders and parallel to the floor.

2. Slowly push the dumbbells up over your head until your arms are fully extended as you count to 2. Make sure you don't lock your elbows.

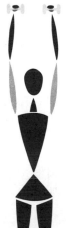

3. Pause. Then slowly lower the dumbbells back to shoulder level as you count to 4, bringing your elbows down close to your sides.

Repeat 10 times. Rest for about 1 minute. Then complete a second set of 10 repetitions.

Exercise 8: Side Hip Raise

This movement should be slow and controlled; you don't need to lift very far.

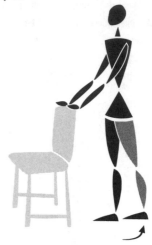

1. Stand behind a sturdy chair with your feet slightly apart and toes facing forward. Keep your legs straight without locking your knees.

2. Slowly lift your left leg out to the side as you count to 2. Keep your leg straight but don't lock your knee.

3. Pause. Then slowly lower your left foot back to the ground as you count to 4.

Repeat 10 times with the left leg and 10 times with the right leg. Rest for about 1 minute. Then do a second set of 10 repetitions with each leg.

PART III

Rounding Out Your Program

By now, you may be getting a little bored. Add these exercises for variety—and to increase your strength. If you're using ankle weights, start out light (1 to 3 pounds per leg), then increase the weight as you get stronger.

Exercise 9: Knee Extension

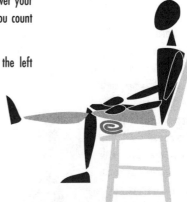

1. Sit all the way back in a sturdy chair so that your feet barely touch the ground. If your chair is too low, place a rolled-up towel under your knees. If you're using ankle weights, put them on snugly.

2. Point your toes forward. Flex your left foot and slowly lift your left leg as you count to 2. Extend your leg until your knee is straight.

3. Pause. Then slowly lower your foot to the ground as you count to 4.

Repeat 10 times with the left leg and 10 times with the right leg. Rest for 1 to 2 minutes. Then do a second set of 10 repetitions with each leg.

Exercise 10: Knee Curl

1. Keep your ankle weights on and stand behind a sturdy chair. Face forward and place your feet a little less than shoulder-width apart.

2. Slowly bend your right leg, keeping your foot flexed, and bring your heel up toward your buttocks as you count to 2.

3. Pause. Then slowly lower your foot to the ground as you count to 4.

Repeat 10 times with your right leg and 10 times with your left leg. Rest for 1 to 2 minutes. Then do a second set of 10 repetitions with each leg.

Note that the thigh of the working leg should always be in line with the supporting leg. Also, the foot of the working leg should remain flexed throughout the move.

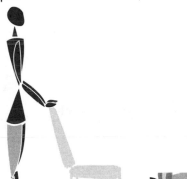

Exercise 11: Pelvic Tilt

It's tempting to lift your upper back or shoulders off the ground. Don't! And remember to breathe.

1. Lie flat on your back on the floor or on a firm mattress. Keep your knees bent, feet flat, and arms at your sides. The palms of your hands should face the ground.

2. Slowly roll your pelvis toward your abdomen so that your hips and lower back are off the floor as you count to 2. Your upper back and shoulders should remain in place.

3. Pause. Then slowly lower your pelvis all the way down as you count to 4.

Repeat 10 times. Rest for 1 to 2 minutes. Then do a second set of 10 repetitions.

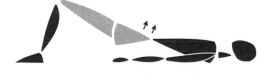

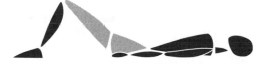

Exercise 12: Floor Back Extension

This exercise will only work if you keep your head, neck, and back in a straight line.

1. Lie facedown on the floor. Extend your left arm straight overhead so that it aligns with your body. Keep the other arm at your side.

2. Slowly lift your left arm and right leg off the ground as you count to 2. Keep your arm and leg at the same level.

3. Pause. Then slowly lower your arm and leg to the ground as you count to 4.

Repeat 10 times with the left arm and right leg, then switch to the right arm and left leg for another 10 repetitions. Rest for 1 to 2 minutes. Then do a second set of 10 repetitions in each position.

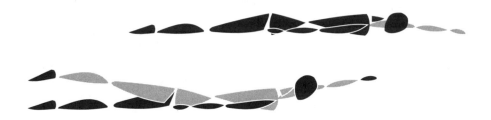

COOLDOWNS

Stretching for Flexibility and Relaxation

Here's something else you should know—stretching after any exercise is just as important as warming up. So don't be tempted to skip it. Besides, stretching and breathing deeply will make you feel better—less tense, more eager to face the day.

Cooldown 1: Chest and Arm Stretch

1. Stand with your arms at your sides and your feet shoulder-width apart.

2. Extend both arms behind your back and clasp your hands. Retract your shoulders if possible.

3. Hold the stretch for a slow count of 20 to 30 seconds, breathing throughout.

Release the stretch and repeat. Remember to keep your back straight, your shoulders relaxed, and your eyes straight ahead.

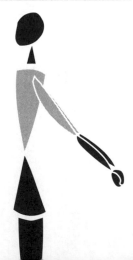

Cooldown 2: Hamstring/Calf Stretch

Just be sure to bend at the hips and keep your back straight.

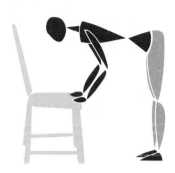

1. Stand facing a sturdy chair.

2. Slowly bend forward at the hips, keeping your legs straight without locking your knees. Rest your hands on the chair seat with your elbows slightly bent, feeling a stretch in the backs of your upper and lower legs. Keep your back flat.

3. Hold the stretch for a slow count of 20 to 30 seconds, breathing throughout.

Release the stretch and repeat. If this stretch is too easy, try bending your elbows more. (Some flexible people may want to rest their forearms and elbows on the seat of the chair.)

Cooldown 3: Quadriceps Stretch

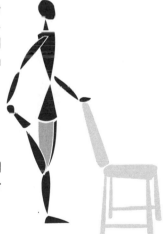

1. Stand next to a sturdy chair or a counter with your feet shoulder-width apart and your knees straight but not locked.

2. Hold on to the chair or counter for balance with your left hand. Bend your right leg back and grab your foot or ankle in your right hand so that your thigh is perpendicular to the ground. Make sure you stand up straight—don't lean forward. (If you can't grab your ankle in your hand, just keep your thigh as close to perpendicular as possible and hold the bend.) You should feel a stretch in the front of your thigh.

3. Hold the stretch for a slow count of 20 to 30 seconds, breathing throughout.

Release your right ankle and repeat the stretch with the other leg.

Cooldown 4: Neck, Upper Back, and Shoulder Stretch

Don't wait for an exercise session to do this easy stretch. It will make you feel better whenever you're stiff or just when you've been sitting at your desk too long. Remember to breathe, and be sure not to curve or arch your back.

1. Stand (or sit) with your feet shoulder-width apart, your knees straight but not locked and your hands clasped in front of you. Rotate your wrists so that the palms of your hands face the ground. Then raise your arms to about chest height.

2. Press your palms away from your body and feel a stretch in your neck and upper back and along your shoulders.

3. Hold the stretch for a slow count of 20 to 30 seconds, breathing throughout.

Release the stretch and repeat.

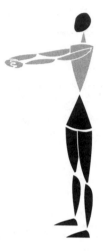

CHAPTER 11

Eyes and Ears

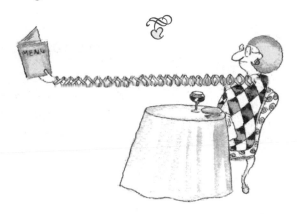

You're out to dinner with a group of your girlfriends, but when you open the menu, something strikes you as odd. Why is the type so small? You hold the menu at arm's length and then bring it closer. While you're busy imitating an accordion, one of your friends looks over and laughs. She reaches into her bag and hands you a pair of designer reading glasses. Since when did she need glasses?

Another friend is complaining about her contact lenses. She's been wearing them since she was 13 years old, and now, suddenly, her eyes are so dry that she feels as if she has two little plastic plates sitting right on her irises. Constantly putting in artificial tears has become a real pain, she says. She hates the way she looks in glasses, but what's the alternative?

A third friend chimes in. Her eyes are fine, but her hearing is driving her crazy. A few weeks after starting combined hormone therapy to treat hot flashes, she was straining to make out conversation at a cocktail party. Everyone seemed to be mumbling.

While none of these problems is "caused" by menopause, some of them (the dry eyes and the hearing problem) have a hormonal connection, and all of them are common at midlife. We have lots of ideas to help you adapt.

EYES

Whether you've always worn glasses or contact lenses or have always had perfect vision, midlife is a time when eye change is common. Sometimes the change is subtle—call it a slight blurring around the edges—and other times it's downright irritating. But whichever the case, you need to pay attention and get things taken care of.

What Can Happen

❖ Your eyes may become drier because of hormone changes as you move through the menopause transition. You may find it increasingly (and irritatingly) difficult to wear contact lenses.

❖ The clear lenses inside your eyes will become less flexible as you age, which will make it harder for you to focus on small print and tiny details. This is called presbyopia. Some women find that their distance vision improves as a result.

❖ The lenses of your eyes slowly start to yellow. You need to put brighter (75 watts and higher) and more direct light on the pages you're trying to read.

❖ Even if you've never had vision problems, at age 45 you'll need to start scheduling regular eye exams to ensure early detection of eye diseases associated with aging.

❖ You may find it more difficult to hear at crowded parties or noisy restaurants, particularly if you're taking an estrogen-progestogen combination.

DRY, IRRITATED EYES

Q *I'm only 45, and my eyes are really bothering me these days. They feel super dry and gritty, and they hurt. I've used a variety of over-the-counter eyedrops, but nothing helps for very long. What's going on?*

A As you get older, dry eyes can become increasingly annoying, even painful and debilitating. A decade ago, eye doctors tended to dismiss complaints about dry eyes without much thought. These days, however, doctors are recognizing that dry eye syndrome can lead to more serious problems, such as chronic inflammation, increased risk of infection, blurred vision, scarring, and, in rare cases, corneal damage and vision loss. More commonly, this eye problem interferes with daily life, making it more difficult for you to read, drive a car, wear contact lenses, work at a computer, or even go out into the sunlight. The discomfort often worsens as the day goes on.

Dry eye syndrome disproportionately affects women. An estimated 6 million American women and 3 million men have moderate to severe symptoms;

When to See the Doctor

Call your eye doctor or your internist if you experience any of these problems with your vision:

❖ DIFFICULTY SEEING, FOCUSING, OR READING

❖ DOUBLE VISION (SIDE BY SIDE, UP AND DOWN, OR SIDEWAYS)

❖ DIFFERENCES IN VISION IN ONE EYE COMPARED WITH THE OTHER (CAN BE CHECKED BY COVERING ONE EYE AT A TIME)

❖ THE APPEARANCE OF ANYTHING UNUSUAL IN YOUR FIELD OF VISION, SUCH AS A BLACK CURTAIN, A WALL, DOTS, WEBS, FLASHING OR FLICKERING LIGHT, OR FLOATING MATTER

❖ A REDUCTION IN YOUR PERIPHERAL OR CENTRAL VISION

❖ BLURRED VISION, OR STRAIGHT LINES THAT APPEAR TO CURVE OR OTHERWISE SEEM DISTORTED

❖ ANY TYPE OF EYE PAIN

❖ A PERSISTENT SENSE THAT SOMETHING IS IN YOUR EYE

❖ CHRONIC DRY EYE THAT DOESN'T RESPOND TO OVER THE COUNTER ARTIFICIAL TEARS, OR SIMULTANEOUS DRY EYES AND MOUTH

❖ A PERSISTENT DISCHARGE FROM THE EYE, ESPECIALLY IF ACCOMPANIED BY CRUSTING OR PAIN

---

another 20 to 30 million have a milder version of the syndrome. Hispanic and Asian women are especially vulnerable to severe symptoms but less likely to seek treatment.

Eyes feel gritty or sandy when you don't produce enough tears or when the tears you have evaporate too quickly. Sometimes this happens because the composition of your tears has changed. Tears have three layers: an oily outer layer (which reduces evaporation), a watery middle layer (which washes the eye and keeps it clean and moist), and a mucus like inner layer (which helps the others stick to the eye surface). All three layers are produced by different glands in the eyelids. As you age, malfunction or illness messes with your tear production and your eyes are less likely to feel comfortably moist, clean, protected, and lubricated. Tears also contain a dose of antibodies. When tear volume is down, your eyes are more vulnerable to infection.

There's lots of evidence that dry eye is related to fluctuations in hormones, especially androgens, which affect the production of the watery and oily layers of your tears; as that happens, your eyes also become less protected against inflammation. In about 10 percent of all cases, chronic dry eye is associated with autoimmune diseases. Dry eye can also accompany diabetes, Parkinson's, and thyroid disease. You should talk to your doctor about the medications you're taking. Antihistamines, decongestants, diuretics, and antidepressants can contribute to eye dryness.

Schedule an appointment with your eye doctor, who will run some tests to determine exactly why your eyes are drying out and the best way to treat them. Typically, the doctor will monitor your tear production and will also measure the thickness of your tears and their chemical composition. More severe cases may require the use of nighttime treatments designed to lubricate your eyes while you sleep. You may benefit from a procedure called punctual occlusion, in which tiny plugs are inserted into your tear drainage ducts to help keep tears on the surface of your eyes. Depending on the need, your doctor has the choice of inserting a temporary (and dissolvable) collagen plug or a permanent silicone plug.

While most treatments are designed to reduce symptoms, one medication has been approved by the Food and Drug Administration to treat an underlying cause of dry eye. Called Restasis (cyclosporine ophthalmic emulsion), it's available only by prescription and is

What to Tell Your Daughter

Wearing sunglasses is smart *and* cool. Research suggests that prolonged exposure to bright sunlight may cause cortical cataracts to develop sooner. This may be especially true for kids, because the sun's damaging rays appear to go deeper into their eyes. Children should wear shades or hats with brims. Even baseball caps offer some level of protection.

designed to decrease inflammation on the eye's surface. It's very effective for some, but doesn't work for everyone. Some people find the drops painful; putting the bottle in the refrigerator seems to help. It takes at least a month for Restasis to work, so keep using your artificial tears until you start feeling a difference.

HORMONE THERAPY AND DRY EYE

Q *If dry eye is related to drops in hormone levels, will hormone therapy make my eyes feel better?*

A Estrogen (especially the oral version) and birth-control pills tend to make dry eye symptoms worse (although a few women say the pills have the opposite effect on them). Some women find that their dry eye improves if they try a different delivery method of hormone therapy, such as a patch or cream.

SELF-HELP FOR DRY EYES

Keep a dryness diary. Determine how often and under what conditions dryness tends to occur. Many women find that environmental and lifestyle changes can make a real difference. For example, you may experience significant relief by reducing your exposure to pollution, air-conditioning, blow-dryers, and over-heated rooms and cars.

Increase your fluid intake. At the same time, reduce your intake of caffeinated beverages (which are diuretics). Try using a humidifier indoors and switching from contact lenses to eyeglasses.

Take a break from your computer. People who spend long hours in front of a screen tend to blink less, which can leave their eyes dry.

Use hypoallergenic makeup. Allergens can contribute to the problem, as can new sensitivities. Even if you've been using the same eye makeup for years, try switching to a hypoallergenic brand of eyeliner and mascara.

Change your diet. A 2003 analysis by Harvard's School of Public Health of the eating habits of 32,470 women revealed that those whose diets were richest in omega-3 fatty acids were the least likely to develop dry eye syndrome. Omega-3 foods are believed to help boost the oily layer of your tears. Natural sources of omega-3 include many types of fatty fish, such as mackerel, and canola, walnut, and flaxseed oils. You might also want to consider omega-3 fatty acid eggs, developed by feeding flaxseed to chickens. These eggs contain 100 milligrams or more of omega-3 fatty acids per yolk, three times more than regular eggs, and are often lower in cholesterol than other eggs. (Because of cholesterol's association with heart disease, talk to your doctor before you increase your intake of eggs.)

You can easily slip these foods into your diet. Sprinkle some ground flaxseed onto your oatmeal or eat sushi or sashimi if you don't like baked or broiled fish. Some doctors say that supplements high in omega-3s seem to make a difference, but this hasn't yet been proven by any high-quality published studies. In the meantime, many feel it's probably best to increase your omega-3 intake through diet (aim for one or two servings per week). If you prefer supplements, you might want to start with flaxseed oil; some doctors are concerned about the possible presence of toxins in fish oil capsules. Keep in mind that flaxseed oil can affect absorption rates of some drugs, so let your doctor know if you're taking any medications.

Try artificial tears. Over-the-counter preservative-free artificial tears can provide relief. (Products with preservatives have a longer shelf life and usually cost less, but they can also be more irritating to your eyes.) Viscosity varies among products; some are more liquid, others are formulated as gels. You may need to experiment to find the one that works best for you. Avoid drugstore eyedrops designed simply to refresh tired eyes and reduce redness. Such products are fine for occasional use, but they aren't made to treat chronic conditions like dry eye. They can even make the problem worse.

ANDROGENS TO THE RESCUE?

Q *I've heard that putting testosterone in your eyes helps. Is this true?*

A Androgen eyedrops may offer women relief without exposing them to the risks associated with hormone therapy. Harvard researchers are studying this and hope to bring a product to market soon. In the meantime, the Eye Center at the Southern College of Optometry in Memphis has been looking into the effectiveness of applying testosterone cream to eyelids to combat dry eye, especially in patients who wear contact lenses. No formal study data have yet been published and the Food and Drug Administration has not approved this treatment, so it remains unclear how effective or safe it is. If you decide to experiment with this idea, do it under a doctor's supervision. Getting the dosage right can be tricky, and overuse can cause you to develop side effects such as excessive facial hair, male pattern baldness, and other masculine traits. You don't want your eyes to get more comfortable just in time to see your mustache come in!

CONTACT LENSES AND DRY EYE

Q *I've been wearing contact lenses since I was a teenager, but my eyes are so dry now that it's torturous to wear them for long. Help! I look awful in glasses.*

A There may be a solution to your problem, but you may have to be tenacious to find it. First, see your eye doctor. If you haven't had your lenses professionally fitted in several years, your prescription may be out of date. It's also possible that the preservative in your wetting and cleaning solutions is irritating your eyes. A good eye doctor will give you a thorough exam and quiz you closely to pinpoint changes you can make in your environment or lifestyle. For example, if you currently sleep in soft lenses, try taking them out before bed; overnight lenses tend to act like little sponges, soaking up moisture. You might also want to try contacts made from a different type of polymer. Proclear Compatibles soft contact lenses (made by CooperVision) have an FDA-approved claim to be more comfortable for people with mild dry eye because they're made to resist lipid deposits and protein buildup, which create dry spots on the eye lenses. Others that promise increased comfort include: Extreme H_2O (Benz); CIBA Vision Focus Dailies with AquaRelease; CooperVision's PC Hydrogel; and Acuvue Oasys. So far, none of the rigid gas-permeable lenses (GPs) are designed to reduce dry eye. But the good news is that a lot of research money is aimed at this problem. Dry eye is the number one reason people stop wearing contact lenses. (If you're having trouble removing your gas-permeable lenses, ask your doctor about mini plungers, which solve the problem painlessly.)

Try using lubricating eyedrops or artificial tears before inserting your lenses. Since the reasons for dryness vary, talk to your doctor about what might be the best drops for you if over-the-counter solutions aren't doing the trick. While there are artificial tear products that are marketed to contact lens wearers with dry eye, no good data show that they are better than the others. You may also be able to reduce irritation by using preservative-free contact lens care products.

If none of these ideas helps and you're still unhappy with the prospect of wearing glasses, talk to your doctor about having plugs placed in your tear ducts. This sometimes increases the moisture level of your eyes enough to make your contacts comfortable again. Insurance will usually cover the procedure if it's medically required.

DROPS OF BLOOD

Q *I've read online that you can use your own blood to make an effective treatment for dry eye. It sounds kind of creepy, but does it work?*

A This treatment, promoted by a well-respected ophthalmologist in Japan, continues to be studied around the world. The drops are typically made from a mix of blood fluid (after red cells have been removed) and sterile saline (dilutions vary), which is then bottled and frozen until needed. Called autologous serum, it has been shown to be an effective treatment for some people with persistent dry eye and other eye surface problems, possibly because the serum includes a mix of vitamins and hormones.

There is no FDA-approved laboratory protocol for doing a large-scale study of this kind, so much of the research has been done outside the United States; the quality of the studies is mixed, and the data on safety and long-term effectiveness are limited. While some ophthalmologists are enthusiastic about the potential of this treatment, others argue that it offers nothing more than the kind of temporary relief already available in currently approved treatments. As a result, your doctor is likely to recommend something more conventional first. However, if you contact dry eye specialists, you'll likely find a few around the country who offer this treatment.

What About LASIK Surgery?

Q *I can't wear my contacts anymore because of dry eye. Could LASIK surgery be a solution for me?*

A No reputable eye surgeon will do LASIK or any other type of refractive laser surgery on someone with chronic dry eye unless the tear problem is solved beforehand. Laser surgery often makes normal eyes feel drier during the recovery period, and having dry eyes to begin with puts you at higher risk for more problems afterwards. If you seek a laser surgery consultation, make sure you're dealing with a licensed eye doctor and mention your dry eye problem up front. If you're told that you'll have to

---

Fitting Frames

If prescription glasses or nonprescription reading glasses suddenly become a part of your fashion statement, you'll need to figure out how you want to frame your face. Sophisticated, stylish, or whimsical frames are easier than ever to find. While designer prescription frames can get pricey, reading glasses can be so inexpensive that you'll be able to buy a handful in different colors, designs, and shapes. Have some fun with this. Pick up at least one pair that qualifies as outrageous. After all, no one looks (or feels) like an old lady in Matisse-inspired hot pink cat-eye frames. Extra advantage: You'll always be able to find them!

See below for some additional tips from the Vision Council of America.

Top Three Rules

◆ The frame shape should contrast with your face shape. (For example, if your face is round, try angular frames to offset rather than emphasize its shape.)

◆ The frame size should be in proportion to your face size.

◆ Your eyes should appear centered within the frames.

Ideas for Downplaying Your "Negatives"

A long nose. A low, dark, straight bridge shortens the nose.

Close-set eyes. A clear bridge makes close-set eyes appear wider apart.

Wide-set eyes. A dark bridge makes wide-set eyes appear closer together.

Thick Rx. Oval shapes and high-index lenses minimize the thickness of the lens.

Long profile. Low temples shorten a long profile.

Short face. High temples lengthen a face.

High forehead. Try frames that are even with or slightly higher than your brow.

Narrow face. Decorative or contrasting temples can make a face look considerably wider.

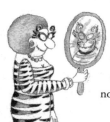

Wide jaw. Narrow frames with a pronounced horizontal line offset a pronounced jaw.

pay a nonrefundable deposit before the doctor will spell out all the risks associated with this kind of elective surgery, find another doctor.

DÉJÀ VU ALL OVER AGAIN

Q *When I was pregnant, I had a lot of trouble wearing my contact lenses. My doctor said it was related to the hormonal changes that occur during pregnancy and it would get better after the baby was born. Am I likely to experience problems when I go through menopause? And will they be permanent this time?*

A It's unclear if you're more likely to have eye problems now because you've had them in the past. But we do know that lots of women who have never had problems with their contacts start having them during the transition. As to what will happen after menopause, it's anyone's guess. Some women say things improve once they're postmenopausal; others find they stay the same; still others report that their problems come and go. Weather and geographic location also have an effect. Your eyes are more likely to feel good in humid places, less comfortable in dry areas.

SJÖGREN'S SYNDROME

Q *I've heard that menopause can make you feel "dried up," and I think that's exactly what's happening to me. First it was my eyes; now it's my mouth. Does this happen to everyone?*

MAKE UP THE DIFFERENCE

These days, you find your reading glasses perched on your nose more often than not. Or maybe you just got your first pair of eyeglasses. In any case, the addition of spectacles means that you need to rethink your makeup routine.

Start at the cosmetics counter of your local department store, especially if there's a brand you particularly like. Some companies offer appointments for a personalized consultation; in exchange, they expect you to buy a few things. If they're running a promotion, you get a goody bag, too. Or you can experiment on your own. Even a few small changes can make a big difference. Here are some tips (you'll find more on page 432):

◆ Make sure your brows are well defined. This will help to frame your look.

◆ Use matte shadows instead of slick creams.

◆ Use bone or white all over the eye (banana or shell for deeper skin tones) to provide a uniform base for your shadow.

◆ Line eyes with dark gel liner or damp shadow liner. You want a clean look—not smoky.

◆ Use mascara for more definition.

◆ Balance lip and eye makeup. If you have a strong lip color, make the eyes more natural. If you like more natural lip tones, you can go stronger on the eyes.

A Menopause does have a tendency to make your skin feel dry, but dryness in both your eyes and your mouth is a signal that you need to get tested for Sjögren's syndrome, an autoimmune disease. While there's no evidence that Sjögren's is menopause-related, it usually becomes apparent in your late 40s and is nine times more common in women than in men. The Sjögren's Syndrome Foundation estimates that as many as four million Americans have this disorder.

Sjögren's begins when the immune system starts attacking the glands that produce moisture and may also cause dryness in the liver, lungs, kidneys, vagina, gastrointestinal tract, pancreas, blood vessels, and central nervous system. About half the time, Sjögren's appears on its own. The rest of the time, it pairs up with disorders like rheumatoid arthritis, systemic lupus, systemic sclerosis (scleroderma), or polymyositis/dermatomyositis. Besides dryness of the eyes and mouth, symptoms include joint pain, fatigue, and almost continual yeast infections. It's not unusual for Sjögren's patients to experience a noticeable increase in tooth cavities and other dental problems related to a drop in their saliva volume. (Saliva contains minerals that help keep your teeth clean.) The syndrome is often overlooked by doctors because patient profiles vary so widely and seemingly unconnected symptoms aren't mentioned to specialists.

TOO MANY TEARS

Q *My eyes often feel dry, but in the winter I have the opposite problem. When I go out in the cold, my eyes suddenly get too teary. It feels and looks ridiculous.*

A At midlife, it's often one extreme or the other when it comes to eyes and moisture. When you're out in the cold, dry air, the watery layer of your tears evaporates faster than normal and your tear-producing glands may overcompensate. Artificial tears can prevent further "reflex" tearing, but be sure to mention this to your doctor, especially if it's a chronic problem. It could be a sign that your eyes' drainage system isn't working right or that there's a problem with your eyelids or corneas.

SHRINKING TYPE

Q *I've never needed glasses, but now that I'm in my 40s it seems so much harder to read small type.*

A The focusing problem you're having is called presbyopia, and just about everyone gets it eventually. It typically pops up around age 45. The lenses of your eyes become less flexible as you age, making it more difficult to focus on things right under your nose, like a book or a map. A pair of inexpensive reading glasses may be enough to fix the problem. Some people just pick up a pair at the drugstore, but it's smarter to go to an optometrist or ophthalmologist for professional advice on the magnification level you need. If you don't get it just right, your eyes will still be straining to read, which can lead to headaches. If you're having trouble seeing things near and far, talk to your eye doctor about bifocal glasses or contact lenses. Some people are able to get a bifocal effect with a different prescription for each eye.

TAKE THEM OFF

Q *Do I really need bifocals? If I take off my glasses and hold the type close, I can read just fine.*

A That may be true, but bifocals were developed so that people didn't have to keep taking off their glasses to read small type. Over time, you may decide that bifocals are more convenient.

WHAT'S IN A NAME?

Q *Does it matter whether I go to an optometrist or an ophthalmologist for an eye exam?*

A Both doctors are trained to give you a complete eye exam. Optometrists treat vision problems and prescribe eyeglasses and contact lenses; in most states, they can prescribe medicine. Ophthalmologists are medical doctors, either M.D.s or D.O.s (osteopaths), who specialize in the eye; they also have training in eye surgery. If you go to a big ophthalmology practice, chances are that an optometrist will do most of the actual eye exam and the ophthalmologist will come

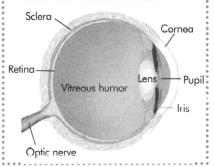

YOUR PRIVATE EYE

L ight enters the eye through the pupil (the black spot in the center of your eye) and travels to a clear, flexible lens located behind the iris. Tiny muscles attached to the lens allow it to change its shape, letting the eyes focus on things near and far. It does this easily at age 20, but by about age 40 to 45 most lenses become more rigid and have increasing trouble making the necessary adjustments. This change often prompts people to get reading or prescription glasses at midlife.

Sclera · Cornea · Retina · Lens · Pupil · Vitreous humor · Iris · Optic nerve

in at the end to review the results and talk to you. An optician, by the way, is someone who grinds prescription lenses and typically dispenses contact lenses.

A CLOUDY FUTURE?

Q *I've heard that if you live long enough, you will eventually need cataract surgery. Is there anything I can do now to prevent this problem?*

A Cataracts are an extremely common problem for people over 60. (Occasionally, an infant is born with them, too.) Very slowly, over time, most

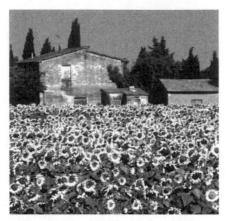

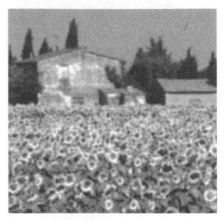

Normal vision.   Vision through a cataract.

NOT-SO-PERFECT VISION

As you age, you'll probably develop cataracts at some point in your life. The first signs are often noticeable after age 50, as the clear lenses in your eyes begin to yellow and you find it harder to read without a bright light. By the time people need cataract surgery, their vision is significantly impaired, as illustrated in the image at the right above.

people develop a fogginess in the lens of the eye that focuses light onto the back of the eye. As the condition worsens, you may notice that colors don't seem as robust, halos may appear around lights at night, and you may find yourself needing increasingly stronger glasses or brighter reading lights.

Little can be done to prevent this disorder, but its progress may be slowed by not smoking and by watching your weight. A few studies show that estrogen helps prevent the formation of cataracts, but there's no research showing that cataracts won't occur eventually. Diabetics tend to develop cataracts earlier, as do people who take steroids for long periods of time.

What can you do? Making sure your diet is rich in vegetables (especially green leafy ones) and fruit may help delay the damage. And don't forget to protect your eyes against bright sunlight.

When a cataract gets to the point where it impedes your vision, it can be surgically removed and a new clear synthetic lens can be inserted in its place. Typically, this surgery results in a fast and safe fix.

SEE THE LIGHT

Q *Reading is my life, but it's increasingly difficult for me to read the print in books and on the pages of newspapers and magazines. I can't make out the words on paper, although I can see things just fine on my computer. Is this somehow connected to menopause?*

A While some menopausal women experience reading problems that may be related to decreased estrogen levels (see Chapter 9), the problem you're describing is probably due to aging. Starting around age 50, the lenses of your eyes start to yellow. At the same time, the number of light-sensitive cells (photoreceptors) in your retinas begins to decline. The earliest stages of cataract development could also be starting. While you're probably a long way from needing cataract surgery, these changes make it harder for light to reach the retinas. The result is that print may look blurry and become hard to read.

You may be able to solve your immediate problem by increasing the amount of light hitting the page you're trying to read. A well-designed reading lamp with a high-wattage bulb can do a lot to alleviate the problem. You should also think about increasing the wattage (75 to 150) throughout your home; aging eyes are responsible for a lot of stumbles and falls. If you have eyeglasses with tinted lenses, you may want to stop using them indoors. Finally, it's very possible that you need a new prescription, bifocals, or reading glasses. The best way to prevent problems from creeping up on you is to get your vision checked regularly.

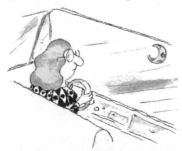

ONCOMING HEADLIGHTS

Q *Driving at night, especially when there's a lot of glare from oncoming cars, is becoming a problem for me. What's going on?*

A Noticing problems with nighttime driving is further evidence that your vision is changing. You may not have realized it, but all through your life you've been a little more nearsighted in the dark. When you were 20, your eyes compensated nicely by bringing in more light. But as you move through your 40s and 50s, your pupils become smaller and your lenses become more opaque, so less light reaches your retinas. (Some scientists estimate that by age 60 only about a third as much light reaches your retinas as when you were 20!) As a result, doing things at night becomes more of a strain for your eyes. You're likely to become more sensitive to both the glare from oncoming headlights and the reflection of lights in your rearview mirror. You'll notice more of an aura or halo or distortion around lights. You'll strain more to see your way on poorly lit or marked roads.

There are things you can do to make nighttime driving easier. If you're bothered by the glare of oncoming headlights, temporarily shift your gaze to the lower right side as a car approaches. If your car has a rearview mirror that automatically filters out nighttime glare, use it. Make sure you're sitting high enough in the driver's seat to see 10 feet in front of you; if you can't, give yourself a boost with a cushion. All windows (as well as your eyeglasses) should be clean and clear, especially in snowy weather. Keep a flashlight in your car to help you read signs and maps. A navigation system (either portable or permanently installed in your car) may be a good investment. Not only can it help you find your way in unfamiliar territory, but its illuminated screen shows upcoming curves in the road.

Finally, see your eye doctor annually. It's important to keep your prescriptions up-to-date, but you'll also want to give him a chance to detect other eye problems that could impact your nighttime vision early on. Even if you don't need glasses during the day, your doctor may recommend a pair for nighttime driving.

DRY AT NIGHT

Q *My contact lenses seem to get super dry when I'm driving at night. Why is this happening?*

A If you're straining to see, you're probably keeping your eyes open more and blinking less. As a result, your eyes get three times drier at night.

AT RISK FOR GLAUCOMA?

Q *I've been told that as a 40-year-old African-American woman I need to start seeing an eye doctor every other year. Why?*

A No one knows why, but African-Americans 40 and older are at greater risk for developing glaucoma,

which is believed to be caused by increased pressure inside the eye. Glaucoma causes no pain and exhibits no symptoms, but it can slowly destroy the optic nerve fibers. Usually, the only way it can be detected and treated early is with regular eye exams. Those with a family history of this disease, as well as those with diabetes, severe nearsightedness, or a history of significant steroid use, are especially vulnerable.

THE PRESSURE IS ON

Q *Does high blood pressure put me at greater risk for glaucoma?*

A That's a widespread misperception. However, high blood pressure can put you at greater risk for a condition called hypertensive retinopathy, which can lead to swelling of the optic nerve and the macula (the visual center of the retina) and eventually to vision loss. To reduce your chances of developing this condition, control your blood pressure through diet and/or medication and have your eyes checked regularly.

AT RISK FOR AMD?

Q *I've never been to an eye doctor, but during my last physical my internist told me to start getting regular eye exams. He's also really pushing me to stop smoking. What's the connection?*

A Menopause, by itself, does not weaken your vision, but the combination of smoking and aging puts you at greater risk for serious vision problems. Smoking doubles your risk of developing age-related macular degeneration (AMD), a retinal disorder that gradually blurs and can eventually destroy your central vision (what you see when you look straight ahead). A family history also increases your chances of developing AMD, currently the leading cause of blindness in the United States; so does being female, mainly because women live longer. People with light-colored irises tend to be more at risk, and there is some evidence that the same may be true for those with worrisome cholesterol counts (especially high LDL cholesterol and triglycerides). If your doctor wants you to take medication to bring your cholesterol down, concern about eye health may be another reason to do so.

As the name implies, age-related macular degeneration is much more common in those over age 60. Since there are no obvious symptoms during its initial stages, the disease is only picked up through regular eye exams. Regular monitoring detects whether the disease is worsening and whether interventions, including laser surgery, are needed to slow its progress. Even if you've never needed to go to an eye doctor in the past, annual eye exams are recommended once you hit 60.

As is true with other eye disorders, sun exposure may put you at greater risk of developing this disease and smart eating might help protect you. Increasing your intake of lutein and zeaxanthin (potent antioxidants found in red, yellow, and orange vegetables and fruits) may offer significant protection against AMD and may even reverse some of its damage. Lutein is available as a supplement, but it may be more effective when it's part of a healthy diet. Good food sources include egg yolks and dark green leafy vegetables such as spinach and collards. (Cooking spinach in oil increases the body's ability to absorb it.) Zeaxanthin is abundant in corn (yellow only, not white), egg yolks, orange peppers, and orange-colored fruits (oranges, tangerines, peaches).

VITAMIN PROTECTION

Q *I've read about a certain mix of vitamins that's recommended for people with AMD. If I take these vitamins now, will they protect me from getting this disease?*

A A specific mix of vitamins and minerals (vitamin C, 500 milligrams; vitamin E, 400 IUs; beta-carotene, 15 milligrams; zinc oxide, 80 milligrams; cupric oxide, 2 milligrams) is recommended for nonsmokers who have intermediate-stage AMD. This combination, used in AREDS (the Age-Related Eye Disease Study, funded by the National Eye Institute), slowed the disease's progression in 25 percent of the participants. Vision loss was also reduced by 19 percent. However, it offered no protection to those who had mild AMD or to those without symptoms.

PROTECT YOUR PEEPERS

The right sunglasses can do a lot to protect your eyes from diseases like cataracts and age-related macular degeneration. If you spend a lot of time in the sun and snow, they're essential for protecting your corneas against sunburn and sun blisters. (Not only are these conditions painful, but they also increase the chance of infection, which in turn can cause irreversible damage to the eye.) Surprisingly, even if you're sitting in the shade, walking outside on an overcast day, or riding in a car with the windows closed, you're vulnerable to the effects of damaging ultraviolet rays. UV exposure is increased when you're near sand, water, or snow, as well as at higher altitudes or near the equator. You also need to be very careful in summer and spring, especially between 10 A.M. and 4 P.M., when the sun's rays are most intense. People who have had retinal problems or cataract or laser surgery, or who take certain medications (including tetracycline, sulfa drugs, birth-control pills, diuretics, and tranquilizers) are at increased risk of UV eye damage.

Sunglasses are an easy way to get the protection you need. Here's what to consider before you head to the cash register:

Ultraviolet rays. The Food and Drug Administration has not established labeling requirements for sunglasses, but most manufacturers adhere to voluntary standards. Before you try on a new pair, look for labels that say full (or 100 percent) UV protection (or UV 400). What you want is full protection against both types of ultraviolet radiation, UVA and UVB, which can damage the eye's cornea, lens, and retina. These types of sunglasses are available at all price points; you don't have to buy expensive ones to be protected.

It's also worth mentioning that you can now order regular (untinted) eyeglasses and contact lenses (soft lenses and gas-permeable hard lenses) with full UV protection. Ophthalmologists are not unanimous about whether this is necessary or even a good idea, since all glass and plastic (including the types used in glasses or contacts) offer a significant defense against UV. However, if you have intraoc-

FLOATERS

Q *This probably sounds weird, but I seem to have some substance free-floating on the surface of my eye. Is this possible?*

A As we get on in years, little pieces of the clear gel (vitreous humor) inside our eyeballs can liquefy into strands of protein and become what are commonly called floaters. Typically, these bits of debris look like little dark

ular lenses surgically implanted after cataract surgery, be sure they have full UV protection.

Coloring your world. The lens color of your sunglasses makes a difference, but not in the way you might think. UV protection is clear, so very dark-colored lenses add no extra UV protection. Most experts recommend gray or amber lenses. Gray distorts colors less; amber blocks out blue light, which has been linked to macular degeneration. Blue-colored lenses permit more blue light to reach your eyes, so avoid them.

Those glare-reducing colors are now available in contact lenses as well. Nike MaxSight contacts, made by Bausch & Lomb, were originally designed to help baseball players see the ball better. The amber tint is recommended for those playing sports with fast-moving balls in variable light: soccer, tennis, and baseball. A gray-green lens is suggested for sports that are usually played in bright sunlight: golf, football, and running.

The right frames. When it comes to frames, most of us look for something that makes us look as stylish as Jackie O or, at least, not like a giant fly. But some styles are safer than others. Try to find frames that fit snugly against your eyebrows and

temples, protecting your eyes as well as your eyelids. For maximum protection, try wraparound frames.

Reducing glare. Polarized lenses are a good idea for those who spend a lot of time at the beach or on the water. They reduce the glare from water and sand as well as surfaces like blacktops. Not all polarized lenses have full UV protection; you'll need to check the label.

Shatter resistance. You may want to spend extra to get polycarbonate lenses, which are impact- and shatter-resistant. The money will be well spent if you're in a car when an airbag is deployed, particularly if you have vision in only one eye or you've had eye surgery or laser vision correction. Polycarbonate lenses always come with UV and scratch protection, so don't get lured into paying extra for those features.

Sunscreen for the eyes. Sunglasses and a wide-brimmed hat can help protect your eyes from cancer, which can develop on the eyelid, on the skin around the eye, or on the eye surface. Look for moisturizers or eye creams with sunscreen that can be used on the skin around your eyes for extra protection.

clouds or shadows moving across your field of vision. You should have your eyes checked for your own reassurance, but most of the time floaters are benign.

If the gel detaches from the back of your eyeball, you may also notice an

unnerving flash of light or a diminished field of vision. In this case, see your eye doctor immediately and have it checked out. It could indicate that your retina is in danger of detachment and may require a surgical repair.

EARS

What's that you say? Your hearing isn't as good as it once was? This could be hormones, aging, or proof that you once had just a little too much fun.

HORMONES AND HEARING LOSS

Q *Is there any connection between menopause and hearing loss? I'm 52 and taking combined hormone therapy. My hot flashes are better, but now my hearing seems to be deteriorating.*

A The natural menopause transition doesn't seem to have a negative effect on hearing, but taking a progestogen as part of your hormone therapy might. Funded by the National Institutes of Health, researchers at the National Technical Institute for the Deaf at the Rochester Institute of Technology conducted two high-quality studies (200 participants in total) comparing the hearing of three groups of women aged 60 to 86. One group was taking a combination of estrogen and a progestogen, the second was taking estrogen alone, and the control group was taking neither. Each group's composition was carefully matched. While the NIH-funded researchers expected the women taking only estrogen to score higher on hearing tests (because earlier studies conducted on animals had found that estrogen aided nerve cells in the brain and ears), it turned out that estrogen alone made little or no difference. Unexpectedly, those taking combined hormones did 10 to 30 percent worse on every hearing test—from the standard "pure tone" test (where you raise your hand to signal that you've heard something) to more sophisticated tests that measure sound echoing out of the ear. They had a particularly hard time hearing when there was a lot of background noise, the kind of situation you might encounter at a cocktail party or restaurant.

The hearing loss seems to occur pretty rapidly. Women usually notice it within a few weeks of initiating hormone therapy that includes a progestogen. (Anecdotally, women who have taken a supplemental progestogen to maintain a pregnancy have reported the same thing.) Some researchers also hypothesize that a progestogen may have a negative effect on balance, another inner ear function.

PAY LATER

Q *I'm only 45, but I'm noticing that my hearing is not what it used to be. Since I'm also exhibiting some of the signs of perimenopause, I'm wondering if this is all related.*

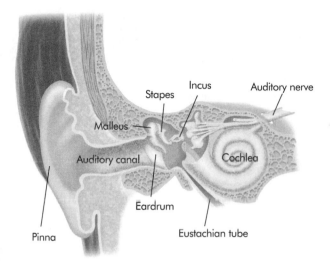

Stapes
Incus
Malleus
Auditory nerve
Auditory canal
Cochlea
Eardrum
Eustachian tube
Pinna

WHAT'S THAT YOU SAY? Sound waves enter the ear through the auditory canal. Vibrations set up when these waves hit the eardrum are magnified by three small bones and passed on to the inner ear. Fluid inside the cochlea catches the vibrations and relays them as electrical impulses along the auditory nerve to the brain's hearing center.

A What you're experiencing probably has more to do with a combination of genetics, age, and life experience than with menopause. Some women are born with great hearing and still have it at age 70 or even 80; however, most people find that their ability to hear well diminishes over time. Currently, there are about 28 million Americans with some degree of hearing loss, and that number is projected to reach 78 million by 2030.

The truth is many baby boomers have sped up this timetable by exposing themselves to a whole lot of noise in their lifetimes. We were the first generation to have a transistor radio plastered to our ears for days on end. A lot of us spent decades with our stereo systems and car radios blaring. Even today, we crank up our iPods way too loud.

When you expose yourself to steady blasts of noise, you increase your chances of damaging the delicate hair cells that facilitate hearing along the cochlea, the cornucopia-shaped structure in your inner ear. The temporary ringing in your head after a particularly loud concert or the muffled hearing you experience when you leave work may be signs that you've stressed these sensitive cells. If you work at a job like construction, manufacturing, or aviation and can't be heard by people an arm's length away without raising your voice, that's another sign that you're being exposed to too much noise. Repeated assaults of "acoustic trauma" can cause these cells to die. Since they don't regenerate on their own, their loss can mean you'll no longer be able to perceive certain frequencies.

What's unclear is whether daily doses of the kind of noise city dwellers take for granted—beeping horns, jackhammers, screaming ambulances—cause steady

THE FIVE-DECIBEL RULE

The louder the noise, the less time it takes to cause damage. That's the essence of the five-decibel rule. For each increase of five decibels, the amount of time it takes to cause damage is halved. This means that eight hours of 85 decibels (equivalent to the racket made by heavy city traffic) can cause the same amount of damage as one hour of 100 decibels (which could be caused by a screaming baby held next to your ear). Short exposure to a loud noise doesn't usually cause harm, but dealing with it 24–7 could hurt your hearing. Exposure to anything over 116 decibels for *any* length of time is very risky. To put this in perspective, an ambulance siren is 120; sitting close to the speakers at a rock concert is 140. What are the most dangerous? Explosive sounds, including gunshots, fireworks, and bombs. The sound of anything bigger than a .22 going off can easily hit 170 decibels—a level so high that it can destroy ear membranes and hair cells. So keep it down!

HOW LOUD IS TOO LOUD?

Noises that reach 85 decibels and above can damage your hearing.

	DECIBELS
Firecracker	150
Ambulance siren	120
Chain saw; sound at rock concert	110
Personal stereo system played at maximum level	105
Woodshop or snowmobile	100
Motorcycle	98
Power mower	90
Heavy city traffic	85
Normal conversation	60
Refrigerator hum	40
Whispers	30

deterioration or how much quiet is needed to recover from repeated exposure. In any case, it's probably a smart move to give yourself occasional respite by finding some quiet time in your noisy life.

TAKE TWO

Q *After you've been exposed to a loud noise, is there anything you can do to reduce the chance of suffering hearing loss?*

A Scientists believe that loud noises prompt free radicals to attack the delicate sensory hair cells in the ear. Animal studies indicate that ingesting antioxidants, vitamin E, or aspirin within three days can help fight off the free radicals and reduce or prevent hair cell death. In one study involving guinea pigs, the sooner the treatment, the better the outcome. Researchers hope that human studies will show similar results and help them develop dosage recommendations.

A LITTLE VANITY

Q *I find myself straining to hear people's conversations these days, but I'm hesitant about having my hearing checked. Frankly, I'm afraid of what the doctor might tell me. I really don't want to wear hearing aids. They never seemed to help my parents' hearing much, and I'm afraid they're going to make me feel (and look) much older.*

A Chances are, you haven't had your hearing checked since your pediatrician was doing annual screens many, many years ago. If your personal sound system is deteriorating, it's time to suck it up and get tested. Doctors today have more options to help you, including the new generation of digital hearing aids that are a lot better and a lot smaller than the ones your parents used. The best of the new breed offer directional or high-definition sound, utilizing two microphones and an algorithm that makes it easier to hear what's right in front of you (like the friend you're talking to) while reducing background noise. Unfortunately, the really sophisticated ones are pricey. While the older analog aids cost just a few hundred dollars, the high-tech ones are about $3,500 and usually aren't covered by insurance. However, if you have a flexible spending account or medical care spending account through your employer, this will likely qualify for reimbursement.

Many people just don't like the feel of something sitting in their ear and, like you, associate hearing aids with getting older. A solution may be on the horizon: permanent, implantable (and semi-implantable) hearing aids surgically inserted in the middle ear. Early trials indicate that they provide better speech perception and have fewer feedback problems than even the new-and-improved external models. They also have the cosmetic advantage of being invisible. It's unclear how much of this insurance companies will pay for, and

YOUR IPOD AND YOUR HEARING

Those distinctive white earbuds may give great sound, but they can also be hazardous to your hearing. Unlike the old earphones on your Walkman or Discman, earbuds keep sound distortion free even at the highest decibel levels, so they can be blasting your eardrums without your realizing it. The best advice: Never set the volume more than halfway up the meter. If you have to make it louder because the environment around you is too noisy, turn it off instead. Your ears will welcome the relief.

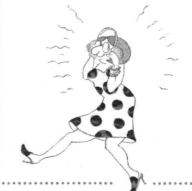

What You Can Do to Protect Your Hearing

There are many ways to reduce your exposure to noise, both around the house and at work.

◆ Fight the tendency to crank up the volume on your television set and stereo. Consider using a vibrating alarm clock or one that wakes you with flashing lights or softer sounds. Run the dishwasher when you're out of the kitchen. Wear earplugs when performing noisy chores like cutting the grass or using power tools.

◆ Be especially sensitive to the volume on your cell phone, which projects sound directly into

VROOOM!

the ear canal. Today's digital technology allows you to increase the volume without sacrificing clarity, making it all the more seductive. Tests have shown that many people using personal listening devices are exposing their eardrums to the equivalent of 115 decibels, a level that can eventually cause permanent hearing loss if exposure lasts more than 28 seconds a day.

◆ Protect yourself against occupational noise. If your workplace is loud, invest in high-quality ear protection or encourage management to provide it. Once you've got it, use it.

the price tag is expected to be steep: $15,000 to $20,000.

Another ray of hope lies in research that is under way to find ways to regenerate new hair cells in the cochlea. Most hearing loss occurs in the upper registers and is related to damage to those sensitive cells, which process thousands of different frequencies of sound. While some vertebrates are capable of replacing damaged hair cells, humans are not—at least not yet.

CHAPTER 12

Heart

What disease scares you most? If you're like many midlife women, breast cancer is probably at the top of your list. Chances are, you have more than one friend who is struggling with that devastating illness. But breast cancer, terrible as it is, pales before the leading killer of women: heart disease. Every year, more women die of heart disease than of all kinds of cancer combined. At this point in your life, you probably know more women who have been diagnosed with cancer than with heart disease, but that will soon change. Before menopause, your odds of a heart attack or stroke are much lower than those of a man your age. After menopause, the odds shift and the risk gap narrows; after age 65, as many women as men die of heart attacks. But here's the good news: Even if you haven't been particularly kind to your heart in the past, you can start healthy habits now.

Let's begin with a brief anatomy lesson. Your heart is a muscle that nestles in the center of your chest. It's about the size of a clenched fist, and it weighs approximately eight ounces—two ounces less than a man's. When you exercise or are stressed, you can often feel the thumping that means your heart is pumping blood through your arteries, delivering oxygen and nutrients to the rest of your body. After performing this vital task, blood returns to your heart through your veins. As a pump, your heart is built to work hard. On an average day, it beats 100,000 times and pumps roughly 2,000 gallons of blood. If you live to be 75, this means your heart will beat more than 2.7 billion times and pump almost 55 million gallons of blood. So—a little respect is in order here!

Your heart has four chambers, two upper (the right and left atria) and two lower (the right and left ventricles). Blood moves from chamber to chamber with the help of four valves that keep it flowing in only one direction with each beat. Electrical signals tell the valves when to open and close. When everything is functioning smoothly, you don't even notice how well your heart works. But when things start to go wrong, you can't ignore it.

THE RISKS OF ATHEROSCLEROSIS

Atherosclerosis, or hardening of the arteries, is caused by plaque: fat, cholesterol, calcium, and other substances from the blood that have built up in your arterial linings over many years, probably starting when you were a child. As you get older and plaque accumulates, you're at risk for diseases and complications of atherosclerosis that are the leading causes of illness and death in the United States and Canada.

Coronary artery disease is atherosclerosis in the arteries that feed the heart itself. A clot that forms in one of these arteries cuts off blood to a section of the heart muscle. Without nourishment, the heart muscle dies. This is a heart attack or, in medical terms, a myocardial infarction (MI). A heart attack may also be called a coronary occlusion or coronary thrombosis.

Angina is the medical name for the chest pain or discomfort you get from coronary artery disease. It's a symptom of insufficient blood to the heart, which means the heart isn't getting enough oxygen because one of the coronary arteries is dangerously narrow. This reduced blood supply is called ischemia. Stable angina is predictable; it occurs only during physical exertion or stress and stops when you rest. If this happens to you, it's critical that you see a doctor for evaluation even if the discomfort goes away. Unstable angina is chest pain that occurs while you're resting. It's an acute symptom of coronary artery disease and should be treated as an emergency.

Strokes occur when blood flow to the brain is blocked by a clot or when there's bleeding in the brain. If a blood clot is the cause, which is the case 80 percent of the time, it's an ischemic stroke. The clot can come from the heart or from atherosclerosis in one of the blood vessels leading to the brain. Bleeding in the brain (hemorrhagic stroke) often occurs when there's a direct injury to the brain, high blood pressure, or a vascular malformation. In other cases, a weakened section of a brain artery balloons out and ruptures. This is called a cerebral aneurysm.

HOW YOUR HEART WORKS Blood from the body descends into the right ventricle, which pumps it into the lungs. The powerful left ventricle receives the oxygenated blood and pumps it out to the body through the aorta.

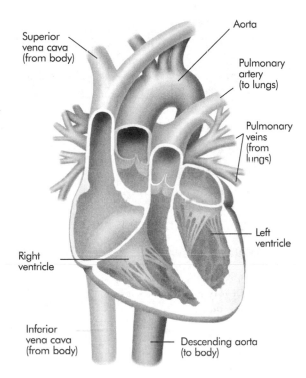

Superior vena cava (from body)

Aorta

Pulmonary artery (to lungs)

Pulmonary veins (from lungs)

Left ventricle

Right ventricle

Inferior vena cava (from body)

Descending aorta (to body)

Brain cells die when they don't get the blood and oxygen they need. Depending on which part of the brain is injured, stroke victims can lose the ability to see, touch, think, or move. More women than men die from strokes, but not enough of us recognize the warning signs. This ignorance can be fatal; more than 30 percent of strokes occur in women under age 65. The sooner you get the right care, the better your chances, so call 911 immediately upon noticing the warning signs (see page 318) and ask for the nearest hospital specializing in stroke treatment. According to a study at UCLA's Stroke Center, every second's delay in treatment costs 32,000 brain cells. Stroke-like symptoms that last only a few minutes may be a sign of a transient ischemic attack (TIA), or "mini-stroke." A TIA is often a warning sign of a bigger stroke to come and requires quick medical attention.

Peripheral arterial disease is atherosclerosis in arteries leading to your arms, legs, and feet. Blockages in these arteries restrict circulation. Early symptoms include cramping or fatigue in your calves or your buttocks when you're active. The discomfort, called intermittent claudication, stops when you stand still. People who have peripheral artery disease are at higher risk for heart attack and stroke because they're more likely to have blockages in the arteries that supply the heart and brain.

When to See the Doctor

Heart attacks and strokes—both the result of cardiovascular disease— are medical emergencies. Below are the most important warning signs:

HEART ATTACK

Common early symptoms:

❖ UNUSUAL FATIGUE

❖ SLEEP DISTURBANCE

❖ SHORTNESS OF BREATH

❖ INDIGESTION

❖ ANXIETY

Symptoms of an acute attack (call 911 if symptoms last more than 10 minutes):

❖ CHEST OR BACK PAIN

❖ SHORTNESS OF BREATH

❖ WEAKNESS

❖ UNUSUAL FATIGUE

❖ COLD SWEAT

❖ DIZZINESS

❖ RADIATING PAIN OR PRESSURE

STROKE (call 911 if any of these symptoms appear):

❖ SUDDEN NUMBNESS OR WEAKNESS IN THE FACE OR AN ARM OR LEG, ESPECIALLY IF IT OCCURS ON ONLY ONE SIDE OF THE BODY

❖ SUDDEN CONFUSION; TROUBLE SPEAKING OR UNDERSTANDING WHAT'S HAPPENING

❖ SUDDEN VISION PROBLEMS IN ONE OR BOTH EYES

❖ SUDDEN TROUBLE WALKING; DIZZINESS; LOSS OF BALANCE OR COORDINATION

❖ SUDDEN SEVERE HEADACHE WITH NO KNOWN CAUSE

ATTACK ALERT

Q *In the movies, you can always tell when a person is having a heart attack because he clutches his chest and falls to the floor. Is that realistic?*

A If only it were so easy to spot trouble. In fact, the symptoms of a heart attack can be much subtler, especially in women. Until recently, doctors didn't know that women's signs of a heart attack can be very different from those presented by men. As a result, many women who sought help for major heart problems were sent home and told they were just suffering from stress or anxiety. Luckily, new research is helping doctors understand the differences between male and female patients.

In a major study of female heart attack patients, 95 percent of the subjects reported noticing some unusual symptoms a month or more earlier. That's significant—paying attention to these warning signs could delay or even prevent an attack. The most common early symptoms were unusual fatigue (70 percent), sleep disturbance (48 percent), shortness of breath (42 percent), indigestion (39 percent), and anxiety (35 percent). Chest discomfort—the classic symptom you see in the movies—struck only 30 percent and was described less as a painful experience than as an ache or a feeling of tightness or pressure.

During the heart attack itself, 43 percent of the women said they had no chest pain. Those who did have pain felt it mostly in their back and high chest. Other symptoms during an attack were shortness of breath (58 percent), weakness (55 percent), unusual fatigue (43 percent), cold sweat (39 percent), and dizziness (39 percent). If you experience any of these for more than 10 minutes and they don't go away when you lie down, you should call 911 immediately. This is especially true if you're having more than one symptom. Acting quickly could save your life.

SHOULD I HAVE WAITED?

Q *When my mother had a heart attack, I drove her to the hospital myself. She did fine, but the doctors told me I should have called 911 and waited for an ambulance. Were they right?*

A Unless you live in a remote area, they were probably right. Many people think they can get to the emergency room faster if a family member

---

WOMEN AND HEART DISEASE

A 1960s conference on women and cardiovascular disease was called "How Can I Help My Husband Cope with Heart Disease?" Now we know that heart disease is just as much a woman's problem. In fact, because women live longer than men and the number of older people is growing, more women than men ultimately die of heart disease. Other stats:

◆ After age 50, more than half of all women will die of some form of cardiovascular disease.

◆ Thirty-eight percent of women will die within one year of a heart attack, compared with 25 percent of men.

◆ Within six years, 35 percent of women will have another heart attack, compared with 18 percent of men. Six percent of those women will die suddenly. Forty-six percent will be disabled with heart failure.

---

drives, but studies have shown that calling 911 and waiting for emergency medical service is usually smarter. EMS personnel are trained to begin treatment immediately, which means you get help even before arriving at the hospital. However, in an area where an ambulance won't arrive for 20 or 30 minutes and if you get to the hospital within an hour of when you first feel symptoms, doctors can do a lot to help. The cardiologist's first rule: Time is muscle. That means the longer you go without treatment, the more heart muscle you lose.

Diagnosing an Attack

Q *I know a number of people who've gone to the emergency room because they thought they were having a heart attack. But when they got there, doctors told them it was something else . . . like indigestion. How can they tell?*

A In the hospital, doctors can tell if you're having a heart attack by looking at your personal medical history, and the results of a physical exam, blood tests, and an electrocardiogram. They also watch your blood pressure and heart rate. If you're having a heart attack, the blood tests will reveal certain enzymes that are markers of damage to the heart muscle.

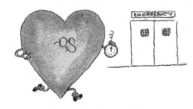

Risk Factors for Heart Disease

Your risk is determined by your age, lifestyle, family history, and overall health. The more risk factors you have, the greater your chances of heart disease. Some factors you're stuck with; others you can change.

Here's how the odds stack up:

What You're Stuck With

Age. Your risk rises as you get older. Before menopause, women are much less likely than men to have a heart attack. After menopause we lose that advantage, and by the age of 65 our chances of developing heart problems are about the same as men's.

Family history. You're at increased risk for heart disease if your father or brother was diagnosed with heart disease before age 55 or if your mother or sister was diagnosed before 65. If you have diabetes, high blood pressure, or high cholesterol in your family, your risk is even higher.

Race. From ages 44 to 64, African-American women are more likely to have a heart attack than Caucasian women. The reason isn't clear, but it could be a combination of diet and higher rates of hypertension and obesity, as well as the fact that African-American women generally do not have access to the same quality of health care as Caucasian women do.

What You Can Change

Smoking. You can't do much about your age or family history, but you *can* stop smoking. More than half of all heart attacks in women under 50 are smoking-related. (Your chances of a heart attack are even higher if you take birth-control pills and smoke.) Quitting smoking lowers your risk by a third within two years.

Diabetes. If you have diabetes, your chances of a heart attack may triple. Diabetic women are likely to be overweight with cholesterol problems and are at greater risk for developing atherosclero-

Different enzymes show up at different times in the attack cycle, indicating what phase of the attack you're in. Other tests measure the level of cardiac muscle proteins released when your heart expands and contracts; this is another marker of an attack. One thing to learn from the sophistication of these tests is that you shouldn't be diagnosing yourself. If you think there's something wrong, get to the E.R. and let the doctors decide whether it's serious or not.

THE CHOLESTEROL TEST

Q *I'm 51 and have never had a cholesterol test, but my new internist wants me to get one. I'm not overweight, I've always exercised regularly, and I feel fine. Why do I need this test?*

A Your internist is following current guidelines, which say you should be screened at least every five years for high cholesterol starting at

sis and blood clots. Diabetes is a more common cause of coronary heart disease among women than among men. After 45, more women than men have diabetes. Losing weight and keeping your diabetes under control improves your odds.

High blood pressure. Hypertension, or high blood pressure, is associated with narrowing of the arteries. It puts extra stress on the artery walls and the heart muscle. Untreated hypertension can enlarge and weaken your heart, which can lead to irregular heartbeats. Before age 55, more men than women have high blood pressure, but women 75 and older have higher blood pressure than men their age. Current recommendations are to keep blood pressure below 120/80. You can get your blood pressure under control through diet, exercise, and medication.

Cholesterol. High cholesterol means a high risk, especially if you're obese and don't exercise. Younger women tend to have lower cholesterol than men of the

same age, but around age 45 a higher percentage of women than men have borderline or high cholesterol. You can lower your cholesterol by losing weight, getting more exercise, eating more wisely, and possibly taking a cholesterol-lowering medication. (See Appendix I.)

Obesity. Too much weight raises your cholesterol and puts an extra strain on your heart. The heavier you are, the higher your risk. In the United States, this is an enormous public health problem. Nearly two-thirds of American women over 20 are overweight and about a third of them are obese. Losing weight reduces your risk dramatically.

Sedentary lifestyle. For women, not exercising is just as bad as smoking or having high blood pressure or high cholesterol levels. You need to get moving! The current recommendation is at least 30 minutes of moderately intense physical activity every day of the week. More is even better. (For suggestions, see Chapter 14.)

Testing for Heart Disease

There are many different tests that doctors can use to see whether your heart is working properly. The four tests below can shed light on the current health of your heart.

Stress test. For this test, you walk on a treadmill or pedal a stationary bicycle. If you can't exercise for some reason, you'll get a medication that increases blood flow to your heart (simulating the effect of exercise). Either way, your doctor will get a picture of what happens when your heart is working extra hard.

Electrocardiograph. This machine produces a graph of your heart's electrical activity. It's often used in the emergency room to detect abnormal heartbeats, problems with blood flowing to the heart, or damage to the heart muscle. Your doctor may also give you this test as part of your annual physical just to establish a baseline.

Echocardiograph. An echo translates sound waves into an image that shows your heart's size, shape, and movement. It's similar to the ultrasound used during pregnancy, but instead of seeing a fetus *in utero*, the patient gets to see her heart in motion.

Halter monitor. Tiny electrodes applied to your chest record your heart's activity over a 24-hour period. The electrodes hook into a monitor that you wear with a strap over your shoulder. It's less cumbersome than it sounds; if you wear a loose sweater, no one will know you have it on.

---

age 20. Until you're tested, you won't know whether you have a problem or not. Cholesterol can be building up in your arteries without any symptoms. Your healthy lifestyle lowers your risk, but it doesn't let you off the hook completely. There might be high cholesterol in your family, which means your levels could be unhealthy even if you're doing everything right. Your age is also a factor. Before menopause, women are much less likely than men to get heart attacks. After menopause, your risk rises dramatically. That's why this is a great time to take charge of your heart health. If your cholesterol is high, your doctor can help you figure out how diet, exercise, and perhaps medication can bring down your numbers. If the test shows that you're doing fine, keep up the good work but don't neglect getting tested on a regular basis.

Cholesterol Demystified

Q *Everybody talks about cholesterol, but I'm not sure what it is and why it's so bad for me. Can you explain?*

A Cholesterol is a lipid: a soft, waxy substance found in all your cells. It does get a lot of bad press, but it's actually critical to your health—helping to make cell membranes, some hormones,

GOOD GUYS AND BAD GUYS

So you just got your cholesterol report and you're seeing numbers that have to do with LDLs, HDLs, and triglycerides. What do they mean?

Your blood tests give your doctor your total cholesterol, which is the sum of your low-density lipoprotein (LDL) cholesterol, high-density lipoprotein (HDL) cholesterol, and triglycerides (blood fats). LDL is the cholesterol that ends up in the lining of your arteries. HDL acts as a kind of scavenger, cleaning up the mess made by LDL and other substances. When you overeat or drink too much, the excess calories are converted into triglycerides, which can be stored as fat; a high triglyceride level raises your risk of cardiovascular disease.

The chart below will help you figure out where you stand. The numbers in the left column are milligrams per deciliter of blood (mg/dl).

	RISK CATEGORY
Total Cholesterol	
Less than 200	Desirable
200 to 239	Borderline high
240 and above	High
LDL Cholesterol	
Below 70	Goal for high-risk patients
Below 100	Optimal
100 to 129	Near optimal
130 to 159	Borderline high
160 to 189	High
190 and above	Very high
HDL Cholesterol	
Below 40	Low
50 and above	Desirable*
Triglycerides	
Below 150	Normal
150 to 199	Borderline high
200 to 499	High
500 and above	Very high

*The most recent research says that women should maintain an HDL of at least 50; even higher is better.

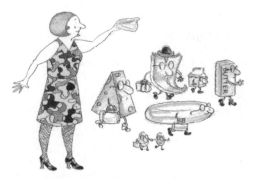

vitamin D, and other vital components. Most of the cholesterol you need is produced by your liver. You get more when you eat food that comes from animals (things like eggs, meat, and whole-milk products). Food from plants does not contain cholesterol. When you eat too much cholesterol-rich food, the excess can land in the lining of your arteries. This builds up into plaque, which narrows your blood vessels. You're at risk for a heart attack or stroke when plaque ruptures and produces a blood clot.

FASTING BEFORE TESTING

Q *My doctor told me I had to fast before my cholesterol test, but a friend of mine ate normally before hers. Are there two kinds of tests?*

A If your friend didn't have any risk factors for heart disease, her doctor probably just wanted to see two numbers: her total cholesterol and her LDL level. Fasting isn't required for that. If her numbers are high, she'll have to get the more detailed test that your doctor has ordered for you, either because you've had high cholesterol in the past or

because you have other risk factors such as smoking, diabetes, or a family history of heart disease. This more detailed test requires that you fast (no eating or drinking) for at least nine hours beforehand. The results include your total cholesterol along with your LDL, HDL, and triglycerides.

GENDER MATTERS: PART I

Q *I know that my risk of a heart attack before menopause isn't as high as my husband's. Why is that?*

A It's true that before menopause women are less likely to suffer a heart attack. Scientists think that estrogen helps to keep blood vessels healthy, although the exact mechanism is not yet completely understood. We do know that premenopausal women produce more HDL cholesterol (the good kind) than men and postmenopausal women and less LDL cholesterol (the bad kind). HDL forages through your blood vessels, scooping up bad stuff (like LDL cholesterol) that can cause plaque. By 10 years after menopause, a woman's heart attack risk has jumped dramatically.

For years, doctors thought taking estrogen would help older women keep the advantage that younger women have. However, that theory was largely dispelled by the Women's Health Initiative, which showed that taking estrogen after menopause did not stop heart disease and may, in fact, have exacerbated it in some women. Current recommendations say that estrogen (either alone or in combination with a progestogen if you have a uterus) should be prescribed only to ease menopausal symptoms like hot flashes.

If you're still pre- or perimenopausal, don't get too complacent. Younger women (especially those who are overweight, who smoke, or who have diabetes) do get heart attacks. And when they do, they die of them more often than men of the same age. One possible reason is that both doctors and women themselves don't expect to see heart disease in a younger woman and ignore or misdiagnose warning signs. Another possibility is that the damage caused by smoking or obesity overrides any advantages you get from estrogen. Bottom line? The best time to think about your heart health in your 60s is when you're in your 40s. Start eating right and exercising now, and chances are you'll have fewer problems in the future.

LOWERING LIPIDS

Q My bad cholesterol is high. How can I lower it without drugs?

A Your doctor may put you on medication immediately if you're at very high risk because of your cholesterol and other factors such as smoking, a family history of heart disease, or a previous heart attack. But if your risk is only moderate or low, lifestyle measures should usually come first (and you'll have to continue them even if you do eventually take cholesterol-lowering medication).

Start with your diet. Limit your fat intake to less than 35 percent of your total calories and your saturated and trans fats to less than 10 percent of the total. Your total daily cholesterol should not exceed 300 milligrams. Saturated and trans fats are found in hard margarine and cheese, shortening, some cooking oils, fatty meat, egg yolks, and full-fat dairy products. Foods that are low in cholesterol and saturated fats include lean meat, fish, skinless poultry, whole-grain foods, and fruits and vegetables. Many food products have labels that you can check to see how much fat and cholesterol you get in each serving. You should also look for certain foods, like cholesterol-lowering margarine, that will reduce your LDL levels. Another way to lower cholesterol is to increase the amount of soluble fiber you eat. You get that from oats, fruits like oranges and pears, and vegetables such as Brussels sprouts and carrots, as well as dried peas and beans. If this change in diet doesn't lower your LDL in three months, your doctor may recommend that you go even further, lowering your total daily cholesterol to less than 200 milligrams and your saturated fat intake to less than 7 percent of your total daily calories.

You should also try to lose weight and increase your level of physical activity. Being overweight increases your cholesterol and is a major risk factor for heart disease. Losing weight can lower your LDL, raise your HDL, and lower your triglycerides. This doesn't necessarily mean dropping 40 or 50 pounds. Even a 10 percent weight loss could lower your cholesterol levels. A sedentary lifestyle is another major risk factor even if you're not overweight. So start exercising! Thirty minutes of moderate to intense physical activity every day is good, and, as we keep reminding you, more is better. You don't have to lift heavy weights or run a marathon, although you might consider signing up for classes you'd enjoy, such as dancing or skating. If time is your problem, remember that walking briskly, climbing stairs, even heavy housecleaning all count. You might also invest in a pedometer. They're not expensive (about $25). Aim for 10,000 steps a day. The main thing is to pick something that you enjoy enough to do regularly.

If none of these efforts is adequate, medication is probably the next step.

GENDER MATTERS: PART II

Q *What about the risks after menopause? Should my cholesterol levels be the same as those of a man my age?*

A The research is ongoing, but there is evidence that HDL cholesterol is more important for women than for men. That's why the American Heart Association recommends that women's HDL levels should be at least 50 mg/dl,

compared with 40 mg/dl for men. In any case, the more HDL cholesterol you have, the better it is for your arteries, because HDL gets rid of the bad stuff that can get into your arterial lining. In premenopausal women, a high level of total cholesterol is a major risk factor. After menopause, the combination of high triglycerides and low HDL is more dangerous. You can see why it's important for you to understand your total cholesterol picture if your doctor tells you you're at risk.

HOT FLASH RELIEF

Q *If there's a history of heart disease or stroke in my family, can I use hormone therapy to relieve my hot flashes?*

A This is something you should discuss with your doctor. The answer depends on your age, your overall health, and the age at which your family members suffered from heart disease. If they were older (over 65 in women, over 55 in men), family history may be less of a factor. However, if your cholesterol is high and you're a smoker, have a significant problem with overweight, or have diabetes, your doctor probably will not want you to take hormone therapy. Fortunately, there are a number of lifestyle changes you can make to get relief from hot flashes (see Chapter 3).

The Women's Health Initiative did not test the short-term risks and benefits of using hormone therapy to treat menopausal symptoms like hot flashes. Most of the women in the study were also older (the average age was 63) and 12 years past menopause (when they would be unlikely to get hot flashes). More research is currently underway to test the effects of short-term hormone therapy in younger women during the menopause transition. Some scientists think that estrogen may be helpful when you're younger but harmful when you're older. Until researchers know more, women have to make this decision on an individual basis with their doctors.

FOOD LABELING

Q *It's bad enough that my eyesight is going. Now I have to struggle to read those labels on food packages to find out the kind of fat I'm about to eat. Save my eyes! What do I really need to look for?*

A Saturated fats and trans fats are your targets. Saturated fats have been on food labels in the United States for some time, but trans fat wasn't required until 2006. It's now right below saturated fat on the label. Together, they make up the "total fat" component.

Trans fat is formed when manufacturers add hydrogen to unsaturated vegetable oils to make them more solid and increase their shelf life. This is called hydrogenation,

and it's part of almost all commercial food processing. You'll find trans fat in everything from frozen pizza to chocolate-chip cookies. It also occurs naturally in some dairy products, as well as beef and pork.

Trans fat is bad because it raises LDL and lowers HDL. A high level of trans fat in your diet significantly increases your chances of having a heart attack. The connection is so clear that Denmark has banned all hydrogenated food. Imagine—banned by an entire country! There is *no safe level,* so cut out as much as you possibly can. If you're not at high risk for heart disease, you should have no more than 20 grams daily of both kinds of fats. If you *are* at risk, stick to less than 15.5 grams a day. We know squinting at those labels is a pain, but your heart will thank you.

WHAT ABOUT WINE?

Q *I don't normally drink wine, but I keep reading stories about how red wine wards off heart disease. Should I be drinking a glass a day?*

A When this idea first gained currency, it was often called "the French paradox" because it appeared to explain why French people, who regularly drink a glass of wine with meals, have a lower rate of heart disease than Americans do. But subsequent research has yet to show any special cardiovascular

ANTIOXIDANTS AND FREE RADICALS

Today, it seems that just about every product on supermarket shelves is advertising its antioxidants. But what exactly are they? And why do you need them?

These natural compounds, which include some vitamins and minerals, are needed to fight free radicals, oxygen-based substances that are formed naturally in your body as a by-product of normal cellular function or that hit you from environmental sources such as cigarette smoke. If their effects aren't balanced by adequate antioxidants, they roam through your body and damage cells. How is this related to heart disease? Oxygen added to LDL cholesterol promotes plaque in your arteries.

Research is ongoing, but the current thinking is that the best way to get antioxidants is from food (not supplements), especially fruit, vegetables, and whole grains. The table below lists some good food sources of antioxidants.

ANTIOXIDANT	FOOD SOURCES
Vitamin C	Citrus fruits and their juices, berries, dark green vegetables (spinach, asparagus, green peppers, Brussels sprouts, broccoli, watercress, other greens), red and yellow peppers, tomatoes and tomato juice, pineapple, cantaloupe, mangoes, papaya, guava
Vitamin E	Vegetable oils (olive, soybean, corn, cottonseed, safflower), nuts and nut butters, seeds, whole grains, wheat, wheat germ, brown rice, oatmeal, soybeans, sweet potatoes, legumes (beans, lentils, split peas), leafy dark green vegetables
Beta-carotene	Carrots, squash, broccoli, kale, sweet potatoes, tomatoes, red and yellow peppers, collard greens, cantaloupe, mangoes
Selenium	Many vegetables, fish, shellfish, red meat, chicken, garlic, Brazil nuts, brewer's yeast, oatmeal, brown rice, dairy products, molasses, onions, wheat germ, whole grains

benefits from drinking red wine. In fact, all kinds of alcohol can hurt your heart if you drink too much, which is currently defined as more than one drink a day for women. (A drink is one 12-ounce beer, 4 ounces of wine, 1.5 ounces of 80-proof spirits, or 1 ounce of 100-proof spirits.) When you drink, you're taking in calories with no nutritional value. Moreover, too much alcohol can lead to high blood pressure, heart failure, and increased levels of triglycerides.

There's even evidence that excess alcohol increases your risk of breast cancer. For all these reasons and more, the American Heart Association says that nondrinkers should *not* start drinking alcohol of any kind in order to receive cardiovascular benefits.

That said, the French paradox may not be entirely wishful thinking. A number of studies have shown an association between moderate drinking and lower chances of death from heart disease. What could explain this link? Flavonoids (naturally occurring compounds in food that comes from plants) and other antioxidants in red wine may help lower the formation of plaque in arteries. Before you start guzzling, however, consider that you can get some of these same benefits from grapes or grape juice. Lifestyle factors may also explain why wine drinkers in France and elsewhere have healthier hearts. Maybe they're more physically active or eat more fruit and vegetables. A few studies have shown that alcohol (not necessarily wine) can slightly raise HDL cholesterol (the good kind) and possibly reduce the risk of blood clots. But again, the evidence isn't strong enough for the American Heart Association to recommend drinking for those goals. You're much better off sticking to the tried-and-true methods of exercising regularly, eating a healthy diet, and controlling your blood pressure, weight, and cholesterol. And if you decide to go ahead and drink a glass of wine occasionally with dinner, that's fine, too.

WEIGHTY MATTERS

Q *What's the connection between weight and heart disease? And how can I tell how much I need to lose to lower my risk?*

A The bigger and heavier you are, the harder it is for your heart to pump blood to the rest of your body. Obesity also raises your risk of heart disease by increasing your chances of getting diabetes, elevating your blood pressure, increasing your LDL cholesterol and triglycerides, and lowering your HDL cholesterol.

But your weight doesn't tell the whole story. Where your body stores excess fat is also important. If you carry weight around your abdomen (in other words, you're apple-shaped), you may have a higher risk of heart disease than a woman who's heavy in the hips and thighs (pear-shaped). That's why you should pay attention to your waistline. If it measures more than 35 inches, you're considered at risk for heart disease. That number should probably be lower if you're petite, so doctors also look at the hip-to-waist ratio. If your waist is almost as large or larger then your hips, you need to lose weight.

WHY WE LIKE CHOCOLATE

Q *I know this sounds nuts, but I read in a magazine that chocolate might be good for your heart. Is that possible?*

A As certified chocoholics, we're happy to say yes! Of course, that doesn't mean you can gorge on a boxful of bonbons. Chocolate contains flavonols, which are also found in apples, onions, and green tea. Flavonols help to relax blood vessels, improve blood flow, and decrease blood clotting. They have also been shown to reduce inflammation. Researchers think that someday cocoa flavonols might even be used to treat diabetes, stroke, and a kind of dementia. Of course, there's a catch! Flavonol is the reason chocolate is bitter. Not so great for those of us with a serious sweet tooth. Your best bet is to choose a dark chocolate (like a semisweet or bittersweet) that is high in cacao and lower in fat and sugar. For example, Dove dark chocolate has 150 milligrams of flavonols in 1.3 ounces, compared with 42 milligrams in the same amount of milk chocolate. Even with its health benefits, chocolate should still be considered a treat. Limit yourself to no more than an ounce a few times a week.

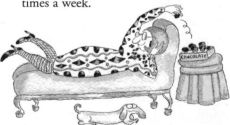

NO SMOKING

Q *I'm trying to get my sister to quit smoking, but I can't seem to get through to her. What can I tell her about the relationship between smoking and heart health?*

A Your sister probably knows that smoking is bad for her, but maybe she doesn't realize just *how* bad it is. Tell her the facts. Women who smoke are two to six times more likely to have a heart attack than women who don't smoke. And she doesn't have to finish the pack. Even smoking just one to four cigarettes a day could triple her risk of heart attack. According to one study, 72 percent of women who had a heart attack in their early 30s were smokers. When you smoke, the chemicals in cigarettes damage your coronary arteries, leading to atherosclerosis. Smoking makes the blood more likely to form the clots that lead to heart attacks. Smoking can also trigger coronary spasms that constrict the heart's blood vessels, again causing heart attacks. The nicotine in cigarettes can raise your blood pressure, adding to the risk. Smokers tend to have an unhealthy cholesterol profile: high triglycerides and LDL cholesterol (the bad kind) and low HDL cholesterol (the good kind). Cigarette smoking even reduces women's levels of estrogen, which protects us against heart and bone disease before menopause.

And if none of those arguments works, try this one: Women who smoke look older prematurely. They're more likely to get wrinkles at an early age, especially lines around the mouth. Maybe vanity will do the trick.

GET MOVING

Q *I know exercise is good for you, but how exactly does it help your heart? And how much is enough?*

A Exercise not only decreases your chances of a first heart attack by strengthening your heart muscle, but controls weight gain, lowers blood pressure, and improves cholesterol levels as well. It also reduces stress, another risk factor we're all very familiar with at midlife. But only *regular* exercise delivers these benefits. See if you can incorporate physical activity even short bursts—into every aspect of your life.

If you're at high risk for heart disease and have been inactive for many years, consult your doctor before starting any exercise plan. In rare cases, excessive exercise after years of inactivity can trigger a heart attack. Your doctor will suggest ways to slowly increase your fitness level.

STILL ON THE PILL

Q *I'm perimenopausal and still ovulating, so I'm on the pill. Does this increase my risk of a heart attack?*

A Today's birth-control pills have a lower dose of estrogen (35 micrograms) than in the past and are generally safe. However, if you smoke, you should quit or get off the pill, especially if you're

THE BENEFITS OF ASPIRIN

A ccording to the Women's Health Study, a 10-year study of nearly 40,000 healthy women aged 45 and older, aspirin doesn't protect women the way it does men. This came as somewhat of a surprise to researchers when the study results were published in 2005. Before then, many doctors had been advising women to take aspirin based on the results of studies on men. Now they know that a woman's age makes a difference in the effectiveness of aspirin against cardiovascular disease. In women 45 and older, aspirin did slightly lower the risk of ischemic stroke (the kind of stroke caused by a blood clot). Men don't get that benefit. However, women in the study got no significant protection from heart attacks until they reached age 65. The researchers found that between ages 45 and 65, aspirin's benefit for women doesn't outweigh the risk that it can cause gastrointestinal bleeding. Whether or not aspirin is a good idea for you depends on your heart disease risk factors and your medical history. Even though aspirin is an over-the-counter medication, don't start taking it without talking to your doctor about how it might help or hurt you.

over 35. If you've had blood clots, a heart attack, a stroke, or any cardiovascular disease, you shouldn't be on the pill. If you have high blood pressure, you need to get it checked regularly if you're on the pill. Your risk for hypertension while on oral contraceptives or the patch also increases if you're over 35, are obese, have a family history of high blood pressure, or have mild kidney disease. You need to talk to your doctor about whether the pill is the best form of birth control for you at this point in your life, considering your own particular medical history.

FAMILY HISTORY

Q *My mother, who was a smoker, died of a heart attack at 48. I'm 46, and my doctor says I'm doing fine. I don't smoke, I'm not overweight, and I exercise fairly regularly. Still, I worry. How important is heredity in heart disease?*

A Even if you don't smoke, your mother's early death could make you twice as likely to have a heart attack as someone without that history. Heredity can play a role in the way you metabolize cholesterol, especially how fast LDL cholesterol is removed from your blood. Unfortunately, your family history is one risk factor you can't control. It should, however, give you extra motivation to keep yourself on track by exercising, eating well, and getting regular heart checkups.

THE EYES HAVE IT

Q *I recently went to have my eyes checked, and my ophthalmologist said I should be checked for high blood pressure. What could he have seen that concerned him? My vision is fine.*

A Your ophthalmologist may have seen some early warning signs of hypertension in your retinas at the back of your eyes. High blood pressure can cause small blood vessels in the retinas to become constricted. If the pressure is very high over an extended period of time, the blood vessels can leak and ultimately hamper your vision. As long as the damage is mild, you probably aren't noticing anything. This condition, called hypertensive retinopathy, is linked to a higher risk of heart failure, especially in women. You're lucky your ophthalmologist caught it early. Now, with your regular doctor's help, you can get your blood pressure under control.

STRESSED OUT

Q *Everyone I know feels some stress at this point in life, but I assume we don't all have the same risk for heart disease. Are some kinds of stress more dangerous than others?*

A Women respond to stress in different ways. Some feel anger and hostility; others get depressed. Neither response is good for your heart. When you're stressed, your blood pressure rises. When your stress level stays high, your blood pressure stays high, too. And that's what causes problems for your heart. Prolonged hypertension damages your blood vessels, making them vulnerable to atherosclerosis. Stress hormones also increase your cholesterol levels, affect your blood clotting, and raise your level of homocysteine, an amino acid that has been linked to damaged arteries. And now most women work outside the home, adding even more potential stress. Some studies say the greatest stress is on women in low-paying jobs where they feel they have no control. But other studies say women executives are three times more likely to get heart disease than women in jobs with low authority. One thing is certain: Women who work outside the home also work inside the home, which means they're doing a double shift. And speaking of shifts, women who work the night shift have a higher risk of heart disease because of stress.

So what can you do about too much stress in your life? Relaxation exercises and meditation can work. Exercise also reduces tension. Anything you can do that gives you a break from your regular routine—even for just a little while—can be helpful. Instead of feeling that your life is out of control, take charge of making yourself feel better.

DEPRESSION AND THE HEART

Q *I'm 56, and I've had several bouts with depression—all treated with medication. Does this have any effect on my risk of heart disease?*

A Your treatment for depression could literally make a lifesaving difference, since postmenopausal women with a history of depression do appear to be at increased risk for cardiovascular disease. And then, after being diagnosed with heart or circulatory problems, they're more likely to die within a relatively short period.

Since studies of depression and heart disease have focused mostly on men, researchers are still trying to figure out the connection in women, but certain links have been successfully identified. To begin with, depressed women weigh more, and obesity is a known risk factor for heart attacks. Also, a 2004 study at the Duke University Medical Center found that depressed women with heart disease are more likely to have variable heartbeats, a risk for potentially fatal heart arrhythmias. Lack of exercise is another factor, which makes sense since depressed people are more likely to be sedentary.

In the Duke study, depressed patients woke up more often at night, raising the possibility that stressful sleep might be contributing to their heart problems. Also, after a heart attack, depressed women report getting less social support from those around them (perhaps because their emotional problems strained their relationships). A strong social network improves the chances of recovery in both men and women.

All of the above should reinforce the message that depression is a real disease with significant consequences for overall health. Treating it is essential. (For more detailed information on this subject, see Chapter 8.)

Affairs of the Heart

Q *Most of the time, I consider myself happily married, but every once in a while I get so mad at my husband that I feel like my blood pressure is skyrocketing. Is that possible?*

A It certainly is. Even brief periods of marital strife can raise your blood pressure. If the rocky times persist, you could be at increased risk of heart disease. Persistent hypertension damages blood vessels and ultimately heart muscle. A 2005 study offered more evidence of the dangers of an unhappy relationship. Researchers found that arguing a lot could slow healing. That delay, they suggest, was caused by prolonged changes in levels of certain proteins necessary for wound healing. A long-term lack of these proteins has been linked to heart disease as well as cancer, arthritis, type 2 diabetes, and depression.

Long-term unhappy marriages can be responsible for serious health consequences. Researchers from the University of Pittsburgh and San Diego State University looked at data for more than 400 healthy women who were followed for 13 years before and after menopause. They found that marital dissatisfaction tripled a woman's chances of having metabolic syndrome, a group of heart risk factors. Only widows were more likely to have metabolic syndrome than the unhappy wives; even divorced and single women had better health risk profiles.

Unhappiness at home can even be fatal after a heart attack. A Swedish study found that women with coronary heart disease had a greater risk of recurrence if they had severe stress in their marriages or live-in relationships. The researchers said that emotional strain and lack of support from a partner may mean that a woman is less likely to stick with heart healthy behavior and may not seek essential medical support.

Before you kick your husband out, consider this: Several studies have shown that good marriages help keep women healthy. It's not just the absence of relationship stress (although that's certainly a factor). Women in happy marriages have strong social support, which generally encourages healthier behaviors. In fact, researchers have found that women in positive relationships actually benefit from spending more time with their partners.

What should you take away from all this? Keep hostility in check. All couples argue, but when you engage in "tit-for-tat" behavior, things really escalate. Cut that off early. One marital stress expert suggests that when you reach an impasse, you might say, "We really see this differently" rather than "You idiot! How could you possibly think that?"

CHAPTER 13

Cancer

Nobody likes to think about cancer. And the fact that this disease becomes more common as you get older (about 80 percent of all cancers are diagnosed after age 54) isn't making you feel any better. But your best defense against "the big C" is knowledge. While most women know that a lump is a warning sign of breast cancer, 47 percent of the women surveyed by the Women's Cancer Network could not name *a single symptom* of gynecological cancer, and 58 percent didn't know of any way to decrease their risks.

Perhaps you'd like to take a moment and read that last sentence again, because the information in it is shocking. And then, when you've had a chance to absorb it, you should start reviewing your cancer facts and getting current about prevention strategies. Make sure you understand your specific cancer risks, based on your personal and family history. Learn more about the complicated relationship between hormones and cancer. Read up on the warning signs of cancer (all detailed in the following pages) and know what screening tests are available. Realize that this is an excellent time to make changes in lifestyle and diet, which are related to an estimated 50 to 75 percent of all cancers. While no one can (or should) offer you guarantees, you can do a lot to lower your risk of getting cancer.

WHAT YOU NEED
TO KNOW

Let's start with the basics. Menopause doesn't cause cancer. It doesn't even increase your risk of getting cancer. But the levels of hormones in your body (what your ovaries produce naturally, as well as what you take via pills and patches) have a relationship to cancer . . . and a complicated one at that. Over the course of your life, hormones appear to be protective against some cancers, while increasing your risk of developing others.

BREAST CANCER. A woman's risk of developing breast cancer is related to her cumulative exposure to estrogen, as well as her breasts' sensitivity to the hormone. For example, women who started menstruating at a young age (before 12) as well as those whose menopause came late (after 55) have about a 50 percent higher chance of developing breast cancer than women whose periods started later or who reached menopause earlier. Women who have never been pregnant (or who got pregnant for the first time after age 30) are also at increased risk for breast cancer, presumably because they were exposed to more estrogen when they were young. In addition, breast tissue has the ability to concentrate, produce, and metabolize estrogen, which means there is often 10 to 40 times more estrogen in the breasts than the level circulating in the blood.

Estrogen interacts with breast tissue through estrogen receptors—proteins in

What Can Happen

◆ As cells get older, they become more vulnerable to cancer. This is not the time to get sloppy about annual checkups or to stop getting your mammograms and Pap smears. It *is* the time to add a colonoscopy to your screening list.

◆ If you're not using menopausal hormone therapy, mammograms will become more effective since breasts become less dense as estrogen levels drop.

◆ Fluctuating hormone levels may cause you to have more breast cysts, which can easily be confused with tumors. All lumps need to be checked out.

◆ A typical menopause transition includes changes that mimic some of the warning signs of cancer (such as abnormal bleeding patterns, pain during intercourse, and abdominal weight gain). Don't panic, but also don't assume it's just menopause. Make sure your doctor is aware of the body changes you're experiencing. If symptoms continue, be sure to keep mentioning them.

cells that act like docking stations for the estrogen circulating in your body. When estrogen docks at a receptor, it can encourage the cell to proliferate. Most of the time, cell division produces more healthy breast tissue. But cells that contain cancer-causing mutations can proliferate and grow to become tumors. Cancer cells that grow faster when exposed to estrogen are called "hormone receptor positive." (Not all tumors are sensitive to estrogen. After a biopsy, your doctor will tell you if your tumor fits this description.) Estrogen may also cause changes in cells that can eventually lead to cancer.

That's why breast cancer treatment often includes drugs like tamoxifen and raloxifene, which greatly reduce the effect of estrogen on cancer cells. In addition, surgically removing both ovaries (the body's chief source of estrogen) from pre-menopausal women rivals chemotherapy as an effective treatment for reducing recurrences and mortality in women with estrogen-receptive tumors. The fact that some cancer cells grow more rapidly when exposed to estrogen also explains why doctors discourage most breast cancer survivors from taking supplemental estrogen in the form of hormone therapy to treat hot flashes and night sweats.

Sounds straightforward enough, doesn't it? But it's not. Take, for instance, the confounding data that combined hormone therapy (estrogen and a progestogen) increases the risk of breast cancer for women who still have a uterus but estrogen-only therapy doesn't increase risk for women whose uterus has been removed. (This topic is discussed in greater detail later in this chapter.)

ENDOMETRIAL CANCER. Estrogen encourages growth of the uterine lining (the endometrium) and a progestogen prompts the body to slough off this buildup, a natural process you typically experience as a menstrual period. If you're postmenopausal and taking estrogen to treat hot flashes, you need to add enough progesterone to ensure that your uterine lining doesn't become overgrown and ripe for cancer growth. (If your uterus has been surgically removed, you don't have to worry about this.) Some women with an intact uterus don't want to take a progestogen because they don't like the way it makes them feel. (Common complaints include uterine bleeding, bloating, headaches, and irritability.) However, not taking a progestogen, even for a short time, may triple your risk of cancer. After three years of unopposed estrogen, a woman's risk of developing endometrial cancer increases fivefold; even after she stops the estrogen supplements, the risk persists for years afterwards. While we're on the topic, we should add that a woman with an intact uterus who takes meno-pausal hormone therapy that includes both estrogen and progesterone has a lower risk of developing endometrial cancer than a woman who takes no supplemental hormones at all.

LUNG CANCER. Estrogen may accelerate the growth of lung tumors. (Cells harvested from some women's lung tumors have been covered with estrogen receptors.) This may explain why a recent study published in the *Journal of Clinical Oncology* of 500 women with lung cancer found that those who had used hormone therapy didn't survive as long as those who had never used it.

Some preliminary studies also indicate that women who reach menopause prematurely (before age 40) tend to be at lower risk for lung cancer than women who reach it later. One more thing: Women with a genetic mutation known as K-ras may develop lung cancer that grows more aggressively in response to exposure to estrogen. Such mutations are sometimes inherited, but in other cases they develop as a result of cigarette smoking or secondhand smoke.

OVARIAN CANCER. Taking oral contraceptives premenopausally seems to reduce the risk of developing ovarian cancer, while the effect of postmenopausal hormone therapy is unclear. Using estrogen-only therapy for 10 years or more may increase the risk slightly.

COLORECTAL CANCER. Taking oral contraceptives or combined hormone therapy seems to lower the incidence of colorectal cancer in women. (Estrogen-

When to See the Doctor

If you experience any of these symptoms, check with your physician:

- ❖ ANY SPOTTING OR BLEEDING AFTER MENOPAUSE
- ❖ ANY CHANGES IN THE BREASTS, INCLUDING LUMPS OR THICKENING, DIFFERENCES IN CONTOUR, DIMPLING OF THE SKIN, DISCHARGE FROM THE NIPPLE (EITHER CLEAR OR BLOODY), OR RETRACTION OF THE NIPPLE
- ❖ ABNORMAL BLEEDING, INCLUDING SPOTTING, BLEEDING BETWEEN PERIODS, AND HEAVY BLEEDING WITH CLOTTING
- ❖ PERSISTENT ABDOMINAL DISCOMFORT, INCLUDING CRAMPING, BLOATING, GAS, DISTENTION, PRESSURE, ENLARGEMENT, AND STOMACH UPSET
- ❖ PAIN OR BLEEDING DURING OR AFTER INTERCOURSE
- ❖ PERSISTENT INTESTINAL OR PELVIC PAIN OR DISCOMFORT
- ❖ ANY FOUL-SMELLING OR PINK (OR BLOOD-STREAKED) DISCHARGE
- ❖ PAINFUL URINATION OR BLOOD IN URINE
- ❖ FREQUENT URGE TO URINATE
- ❖ VAGINAL ITCHING AND BURNING THAT DOESN'T RESPOND TO TREATMENT
- ❖ APPEARANCE OF ANY LUMPS OR SORES (RED, WHITE, DARK, RAISED) IN THE VULVAR OR VAGINAL REGION
- ❖ RECTAL BLEEDING
- ❖ UNEXPLAINED WEIGHT GAIN OR WEIGHT LOSS
- ❖ CHEST PAIN THAT DOESN'T GO AWAY
- ❖ A PERSISTENT AND WORSENING COUGH

only therapy seems to have virtually no effect.) However, if tumors do develop, they tend to be larger in women taking combined hormone therapy. It's also worth noting that while hormones may make a difference in the colorectal cancer risk for most women, taking them doesn't seem to lower the odds for those at high risk for the disease because of their family history.

Menopause's Mixed Signals

Scan through the list of cancer symptoms and it suddenly hits you: They include some of menopause's most common markers. Take abnormal bleeding. Just about every perimenopausal woman experiences it. So how do you deal with the fact that it's also the most obvious symptom of endometrial cancer? And what about pain during intercourse or abdominal weight gain? Do they mean you need a cancer scan?

The good news: It's not your job to figure this out. However, it *is* your job to mention these changes to your doctor—and to keep mentioning them if they persist, even if repeated screens or tests or biopsies come back negative. Many gynecological cancers can grow slowly and may take years to get big enough to be detected. Specialists in women's cancers say it's not uncommon for a premalignant growth to be detected on the second, third, or *fourth* round of testing. So you're not being a hypochondriac if you keep mentioning a symptom that isn't going away or has you worried.

Your doctor needs to know what you're experiencing and needs to hear it from *you*—one of the best sources of information about your own body. The partnership you have with your doctor isn't going to work if you don't speak up.

Sometimes it's not fear of being ridiculed that prevents us from mentioning symptoms. It's our fear of what a doctor might ultimately find. Take comfort in the fact that, chances are, whatever you're experiencing is not proof of cancer. Even a worrisome symptom— say, postmenopausal bleeding in a 50-year-old—turns out to be endometrial cancer only about 9 percent of the time. (An infection or fibroid, both of which can be treated, is the usual cause.)

But even if it turns out that you have cancer, it's certainly better to find it as soon as possible. Early detection is the best way to start a successful cancer fight. (For more details, see Appendix I.)

WEB WISE

Worried about your risk of developing cancer? The Women's Cancer Network offers an interactive risk assessment tool on its website that personalizes your odds (low, average, or high) of developing a range of cancers, including breast, ovarian, endometrial, cervical, vulvar, and vaginal, based on your answers to 101 questions. To check it out, go to www.wcn.org and click on "risk assessment."

The Cancer Detectives

Screens are tests given by doctors to look for signs of cancer in people who don't have symptoms. They're often the most effective way of discerning the earliest signs that cancer is developing. While there are no screens yet for many cancers (ovarian, lung, bladder), you'd be wise to take advantage of the screening techniques that are currently available.

Breast Cancer Detection

Mammogram: a type of X-ray that can detect suspicious changes in the breast as well as lumps up to two years or more before they can be felt.

A technician places the breast between two metal plates and then presses them together to get a clear image. The pressure is often uncomfortable but usually not painful. The risk associated with the amount of radiation you're exposed to during a mammogram is very small. Most doctors recommend that women begin to get annual mammograms starting between ages 40 and 50, partly because breasts become less dense as estrogen and progesterone levels fall. That makes it easier for radiologists to detect abnormalities. (Women using hormone therapy maintain denser breasts, even after menopause.) If you are either pre- or peri-menopausal, are under age 50, or have very dense breasts, ask your doctor about digital mammography; it's been known to be significantly more effective in screening these groups of women. Digital mammography also uses X-rays, but its electronic images are stored directly on a computer rather than on film. While mammograms are not foolproof, they do (when combined with regular breast exams performed by a doctor during checkups) reduce the number of deaths associated with breast cancer.

Breast exam during doctor checkup: a thorough manual and visual examination of breast tissue.

Most women get a physical breast exam during their annual checkup with their ob-gyn or internist. (If your doctor doesn't routinely do this, ask for it.)

Ultrasound: high-frequency sound waves used to differentiate cysts from tumors or as a supplement to mammography for women with dense breasts.

It should be noted that ultrasound is *not* a good way to detect tiny tumors or calcifications that can be early signs of cancer.

Thermography: analyzes heat patterns for the presence of suspicious areas; used in conjunction with mammography.

Computer-aided detection (CAD): special software that analyzes mammograms for suspicious-looking areas.

While not foolproof, CAD may increase breast cancer detection by as much as 20 percent.

Cervical Cancer Detection

Pap test: the collection and analysis of cells from the cervix.

Since Dr. George Papanicolaou developed this screen in 1941, deaths from cervical cancer have been cut by more than 70 percent. A swab is used to collect cells from the cervix; if abnormal cells are detected, another Pap test is scheduled a few months later. (It is not uncommon for subsequent Pap smears to be "normal," since atypical cells can revert to "normal" on their own.) You should get a traditional Pap test every year, or every two years if your doctor uses a liquid-based cytology test. Once you've turned 70, you can stop getting Pap tests as long as you haven't had an abnormal screen for 10 years.

HPV test: a swab of the cervix that can be done at the same time as a Pap smear to detect the presence of human papillomavirus (HPV), a sexually transmitted disease that is responsible for almost all cases of cervical cancer.

This test is usually given to women over 30 who have had abnormal Pap test results. Not only does it reduce the chance of getting a false positive on a Pap test, but it's another way to detect precancerous lesions. Women over 30 who have a "clean" HPV test can wait three years before being tested again.

COLORECTAL CANCER DETECTION

Manual rectal exam: a manual check of the contours of the rectum, usually performed as part of an annual physical or pelvic exam.

For this test, the doctor uses a lubricated gloved finger to determine if any lumps or other abnormalities are present.

Stool occult blood test: a take-home kit (usually distributed by doctors as part of annual exams) that requires you to collect a specific number of fecal samples, seal them in a special envelope, and mail them in to a lab, where they are checked for the presence of blood.

To get the most reliable results, you're usually told to avoid red meat, vitamin C

pills, increased iron, turnips, and horseradish before doing the test. If a worrisome amount of blood is detected, you'll need more tests. Most of those (over 90 percent) getting extra scrutiny will not turn out to have cancer, but odds are that 1 in 20 will. Just remember: Letting the kit sit on a bathroom shelf for a year makes the screening pretty ineffective. It should be done every year after age 50.

Sigmoidoscopy/colonoscopy: an examination of the lower half of the large intestine (sigmoidoscopy) or the entire colon (colonoscopy) with an illuminated, flexible scanning tool inserted into the rectum.

Starting at age 50, you should get either a sigmoidoscopy (every 5 years) or a colonoscopy (every 10 years). If you're at high risk because of a family history of colon cancer or a personal history of polyps or ulcerative colitis, your doctor will probably urge you to get screened at a younger age and get follow-up screens more regularly. Doing one of these two internal exams greatly increases the chance that any colorectal cancer will be found early, in part because the scanning device also has the capacity to remove any polyps found during the exam. The procedure itself does not hurt (you'll get a painkiller or anesthesia), but the prep work, which begins the day before, is unpleasant and sometimes messy and uncomfortable. Basically, you drink a liquid that clears out your bowels, requiring lots of time in the bathroom. However, once that's over, you've passed the worst of it. We realize that there is a certain yuck factor that goes along with these tests, but the discomfort is a small price to pay to stay healthy.

BREAST CANCER

Breast cancer is the one that scares us most, probably because it's the most common cancer in women. While many of us have lost a young friend to this disease, its prevalence actually increases as we age to the point where about one in eight women will develop it over the course of a lifetime. The encouraging news is that more and more women are surviving breast cancer, thanks to early detection. When found while still restricted to the breast, the chance of surviving five years or longer is 97 percent. There's also a lot more support and information than ever before to help you find the strength you need to keep fighting and hoping.

Who's at Higher Risk for Breast Cancer?

The cause of most breast cancer is still unknown. On the other hand, there are traits and experiences that appear to put some women at higher-than-normal risk:

• Defective "breast cancer genes" (BRCA1 and BRCA2), which can be detected with a blood test

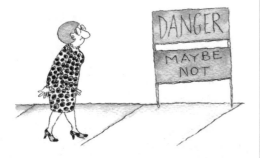

• Exposure to high levels of ionizing radiation early in life (under age 30)

• Development of breast cancer in one breast (increases the risk of developing a new cancer in the other breast)

• A family history of breast cancer, especially a sister or mother who developed it before menopause or in both breasts

• A personal history of benign breast biopsies

• Obesity after menopause

• A history of very early menarche (before age 12) or a very late menopause (after 55)

• Ashkenazi Jewish descent

• Dense breasts

• A family history of breast cancer in a male relative

• Taking combined hormone therapy (estrogen and a progestogen) for more than four years

• A personal history of endometrial or ovarian cancer

• Heavy alcohol use over many years

• Age past 65

Perhaps you scanned the list of high-risk factors above and felt some relief because there was nothing there that applied to you. But don't get too comfortable yet. One of the ironies of breast cancer is that many of the women who get this terrible disease don't identify with anything on that list, either. Most women diagnosed with breast cancer have only two risk factors: They are female and older than 65. Many experts believe that age is actually the biggest risk factor of all. It seems counterintuitive that breast cancer risk increases after menopause, especially since it's clear that estrogen makes malignant cells grow faster. Why would breast cancer become more of a threat just as your body's estrogen levels are plummeting? It turns out that over the course of a lifetime, cells can become more vulnerable to alteration because of exposure to toxins, disease, weight gain, or lifestyle choices. Aging cells are more likely to have DNA damage and, as a result, make more cell division errors and create more abnormal versions of themselves. The immune system may also weaken over time and become less able to fight off cancer. Breast cancer is generally a slow-growing cancer and often takes a while to show itself. So menopause is no time to slack off on your screening schedule. You want to do everything you can, as early as possible, to find any cancer cells lurking in your body. This is also the right time to redouble your efforts to do things that

WARNING SIGNS OF BREAST CANCER

◆ Any change in the nipple or breast

◆ Lumps or thickening of the breast

◆ Any change in a breast's contour

◆ A puckering or rippling of breast skin

◆ Any discharge (clear or bloody) from the nipple

◆ Persistent redness, scaliness, or a retracted nipple

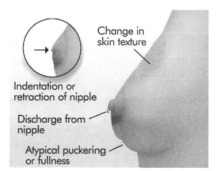

Change in skin texture

Indentation or retraction of nipple

Discharge from nipple

Atypical puckering or fullness

A woman's breast is composed of glands that make breast milk (lobules), ducts (small tubes that link lobules to the nipple), fatty and connective tissue, blood vessels, and lymph vessels. Breast cancer usually begins in the ducts (ductal carcinoma), but it can also originate in the lobules (lobular carcinoma), as well as in other tissues.

WEB WISE

The National Cancer Institute offers a really interesting risk assessment tool (http://bcra.nci.nih.gov/brc/) that projects your five-year and lifetime risk of developing breast cancer, based on a variety of factors.

could make a positive difference, starting with living as healthy a lifestyle as you possibly can.

GEOGRAPHIC DIVERSITY

Q *Is breast cancer more common than it used to be?*

A Yes, but there is a lot of variation from country to country. Europe, the United States, Canada, New Zealand, and Israel have the highest rates in the world. The lowest are in Asia and Latin America. Some 212,920 American women are now diagnosed with breast cancer each year, about double the rate seen in 1940.

One reason for the rise in diagnoses is that more women are living longer and the disease is more prevalent in women 65 and older. Detection of the disease at early stages is also increasing. While race and ethnicity affect prevalence, researchers suspect that environment and lifestyle play the biggest roles. As women emigrate from low-incidence countries to higher-incidence countries, their families' breast cancer risk rises with each generation. Women living in more developed countries spend less of their lives breast-feeding and have their babies later, which limits the effectiveness of two traditional protections. Because of more nutritious diets, they tend to start menstruating earlier, exposing their bodies to more years of high estrogen levels. They may also be exposed to more pesticides and chemical toxins, long suspected to play a role in breast cancer.

It's not all bad news, however. The proportion of women dying of the disease is on the decline in some countries, including the United States, Canada, the United Kingdom, Austria, and Sweden.

ETHNIC DIFFERENCES

◆ Women living in North America and Europe are the most likely to develop breast cancer, but the disease is on the rise in Asia, Australia, and South America.

◆ Caucasian women are more likely than African-American women to develop breast cancer. In turn, African-American women are more likely to be diagnosed with it than are Asian or Hispanic women.

◆ More Caucasian women are diagnosed with breast cancer, but a higher proportion of African-American women die of the disease. For years, doctors suspected that this was due to the fact that women of color tend not to get diagnosed as early as Caucasian women do. However, new data suggest that genetic differences could explain the gap.

Credit goes to earlier and more effective detection through mammograms as well as better treatments.

GENETIC CONNECTION

Q *Is it true that most breast cancer is inherited?*

A While having a close family member (especially a mother or sister) diagnosed with the disease or carrying a defective "breast cancer gene" (BRCA1 or BRCA2) increases your risk, it is estimated that less than 10 percent of all breast cancer is inherited and only about 5 percent is related to a defect in a single gene. About 70 to 80 percent of breast cancer occurs sporadically or is related to gene mutations that occur over a lifetime.

BREAST-FEEDING BONUS

Q *Does breast-feeding reduce the risk of breast cancer?*

A Some studies suggest that breast-feeding for four to six months (cumulatively, over a lifetime) reduces the risk of breast cancer by 20 percent or more. Women who start breast-feeding before age 20, as well as those who breast-feed for longer periods or who

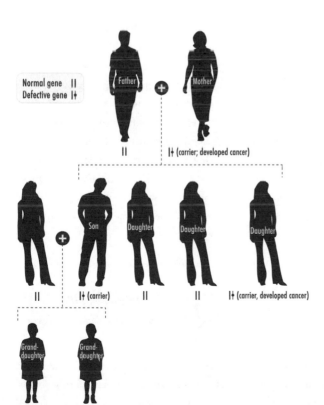

Normal gene ‖
Defective gene ‖+

Father ● Mother

‖   ‖+ (carrier; developed cancer)

● Son   Daughter   Daughter   Daughter

‖   ‖+ (carrier)   ‖   ‖   ‖+ (carrier, developed cancer)

Grand-daughter   Grand-daughter

‖+ (carrier)   ‖

PASSING ON A DEFECTIVE GENE A woman who carries one copy of a breast cancer gene typically passes it on to half of her children. In this example, one daughter and one son inherit the defective gene. The son does not get breast cancer, but he passes the defective gene on to one of his two daughters.

breast-feed multiple children, may further reduce their risk. The theory is that breast-feeding prompts breast cells to fully mature, which may make them less vulnerable to cancer.

PREGNANCY PROTECTION

Q *Why are women who never had children at a higher risk for breast cancer?*

A Pregnancy has a negative effect on short-term breast cancer risk and a positive effect on long-term risks.

During pregnancy, your estrogen and progesterone levels rise, prompting breast tissue to differentiate and mature into a variety of new forms in preparation for breast-feeding. It is believed that this process makes breast tissue more resistant to the stimulating effects of estrogen and lessens your chance of developing estrogen-responsive breast cancer in the long run. But if there are any premalignant cancer cells already in the breast when you get pregnant, the rising levels of hormones associated with pregnancy may accelerate cancer cell growth. This probably explains why there's a slightly elevated risk of developing breast cancer in the 15 years after a pregnancy. (Most breast cancers are slow-growing.) After that time passes, the chance of developing breast cancer appears to be smaller among women who have had a full-term pregnancy than among women who have never been pregnant. If you have a second child, your short-term risks rise again, but not as much as the first time,

What to Tell Your Daughter

Studies suggest that girls who exercise regularly during adolescence have a significantly lower risk of developing breast cancer in their lifetime than their sedentary girlfriends. This is further proof that encouraging young girls to make exercise a priority can literally save their lives.

because you're already benefiting from some of the long-term protection that childbearing offers.

Maternal age also plays a role. Women who have babies when they're younger (under age 30) seem to get extra protection. This may be because they're less likely to have premalignant cancer cells in their breasts or because alpha fetoprotein (a protein that regulates fetal growth) offers some protection. In general, the less time that goes by between your first period and your first pregnancy, the lower your future risk. This is one of the few benefits of a teenage pregnancy.

ANXIETY OVER THE PILL

Q *I took birth-control pills when I was in college. Am I at higher risk for breast cancer as a result?*

A This one isn't clear. Generally speaking, women taking birth-control pills have a slightly increased risk of breast cancer. That risk seems to decline over time, however, and 10 years after a woman stops taking oral contraceptives, her risk appears to be the same as that of a women who was never on the pill.

Some scientists say those higher risks are associated with the high-dose oral contraceptives used decades ago. Because modern formulations use much lower doses, the assumption is that there is little or no increased risk of breast cancer associated with birth-control pills. Still, women who are at high risk of breast cancer because of their family history should consult with their doctor before taking oral contraceptives.

Hormone Therapy and Breast Cancer Risk

If you've read our information about hormones in Chapter 2, you know that most healthy postmenopausal women can use hormone therapy for a year or two to treat menopausal symptoms with minimal risk. But you also got the message that the relationship between menopausal hormone therapy and breast cancer risk is complicated. Take the results of the Women's Health Initiative, for instance. The estrogen-only therapy used by women without a uterus didn't increase breast cancer risk, even after six years of use. However, the combination of estrogen and a progestogen, taken for five years by women who still had a uterus, did. The risk for this latter group increased the longer supplemental hormones were used. This divergence in the results was surprising, since there is so much evidence linking estrogen to breast tumor growth.

Researchers continue to dig deeper into the WHI data, fine-tuning those general conclusions and providing new information that should help women and their doctors weigh the costs and benefits of using hormone therapy. For those interested in all the details, here are some of the newer findings:

• The women who took hormones (either estrogen alone or combined therapy) were much more likely to have abnormal mammograms and as a result required more biopsies than the placebo group. This probably happened because hormones make the breasts denser, which makes it harder to read mammograms accurately.

• WHI participants diagnosed with invasive breast cancer were more likely to have larger tumors that spread to the lymph nodes if they had used hormones (either estrogen alone or combination therapy) than women who took a placebo. Their increased exposure to estrogen presumably made it harder to detect precancerous areas and tumors until they were further along.

• The age at which you start hormone therapy seems to make a difference. If you're younger than 51, the average age of menopause, there's probably little risk associated with combined hormone therapy, but if you're 56 the risks are probably higher. (The same is true if you reached menopause at 51 but don't start taking hormones until 61.)

• Women at *high risk* for breast cancer who took estrogen only were more likely to get diagnosed with breast cancer than were similar women taking the placebo.

• On the flip side, estrogen pills seemed to have a stronger protective effect on women who were at low risk for breast cancer (no family history, no previous breast biopsies, etc.).

• It appears that estrogen-only therapy increased breast cancer risk more among thin women than among heavier ones. This was another surprise, because increased weight is a known risk factor for breast cancer. One possible explanation is that the fat cells of overweight and obese women produce so much natural estrogen that the supplemental estrogen contained in the hormone pills had little additional effect on breast cancer risk. This doesn't mean that heavier women can now take hormones without a care. They remain at higher risk for blood clots, heart disease, and stroke. (In fact, most of the blood clots experienced in the WHI study were concentrated among the obese participants.)

• Women taking the combined hormones had more breast cancer than the placebo group in every age bracket. Several other studies have shown similar results.

Here's the bottom line. Hormone therapy often makes sense for low-risk women with significant symptoms who go into early menopause (younger than age 40). For them, the positives of supplementing estrogen (stronger bones, lower cholesterol) often outweigh the risks. For healthy women who reach menopause around age 50 and are struggling with significant symptoms, hormone therapy can be a very reasonable choice, especially if the lowest effective dose is used for the shortest time necessary to meet their treatment goals. However, the woman who wants to do all she can to reduce her chances of getting breast cancer may decide that the slightly increased risk associated with short-term use of combined hormone therapy is unacceptable. Women of any age with a personal or family history of estrogen-sensitive cancer or other risk factors should think twice (or more) before taking hormone therapy.

THE OTHER HORMONE

Q *If estrogen alone doesn't increase breast cancer risk but estrogen combined with progesterone does, is progesterone the bad guy here?*

A Perhaps. We know that a progestogen combined with estrogen lowers the risk of endometrial cancer. But the combination may have a dark side that includes increasing the risk of breast cancer. We just don't understand why yet. We do know that progesterone has a stimulatory effect on a woman's breasts during the second half of her normal menstrual cycle. And we do know that an estrogen-progestogen combination given to postmenopausal monkeys promotes breast cell proliferation, which can lead to an accumulation of genetic errors, which in turn may increase the risk of breast cancer. But more work on humans needs to be done. Expect to see an increasing degree of scrutiny given to the role of progestogens in breast cancer, as well as to their effect on the metabolism of estrogen. Researchers are also investigating alternative ways to provide progestogens, including versions that can be inserted into the vagina or delivered through an intrauterine device (IUD). The hope is that these latter options might put the progestogens where they're needed without increasing levels in the blood or breasts.

ESTROGEN PROTECTION?

Q *If estrogen-only hormone therapy reduces the number of breast cancer cases, should I use it to prevent the disease?*

A Only if you don't have a uterus and have significant symptoms. While the WHI results are reassuring to women who need hormones for symp-

tom relief, there are still so many unanswered questions about the relationship between estrogen and breast cancer, heart disease, stroke, and blood clots that it's way too early to be popping hormones like calcium pills. Researchers think it's possible that the reduced cancer seen in the estrogen-only arm of the WHI trial was actually misdiagnosed or delayed breast cancer. These women will continue to be monitored over time. The bottom line: No reliable medical authority is recommending hormone use as a preventive strategy.

JUST ESTROGEN

Q *It sounds like the way around the risks of combined hormone therapy is simply to take the estrogen and skip the progestin.*

A If you still have a uterus, you'll have to think carefully about the wisdom of that strategy. We don't know if there's something about progestogens, or the combination of the two hormones, or something else entirely that explains the increased risk. But we do know that the use of estrogen alone by a woman with an intact uterus dramatically increases her risk of endometrial cancer; adding a progestogen reduces her risk to the same level as that of a woman who is not taking hormones.

What do you do for now? As we've said before, doctors sometimes suggest that women who are having a rough time with menopausal symptoms and are against taking a progestogen use it a few times a year instead of monthly or apply it locally. Others might let you try estrogen-only therapy and monitor your endometrium through ultrasound or biopsy. But since none of these alternatives currently meets the "standard of care" (the recommended course of business in gynecology today), your medical insurance may not pay for the associated cost. If you decide to try one of these treatments anyway, it's imperative to get regular checkups and keep your doctor informed of any abnormal bleeding, which could be a warning sign of endometrial cancer.

Long-Term Risks

Q *Am I at increased risk for breast cancer if I took combined hormones between ages 51 and 54 but have since stopped? I'm now 59.*

A That question is under study by the WHI. However, the Million Women Study, an observational randomized study, found that past users did not have an increased risk of breast cancer or breast cancer death. A meta-analysis of 51 epidemiological studies (which included more than 17,000 women who had used estrogen alone or combined hormones at one time) found no increased risk of breast cancer among those who had stopped taking pills more than five years before.

Hot Flash Relief

Q *I had breast cancer four years ago and no longer have a uterus. Can I take hormone therapy consisting of estrogen alone to help deal with hot flashes?*

A Taking supplemental estrogen is generally not recommended for women who have (or have had) an estrogen-responsive breast tumor for fear of spurring a recurrence or the growth of new tumors. One randomized placebo-controlled study followed 434 breast cancer survivors (average age 55) who were assigned to take either estrogen only or combined hormones to treat symptoms, but the trial had to be stopped after only two years because of an increased rate of new breast cancers. Menopausal hormones also increase the density of the breasts, which could make it more difficult to effectively use mammography to monitor tumor growth in the breasts. Instead, breast cancer survivors dealing with severe hot flashes are usually encouraged to take antidepressants, such as Effexor (venlafaxine) or Prozac (fluoxetine), or one of the other alternatives discussed in detail in Chapter 3. Paxil (paroxetine) is also effective, but since it appears to interfere with the antitumor effect of tamoxifen, the two should not be given in combination.

One final note: If significant symptoms continue for

many years, you and your doctor may want to revisit the hormone therapy question at some point. There have been some uncontrolled (i.e., no placebo group) studies indicating that women who had breast cancer more than 10 years earlier were eventually able to take hormone therapy without dire consequences.

ESTROGEN CONFUSION

Q *Since there's so much evidence that estrogen contributes to breast cancer, I don't understand how estrogen-only therapy could possibly reduce the risk of breast cancer in women without a uterus.*

A You're not the only one who's confused! Even research scientists who have been studying hormones for years can only offer us theories. One hypothesis revolves around the fact that the particular estrogen used in the WHI study, conjugated equine estrogen (sold as Premarin), is less potent than the estradiol your body makes. Since both types of estrogen compete for receptors in breast cells, perhaps Premarin displaces enough estradiol that the overall effect of the natural hormone is diluted.

Another possibility is that Premarin reduces the risk of breast cancer in the short term but over time that positive effect wears off. This would explain why the WHI participants who had used hormone therapy in the past had more invasive breast cancer than women who had never used it before. (This was espe-

cially true of women who used estrogen and a progestogen in the past.) If anything, these findings confirm that hormones are wondrous and complicated agents and that we still have a lot to learn about them.

NEGATIVE RESPONSE

Q *What if my cancer was not estrogen-responsive? Can I try hormone therapy?*

A There is limited research on this topic. However, a study conducted by the M.D. Anderson Cancer Center in Houston followed 56 women with estrogen-receptor-negative breast cancer who used estrogen-only therapy for five years and found no increase in recurrence levels.

BETTER MAMMOGRAMS

Q *I'm taking hormone therapy, and now I worry about the fact that this medication makes my breasts more dense and less sensitive to mammography. Is there anything I can do about that?*

A Hormone therapy may reduce the effectiveness of mammography by about 15 percent. As a result, your doctor may recommend that you go off hormones for about two weeks before your annual mammogram in order to maximize the effectiveness of the screening. Be sure to discuss your concerns at your next visit.

What You Can Do

If you're looking for another incentive to put down the butter knife and climb back on the treadmill, here's a good one: Keeping yourself trim is one of the few things you can do to reduce your risk of breast cancer. Fat cells produce estrogen, which can feed the growth of malignant cells in breasts. (In some women, fat is the main source of estrogen after menopause.) When women lose weight, they lose fat and lower their circulating estrogen levels.

The numbers on the relationship between obesity and breast cancer are dazzling. If your body mass index score at midlife qualifies you as either overweight or obese, you have a 50 percent or greater chance of getting breast cancer than that of a thinner woman. Researchers at Boston's Brigham and Women's Hospital recently assessed data from 87,145 women whose weight changes were followed for more than two decades. Among women who never used postmenopausal hormone therapy, about 24 percent of their breast cancers could be attributed to pounds put on after the age of 18. The more weight a woman gains, the greater her risk. For example, women in this group who gained 55 pounds after the age of 18 had double the risk of women who maintained their weight. This is an especially significant finding in light of statistics showing that two-thirds of American women are overweight or obese.

Where to begin? Cutting back on fats is probably a good idea, though the exact correlation between dietary fat and breast cancer isn't known yet. Until more is known, concentrate on increasing your "good fats" (like those found in olive oil and nuts) and reducing your "bad fats" (like saturated and trans fats).

What else can you do? Eat a wide variety of fruits and vegetables (good for your general health and maybe for reducing your breast cancer risk), and cut back on those cosmos and margaritas. They're full of empty calories, but, more significantly, knocking back more than one alcoholic drink a day increases your risk of breast cancer by about 20 percent. And the risk rises with the number of drinks.

If you've put on more than a few pounds since high school, don't lose hope. This same study, which was published in the *Journal of the American Medical Association*, found that non-hormone users who maintained a weight loss of at least 22 pounds since menopause lowered their breast cancer risk by 60 percent compared with women who didn't take off weight. And the secret for taking off weight and keeping it off is, of course, no secret: Pull on those running (or at least walking) shoes. Exercise helps you lose weight. It helps keep you trimmer. And it lowers your percentage of body fat, which, as you now know, means less estrogen circulating in your body to encourage tumor growth. It may also boost your immune system so that it's more capable of beating off cancer.

What else might make a difference? Stop smoking and avoid secondhand smoke. While the link between tobacco smoke and breast cancer isn't certain, a growing number of studies indicate that it may contribute to or cause the disease.

MEDS THAT PROTECT?

Q *Is there a vaccine that can help to prevent breast cancer?*

A No, but a few medications may offer protection to some women. Tamoxifen (Nolvadex), which acts like estrogen in some parts of the body (bones and uterus) but not others (breasts), has been used for more than 25 years by breast cancer survivors to prevent recurrence. Studies indicate that it can also reduce the chance of a healthy woman getting breast cancer by about 50 percent. While tamoxifen does help preserve bone density, it has its downsides. It's only effective for five years, and it can cause menopausal symptoms such as hot flashes, vaginal discharge, and bleeding. It also slightly increases the likelihood of women aged 50 and older developing endometrial cancer (2 additional cases per 1,000 women). Women taking the drug are more likely to develop blood clots in the legs or lungs, but this occurs less than 1 percent of the time. They are also at increased risk of cataracts and stroke.

Raloxifene (Evista), a drug that is usually prescribed to prevent or treat osteoporosis, recently proved itself to be similarly effective. The Study of Tamoxifen and Raloxifene (STAR), a five-year study of more than 19,000 postmenopausal women aged 35 and older at about 400 centers nationwide, recently demonstrated that raloxifene also reduced breast cancer by 50 percent, but with significantly less chance of endometrial cancer, blood clots, or cataracts. But raloxifene isn't perfect, either. Like tamoxifen, it's associated with an increased risk of stroke and menopause-like symptoms (hot flashes and vaginal dryness). It's assumed that, like tamoxifen, it may be effective only in reducing breast cancer risk for five years before losing steam. Unlike tamoxifen, it did not reduce the incidence of noninvasive cancers in the breast.

Some cancer experts and patient advocates have been quick to point out that many healthy women aren't anxious to take a medication to prevent a disease that the vast majority of them will never get, especially when the drug can have significant side effects. However, if you're at high risk for breast cancer or you're looking to do all you can to prevent it, you should discuss these options with your doctor. One bright spot: About 500,000 women already use raloxifene to prevent or treat osteoporosis. If nothing else, this latest round of research indicates that some of them may get breast cancer protection (at least for five years) as an added benefit.

SURGICAL SOLUTION

Q *If I'm at very high risk for breast cancer, could preemptive surgery offer some protection?*

A It sounds pretty drastic, but in some rare cases premenopausal women at very high risk for cancer may decide, after consulting with their doctor, that surgical removal of the breasts (which reduces risk by 90 percent) or ovaries (which reduces breast cancer risk by 50 percent and ovarian cancer risk by 90 percent) makes sense for them.

DEODORANT AND RISK

Q *Someone told me that anti-perspirants are behind the increase in breast cancer. Has anyone looked into those things?*

A Yes. Several high-quality studies have been done on deodorants, and there is no evidence to back up that theory. You may also have heard that wearing underwire bras, having larger breasts, getting stressed out, drinking coffee, and having breast implants increase the risk of developing breast cancer. There is no scientific proof that any of these things are true.

The Latest on Breast Self-Exams

Here's a development that may surprise you. While most doctors still urge their patients to do self-exams, researchers have found that they do not reduce the number of women who die of breast cancer. Even the American Cancer Society now says that it's a woman's personal choice whether or not to do a self-exam. Finally . . . one less thing to feel guilty about. The call is yours. But remember that many women *have* detected their own breast cancer with a self-exam. And it's still a good idea to be familiar with how your breasts normally look and feel.

So, where do you start? If you're still having monthly cycles, pick a date and try to do your exam on that date every month. Since the consistency of breast tissue changes over the course of a month, you're more likely to detect differences. If you're no longer getting periods, a regular schedule makes it more likely that you'll remember to do it.

Begin by visually and manually inspecting your breasts from every angle, looking and feeling for any difference in their appearance, including changes in size, shape, color, and texture. After getting undressed to the waist, look at your breasts head-on in the mirror and:

1. Turn to one side and then the other, with hands on hips, looking for changes on the outside and inside of each breast.

2. Gently pull up each breast and carefully inspect the bottom half.

3. Bend forward, rolling your shoulders and elbows forward at the same time. Clasp your hands behind your head and turn from side to side. Check each

nipple for signs of discharge (clear or bloody) or a change in its direction. Gently use your fingertips to probe every inch of your breast tissue for lumps or thickened areas, moving in a circular motion. Check under your armpits and above your breasts as well.

4. Put your right hand behind your head and use the flat part of your left fingers to gently press into your right breast, in an up-and-down pattern. Then do the left breast with the right hand. Lie down and prop up your right shoulder with a small pillow or towel. Repeat the movements of the last exam. Now press down on your nipple, feeling for changes beneath it. Push your nipple in; it should give way easily. Do the same on the other side. If you notice any changes, call your doctor—but don't panic. About half of the breast lumps found in postmenopausal women turn out to be noncancerous. (Benign lumps are even more common in premenopausal women.) There are lots of things besides cancer that can cause lumps, nipple discharge, and inflammation.

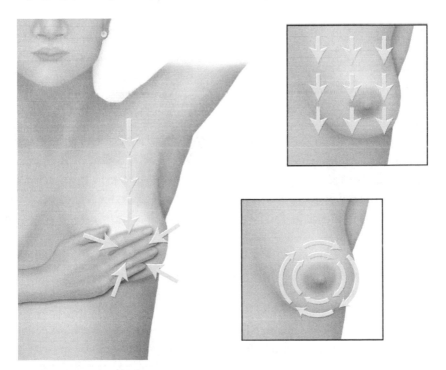

BREAST SELF-EXAM
Use your eyes and fingers to carefully inspect your breasts for signs of any changes in shape or texture, as well as lumps or thicknesses. It's recommended that you gently probe breast tissue in a variety of ways: from top to bottom, from the outer areas toward the nipple, and in a circular motion, ending up at the nipple.

TUMORS VS. CYSTS

Q *So, am I right to think that not all breast lumps will turn out to be malignant?*

A That's right. Some lumps turn out to be benign tumors or cysts. This is especially likely during the pre- and perimenopausal years. The likelihood that a lump is malignant does increase with your age, however. By the time a woman is 70, about three-quarters of breast tumors will turn out to be malignant.

What's the difference between a cyst and a tumor? A cyst is a fluid-filled sac; a tumor is a solid mass. Cysts can usually be moved under the skin; if you have one you may feel a dull pain near the armpit of the affected breast. A tumor feels like a hard pebble or maybe a small rock (sometimes with irregular edges); it may not move under the skin (or may do so only with great difficulty). Cysts, which may be caused by fluctuating hormone levels, are most common in women in their 30s, 40s, and 50s and are more likely to occur as you move closer to menopause.

You should never rely on your own touch to tell the difference, however. Let a doctor do the diagnosing. If you experience any type of lump or thickening of the breast, or any other change in the nipple or breast—perhaps you've noticed some puckering or dimpling of the skin or a discharge—you should call your doctor immediately. Better safe than sorry.

CYSTS AND CANCER

Q *Can cysts ever be a sign of breast cancer?*

A It's unlikely but still possible. For example, recurring cysts can be an early symptom of cancer. That's why many doctors will request that you come in for a follow-up visit a month or two after a breast cyst has been diagnosed and aspirated (withdrawn through suction). They want to make sure that the cyst hasn't come back.

BREAST PAIN

Q *I'm perimenopausal and experiencing breast pain. I am so worried that this might be a symptom of breast cancer. What do you think?*

A Only about 6 percent of breast cancer patients say they experienced breast pain, which is much more usually a sign of fluctuating hormone levels. That's why it's so common an annoyance during the menopause transition and among women using hormone therapy.

A dull pain near the armpit may be caused by a cyst in the breast. Intense pain radiating around the breast and under the arm (sometimes accompanied by raised lesions) could be a sign of shingles. See Chapter 7 for a detailed discussion of breast pain, but in the meantime you might find it helpful to cut caffeine out of your diet.

ENDOMETRIAL CANCER

Endometrial cancer, the most common of the gynecological cancers, develops in the lining of the uterus and will affect between 2 and 3 of every 100 women at some point in their lives. A disease that largely targets postmenopausal women, it's most commonly diagnosed between ages 50 and 70. (However, about a quarter of the diagnoses are made before age 50.) Because the most frequent symptom is postmenopausal bleeding, it's usually caught early and most women survive.

Who's at Higher Risk for Endometrial Cancer?

• Women exposed to a disproportionate amount of estrogen in relation to progesterone (includes women taking estrogen-only hormone therapy who still have an intact uterus)

• Those who experience early menstruation or a late menopause

• Obese women

• Women who have never had a full-term pregnancy

• Young women (under 40) who rarely or never have periods and have symptoms of excessive androgens (a lot of facial hair, deepening voice, etc.)

• Those with liver disease

• Anyone who has had breast or ovarian cancer or hereditary colon cancer

• Women taking tamoxifen to prevent recurrence of breast cancer

• Diabetics

• Women with high blood pressure

• Women who have endometrium cells and other irregularities in their Pap smear

• Caucasian women

Symptoms of Endometrial Cancer

• In postmenopausal women, *any* vaginal bleeding or spotting (requires prompt report to doctor)

• In pre- or perimenopausal women, any abnormal bleeding that ranges from very heavy bleeding to bleeding between periods to spotting

• A clear or pinkish watery discharge from the vagina

• Abdominal pain and discomfort

• Pain during intercourse

WEIGHT AND RISK

Q *Why are overweight women at higher risk for endometrial cancer?*

A As you probably know by now, fat cells produce estrogen. The more fat you have, the more estrogen you produce and the more your cancer risk increases. This is particularly true after menopause, when your body is no longer producing progesterone. Studies indicate that women who are 20 to 50 pounds overweight have three times the risk of developing the disease as thinner women. Those who are more than 50 pounds overweight are 10 times more likely than thinner women to develop the disease. By one estimate, excessive weight accounts for about a quarter of all cases.

PREGNANCY PROTECTION

Q *If women who have never had children are at higher risk, does your risk drop if you've had kids?*

A Yes. And your risk drops dramatically if you've had lots of kids. Women who have breast-fed also appear to be at lower risk.

THE OC

Q *Do oral contraceptives help to protect you against endometrial cancer?*

A Taking combination oral contraceptives (estrogen plus a progestin) reduces the risk of endometrial cancer. Taking the pill for a longer period provides more protection. One review found that women who took oral contraceptives for more than four years reduced their risk by 56 percent; those who took them for 12 years low-

ered their risk by 72 percent. Research indicates that some extra protection lasts for about 15 years after you stop taking them.

ON THE SPOT

Q *I'm taking menopausal hormone therapy, and I was told to expect some bleeding, including spotting. How will I know abnormal bleeding if I see it?*

A Different dosages and types of menopausal hormone therapy result in some bleeding and spotting. Women on cyclic combined hormone therapy have a designated time each cycle when they're not taking a progestogen. They can expect to bleed at that time. (It may seem like a menstrual period, but no ovulation has taken place.) Any bleeding that occurs at other times of the cycle is abnormal and should be reported to your doctor.

If you're taking a continuous combined hormone therapy (meaning that low doses of progesterone are taken every day, as opposed to higher doses taken intermittently), this issue is a little trickier. With certain dosages, it's not unusual to experience some sporadic bleeding and spotting the first year. Ask your doctor to explain exactly what kind of bleeding you should expect and what is considered abnormal. In the meantime, be sure to report any bleeding you're experiencing and keep your annual appointments for pelvic exams.

CANCER SCREEN

Q *Is there a screening test for endometrial cancer?*

A No. Irregularities on a Pap test may signal that you're at higher-than-normal risk for endometrial cancer, but most women diagnosed with the disease have normal Pap smears. A skillful clinician doing a thorough pelvic exam may notice a change in the size of your uterus or signs of an abdominal mass. If anything suspicious is found, a biopsy of your uterus will likely be recommended.

HORMONES AFTER CANCER

Q *I had a hysterectomy as a result of endometrial cancer, and my ovaries were also removed. I'm having terrible hot flashes, I'm not getting any sleep, and I feel awful. Can I use hormone therapy to help me get over the hump?*

A This is a hugely controversial area. Some doctors think that, as a general rule, women who have had an estrogen-sensitive cancer, such as endometrial cancer, should avoid menopausal hormone therapy even if they have severe menopausal symptoms. They worry that taking supplemental estrogen could encourage the growth of any remaining cancer cells. However, two recent retrospective studies on women who took hormones after having had endometrial cancer found that these women did not experience a notable increase in recurrences.

The American College of Obstetricians and Gynecologists recommends that physicians assist patients in making an informed decision in this matter after taking into consideration the specifics of each woman's case and her individual risk factors. If you decide not to use hormone therapy, keep in mind that other alternatives, including a variety of antidepressants, may give you some relief from hot flashes without increasing your risk.

A SHIELD FOR TAMOXIFEN?

Q *I'm taking tamoxifen to reduce my chances of a recurrence of breast cancer, but I'm worried about the associated increased risk of endometrial cancer. Would it make any difference if I added a progestogen?*

A Since adding a progestogen to estrogen protects a woman with an intact uterus from an increased risk of endometrial cancer, some doctors suspect that adding one to tamoxifen may provide a similar shield. However, we have no proof of that yet. In the meantime, your doctor will want you to be vigilant about reporting any abnormal bleeding and scheduling your annual pelvic exams.

PROGESTERONE PROTECTION

Q *How much progesterone do I need to take each month to prevent endometrial cancer? There are so many different combinations.*

A To get the maximum amount of protection, you're looking at 12 to 14 days a month—the same number of days your own body provides progesterone during the typical monthly cycle. Another option is to take it every day as part of a continuous combined hormone therapy. In time, researchers are hoping to figure out how to give progesterone every couple of months, but we're not there yet.

OVARIAN CANCER

About the only good thing you can say about ovarian cancer is that it's rare. Even so, it's the second most common type of cancer found in the female reproductive system (occurring in 1 out of every 70 women over the course of her lifetime and causing more deaths than all the other gynecological cancers combined). But there are some rays of hope. Prevalence has declined since 1990, and more survivors are living longer as better treatments are developed.

Who's at Higher Risk for Ovarian Cancer?

Not much is known about the risk factors for ovarian cancer. While the following links have been established, they fall far short of explaining the cause of most cases of the disease.

• Women born to families with the rare familial ovarian cancer syndrome, which spans multiple generations

(These families have unusually high rates of ovarian, breast, endometrial, and colon cancer.)

• Postmenopausal women with a defective "breast cancer gene" (BRCA1 or BRCA2)

• Women with a first-degree (mother or sister) relative who has had the disease (Those with two or more first-degree relatives are at the highest risk.)

• Breast and colon cancer survivors

• Caucasian women (at greater risk than African-American women)

• Women living in industrialized countries

• Women who have never given birth

• Women with fertility problems

• Smokers

Symptoms of Ovarian Cancer

Most of the time, women experiencing the symptoms of ovarian cancer do not have the disease, but you can't just keep popping Tums hoping that everything turns out fine. If you experience any of the symptoms in the following list, talk to your doctor. If he prescribes a treatment that doesn't work, talk to him again . . . or get a second opinion. There are women who have saved their lives by mentioning persistent and worsening symptoms like these to their doctors.

• Abdominal, intestinal, or pelvic complaints that persist and worsen even after several treatments

• Constant (rather than intermittent) bloating, abdominal enlargement, a sense of fullness or pressure in the abdomen, as well as a vague sense that something just isn't right

• In women over 40, any digestive problems that don't go away, including bloating, gas, distention, pain, constipation, diarrhea, nausea, and stomach upset

• In women over 40, back pain, lack of appetite, pain during intercourse, frequent or burning urination

GENETIC CONNECTION

Q *Do most of the women who develop ovarian cancer have a family member who has had it?*

A No. Estimates are that less than 5 percent of women who are diagnosed with ovarian cancer have a family history.

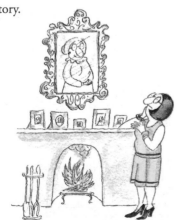

EARLY DETECTION

Q *I know that my chances of getting ovarian cancer are very low, but I still get scared whenever I read about it. Is it usually caught early?*

A No. Part of the problem has been that no precancerous stage (such as polyps in colon cancer) has been identified for this disease. Often, there are few or no noticeable symptoms until it has spread beyond the ovaries to the pelvis, abdominal cavity, and sometimes other organs such as the liver. In some cases, symptoms like persistent and worsening abdominal distress are noticed but are brushed off as nothing special. The disease is most commonly diagnosed after an unexpected and unusual increase in abdominal girth or finding fluid in the abdomen (called ascites).

Ovarian cancer's stealthy nature is one reason that mortality rates are so high. About 80 percent of the time, the disease is not diagnosed until it is at an advanced stage.

Researchers are not even sure that ovarian cancer has a stage 1 or that it progresses through stages 2, 3, and 4 the way other cancers do. They suspect that, in some cases, cancer cells begin to flake off the ovary and are then spread around the abdominal cavity pretty quickly. That's why ovarian cancer is often at a more advanced stage when first diagnosed.

TESTING FOR OVARIAN CANCER

Researchers have spent decades looking for a reliable screening test that would detect ovarian cancer while it is still confined to the ovary. And for decades that goal has eluded them. With nothing else to offer women, some doctors routinely do a blood test called CA-125, which measures the level of a protein associated with ovarian cancer. This test is not reliable for younger patients, since elevated levels of this protein may occur in premenopausal women for a variety of reasons (including fibroids and endometriosis). But in postmenopausal women it's more likely to signal ovarian cancer. Still, there are problems with using it as an ovarian cancer screen. For a long time, doctors were told that any CA-125 score above 35 should be classified as abnormal and surgical removal of the ovaries should be considered. Detection of worrisome growths and other symptoms picked up on a transvaginal ultrasound sometimes resulted in a similar recommendation. But over the years surgeons have found that the vast majority of women who followed their doctor's advice and had surgery did not have cancer. In other words, there were too many false positives. One study found that for every 100 women who had their ovaries removed following an abnormal CA-125 or suspicious ultrasound, only three actually had ovarian cancer. Researchers began to worry that CA-125 was doing more harm than good.

New criteria for "abnormal" findings have been developed, based on early results from more than 28,000 women involved in the ovarian arm of the ongoing Prostate, Lung, Colorectal and Ovarian (PLCO) Cancer Screening Trials.

When detected early, while still restricted to the ovaries, the five-year survival rate is 90 percent.

TAMOXIFEN AND CYSTS

Q *I've been told that tamoxifen, which I'm taking to prevent a recurrence of breast cancer, can cause ovarian cysts. Does that increase my risk of ovarian cancer?*

A There have been studies that have looked at this issue, but none has found an increased risk of ovarian cancer.

WHAT ABOUT FERTILITY DRUGS?

Q *Do fertility drugs like Clomid and Serophene increase risk?*

A While some studies indicate that using fertility drugs for more than a year (without getting pregnant) can increase risk, other studies haven't verified this finding.

THE THREAT OF TALC

Q *Is it true that using talcum powder on your genital area increases the risk of ovarian cancer?*

◆ A CA-125 score of 65 or above. (About one in five, or 21 percent, of the women studied turned out to have ovarian cancer. Only .3 percent of the women with scores under 65 were found to have ovarian cancer.)

◆ A CA-125 score increase of 40 points or more compared with the score one year before. (Among these women, 27 percent were ultimately found to have ovarian cancer. The chance of having ovarian cancer with a smaller increase was only 0.4 percent.)

◆ An ovarian cyst found during a transvaginal ultrasound that is equal to or greater than 3 centimeters in diameter, coupled with a CA-125 score that has increased by 10 points or more compared with the year before. (One in five of the women who met this criterion had cancer.)

◆ An ovarian cyst that has grown more than 6.5 centimeters in diameter in a year. (This was the most reliable predictor, with 60 percent having cancer.)

Does this mean that every woman should now get a CA-125 or transvaginal ultrasound as part of her annual physical? Based on what we know, the answer would be no for asymptomatic women. Even if research eventually proves that this test results in lower mortality rates, it will be only part of the answer. At least 50 percent of the women who are diagnosed with ovarian cancer never exhibit any symptoms or see any increase in their CA-125 during the early stages of the disease. Transvaginal ultrasounds do not catch all ovarian cancers, either. Many women with abnormal ultrasound results end up having a benign cyst or tumor or a fibroid—not cancer.

A Talcum powder once contained asbestos, but this hasn't been so for 20 years. Long-term studies are needed to determine if newer talc products are risky. In the meantime, it's probably wise not to use talc down under or on sanitary napkins. Cornstarch powder is a safer bet.

IMPROVING YOUR ODDS

Q *Is there anything that reduces the risk of getting ovarian cancer?*

A We don't know a lot about the causes of ovarian cancer or what can be done to prevent it. Sometimes a localized tumor can be detected during a physical exam performed by a skillful clinician, so one thing you can do is get an annual pelvic exam.

Women who have used oral contraceptives are about 50 percent less likely to develop this disease than women who have never used them. Giving birth to at least one child is associated with a lower risk. So is tubal sterilization.

Women who have been identified as being at high lifetime risk for the disease (because of family history or the diagnosis of the rare familial ovarian cancer syndrome) may consider having their ovaries removed as early as their mid-30s or as they approach menopause as a prevention strategy. New technologies that allow ovarian tissue to be frozen and later transplanted to other places in the body (under the skin of the arm, for example) are still experimental but someday may permit many of these women to retain their fertility. (For more information about this procedure, see page 18.)

The fact that we still don't have a reliable screening test for this deadly disease is the main reason most surgeons will urge postmenopausal women having a hysterectomy to have their ovaries removed at the same time. But because it's still unclear how the disease spreads and progresses, even an oophorectomy (surgical removal of the ovaries) is not an absolute guarantee that any individual woman will never get ovarian cancer. However, it does reduce risk by about 90 percent.

CANCER IN ONE OVARY

Q *Do both ovaries have to be removed if ovarian cancer is found in only one ovary?*

A If cancer is found in only one ovary, your doctor may recommend the removal of only that ovary. The decision will depend on the extent of the cancer, the type of ovarian cancer, and your age, among other things. A woman with one ovary can continue to produce estrogen and can get pregnant. However, if chemotherapy is part of the treatment plan, a woman may go into early menopause anyway, especially if she's older than 40.

INSTANT MENOPAUSE

Q *If I'm premenopausal, can treatment for ovarian cancer result in menopause?*

A It often does. Treatment typically includes removal of the ovaries as well as the fallopian tubes, uterus, supporting ligaments, and sometimes the pelvic and aortic lymph nodes. Surgical removal of both ovaries in a pre- or perimenopausal woman will result in menopause overnight. Menopausal symptoms like hot flashes can be quite severe. If this happens to you, you may be a very good candidate for menopausal hormone therapy if you're at normal to low risk for breast cancer. However, the latest data from the Women's Health Initiative indicate that women at high risk for breast cancer, blood clots, or stroke should carefully weigh the relative risks and benefits of taking supplemental hormones in consultation with their doctor.

CERVICAL CANCER

The third most common type of gynecological cancer, cervical cancer develops in the cervix, the opening between the vagina and the uterus. In most cases, it's caused by a sexually transmitted disease, the human papillomavirus (HPV).

Before the 1940s, cervical cancer was the number one cancer killer among American women. But thanks to effective screening (the Pap test), it's no longer even in the top 10. And here's more good news: A new vaccine is available that can protect girls and women ages 9 to 26 from getting the most worrisome strains of HPV. Research on two HPV vaccines' safety and efficacy for women 26 and up is now under way. While cervical cancer remains a major threat to women living in developing countries, it's possible that we may see this disease largely eradicated in our lifetimes.

Who's at Higher Risk for Cervical Cancer?

• Women diagnosed with HPV

• Women infected with human immunodeficiency virus (HIV)

• Women with multiple sex partners

• Women with a history of sexually transmitted infections

• Women of African-American, Hispanic, or Native American descent (perhaps because these women tend not to have as much access to regular medical care)

• Women who started having intercourse at a young age

• Women who do not get regular Pap smears

• Current and former smokers

• Women whose mothers took diethylstilbestrol (DES) while pregnant with them

Symptoms of Cervical Cancer

There often are no noticeable symptoms during the early stages of this disease. However, pay attention to any of the following signs and mention them to your doctor:

• Abnormal bleeding (heavy bleeding, spotting, or bleeding after intercourse or between menstrual periods)

• Pain during intercourse

• A foul-smelling or pink-tinged discharge

• Painful urination

• Pelvic, leg, and back pain

HPV AND CERVICAL CANCER

Q *What is the link between cervical cancer and HPV?*

A DNA tests indicate that almost all (99 percent) cases of cervical cancer can be traced back to HPV, especially among women who have had multiple sex partners. Sometimes infected women experience no symptoms; in others, the infection is characterized by genital warts (small, hard, raised growths). Unlike many other sexually transmitted diseases, HPV does not require an exchange of bodily fluids in order to be transmitted; skin-to-skin contact is enough. Healthy women usually shed the infected skin before anything more serious occurs, but not always. If a persistent infection takes hold, cervical cells may eventually begin to develop abnormally, which can lead to precancerous changes and to full cancer if not treated. The conversion from infection to cancer can take about 10 to 20 years to develop.

Current estimates are that more than half of all American women and men have been exposed to HPV, making it the fastest-spreading sexually transmitted disease in the United States.

A MIDLIFE PEAK

Q *Does cervical cancer become more common as you get on in years?*

A No. While it can develop in women of any age, cervical cancer is most often found in women between the ages of 25 and 35. There is a secondary cancer peak around age 60. This is due to the jump in HPV cases that occurs around age 40 and is probably related to midlife dating after divorce or weakening immune systems. (Remember, it can take more than 10 years for HPV to become cervical cancer.) Keep in mind that even if you're not worried anymore about getting pregnant, you can still contract a sexually transmitted disease. (Information on STDs begins on page 132.) And there's

some evidence that cervical cancer may develop more rapidly in women who are over 65.

BEYOND CERVICAL CANCER

Q *Does HPV cause other cancers besides cervical cancer? And do only women get it?*

A HPV is believed to be responsible for about a third of the cancers affecting the penis, anus, tonsils, throat, and larynx, and causes some cases of vulvar, vaginal, and tongue cancer as well. Partners of men with penile cancer (which is quite rare in areas where most men are circumcised) are more likely to develop cervical cancer.

VACCINES ON THE SCENE

Q *How do the new vaccines that protect against cervical cancer actually work?*

A Two vaccines have been developed, but so far only one, Gardasil, has been approved by the FDA. Gardasil protects against the two types of HPV most likely to cause cervical cancer, as well as precursors that can lead to vulvar and vaginal cancer. It also protects against two strains of HPV that cause genital warts in men and low-grade lesions in women. Studies indicate that it's effective for more than three years, but no one knows how long the protection ultimately lasts. Another vaccine, Cervarix, is expected to be before the FDA for approval soon.

The vaccines seem to be especially potent when administered to girls 9 to 14 years old but are recommended for women up to age 26, even if they've had HPV before. Both vaccines are being tested in "older" women (Gardasil in women up to age 45, Cervarix in women up to age 55). Research is also underway to determine if these vaccines are safe and effective for men and boys.

As more women are inoculated, health officials expect that the number of women being diagnosed with cervical cancer will drop dramatically.

HISTORY OF HPV

Q *I have HPV. Does the vaccine make sense for me?*

A Probably. Most people with HPV have only one strain, and this will usually go away on its own. Once you've been vaccinated, you're protected against the other three most worrisome types. The vaccine is not a treatment, however; it will not prevent women already infected from developing cancer.

VACCINE VS. PAP

Q *If I get the HPV vaccine now, will I still need to get Pap smears in the future?*

A Yes, most definitely. A very small percentage of cervical cancer is not caused by HPV, and neither vaccine has been proven to protect against all strains of this virus. Research is currently under way to determine how many types of HPV the vaccines will prevent. Until more is known about that, your doctor will want to continue to monitor you annually for any signs of cervical cancer.

PAP AFTER HYSTERECTOMY

Q *Do I still need a Pap test if I've had a hysterectomy?*

A If you had a hysterectomy that left your cervix intact, you need to follow the same recommendations as everyone else. If your cervix was removed with your uterus, there is a very small chance (about 1 in 1,000) that cancer could still develop. Studies do not indicate that getting a Pap test reduces the mortality rate in these cases. Ask your doctor to confirm the type of hysterectomy you had, and whether you still need to be tested.

HOW CAN I PROTECT MYSELF?

Q *Besides the vaccine and the Pap test, are there other things I can do to protect myself against cervical cancer?*

A Using a condom or diaphragm may be helpful in preventing cervical cancer by reducing the chance of contracting sexually transmitted diseases, including HPV. This is especially important if you have recently become sexually active.

PAP AFTER TREATMENT

Q *If I've been treated for dysplastic (abnormal) cells, do I need to keep getting Pap tests in the future?*

A Yes. Even if all your abnormal cells are removed, precancerous cells can recur. Usually, doctors will order a stepped-up schedule of Pap tests for the next year after treatment and annual Pap tests after that.

FERTILITY AFTER CANCER

Q *If I have cervical cancer, is a hysterectomy usually recommended? I'm 40 and just got married, and I was hoping to start a family.*

A A hysterectomy is usually recommended, but if you're younger than 45 and are still hoping to have children, you may be a good candidate for an experimental alternative called a trachelectomy, in which the cervix and nearby lymph nodes are removed but the uterus is left intact. You and your doctor can decide if this is the right choice for you.

AVOIDING SURGERY

Q *Do most women diagnosed with a precancerous version of cervical cancer require a hysterectomy?*

A Women in that situation do not usually require a hysterectomy. If your doctor suggests it, ask why it's a good idea in your case.

LUNG CANCER

It may not surprise you to learn that lung cancer kills more women than any other kind of cancer (as many as breast, ovarian, and uterine cancer combined). But what may really surprise you is that lung cancer is the third most deadly cancer among women who *do not* smoke, right behind breast cancer and colon cancer. Exposure to secondhand smoke explains part of this remarkable statistic. In addition, the types of lung cancer that are not closely associated with smoking are also much more common among women than among men. More than two-thirds of nonsmokers who get lung cancer are women.

Not that the news is any cheerier for smokers. New research indicates that women who smoke are more likely to get lung cancer than men who smoke. No one is sure why, but one theory is that women are more vulnerable to the carcinogens in tobacco.

Both of these findings may help explain why the number of women getting lung cancer has increased 600 percent in the last 80 years.

Who's at Higher Risk for Lung Cancer?

• Anyone who smokes tobacco, particularly cigarette smokers

• People exposed to environmental carcinogens like asbestos, secondhand smoke, and radon

• People who have had prior lung disease or have lung damage

• People with a family history of lung cancer

• People with poor diets that include few vegetables, fruit, and whole grains, and too much fat and cholesterol

• Genetic mutations that are inherited or are the result of environmental factors like secondhand smoke

Symptoms of Lung Cancer

• A persistent and worsening cough

• Breathing difficulties; wheezing, recurrent pneumonia or bronchitis

• Chest pain that doesn't go away

• Unexplained weight loss or reduced appetite

• Coughing up blood-streaked or pus-colored mucus

• Hoarseness or difficulty swallowing

• Headaches, fever, fatigue

HOW CAN I PROTECT MYSELF?

Q *How can lung cancer be prevented?*

A Stop smoking and avoid the cigarette smoke of others. Secondhand smoke has been proven to be more dangerous than previously thought. Even long-term and heavy smokers can reduce their future risk of lung cancer by half if

they quit smoking and stay smoke-free for 10 years. If you've tried to stop before and failed, your life may depend on your trying again.

WHERE THERE'S SMOKE

Q *How common is lung cancer among women who smoke?*

A About 15 percent of women who smoke will eventually develop lung cancer. Put another way, smoking is involved in about 80 percent of the lung cancer diagnosed in women. Some studies have found that female smokers tend to develop lung cancer sooner than male smokers, even if they smoke less than most men. Women smokers are also much more likely than men to have small-cell lung cancer, a very aggressive form of cancer that often metastasizes before exhibiting any symptoms.

SMOKE SCREEN

Q *Is there an effective screen for lung cancer?*

A There is no screening test that is the equivalent of a mammogram for the lungs. A variety of visualizing technologies have been studied, but so far none has proved effective in reducing mortality and in the past none was studied in women. The National Cancer

Institute has included women in a screening study being conducted to determine the effectiveness of spiral computed tomography, in which an amazing machine spins around the patient's chest, taking as many as 400 images that can be assembled into a 3-D model. While a chest X-ray might detect tumors that are two centimeters big, the spiral CT can pick them up at two millimeters. A recent international study found that 81 percent of the tumors detected through spiral CT were surgically removed at early stages of the disease and 96 percent of the patients were still alive eight years later. Before it can be used widely, researchers need to figure out how to differentiate between the 90 percent of benign lesions detected by the machine and the 10 percent that are malignant. Monitoring the growths over time and operating only on those that change may be the solution. While professional groups have yet to back annual screenings, some physicians are urging high-risk patients over 50 to get an annual CT scan.

COLORECTAL CANCER

Colorectal cancer (cancer of the colon and rectum) is the third most common cause of cancer deaths among women, just behind lung and breast cancers. The rate of death from this disease, particularly among women, has been on the decline since 1950. You can help protect yourself by getting regular screens.

Who's at Higher Risk for Colon Cancer?

• People who have a close family member who has had colorectal cancer

• People with a personal history or a family history of ulcerative colitis or inflammatory bowel disease

• People with adenomatous polyps (a common type of growth found in the bowel that has the potential to become cancerous) or a personal or close family history of adenomatous polyps

• African-Americans

• People with unexplained anemia

• People who eat beef, pork, or lamb on a daily basis

• Smokers

Symptoms of Colon Cancer

• Rectal bleeding (often the result of hemorrhoids rather than cancer, but must be reported to a doctor in any case)

• Changes in size or shape of stool (a common occurrence for healthy bowels as well)

• Abdominal cramping and pain

• Unexplained anemia

• Unexplained weight gain

AGE AND CANCER

Q *Does colon cancer become more common as you age?*

A Diagnoses of colon cancer rise significantly between ages 40 and 45 and peak at about age 70. Between the ages of 50 and 54, about 41 in every 100,000 women are diagnosed with the disease.

POLYPS AND CANCER

Q *If you have a colonoscopy and they find polyps, does that mean you have colon cancer?*

A It can take 10 years or more for polyps (also called adenomas) to become malignant. Removing them early dramatically reduces your chances of getting this disease. That's one reason why it's recommended that you have a colonoscopy every 10 years. Lingering questions about the findings of your specific screening need to be addressed to your doctor.

HOW CAN I PROTECT MYSELF?

Q *What else can be done to prevent colorectal cancer?*

A You might think about cutting way back on the amount of beef, lamb, and pork you eat. The Nurses' Health Study (which followed 90,000 nurses over six years) found that women who ate meat every day had two and a half times the risk of developing colo-

rectal cancer as women who ate it less than once a month. What's unclear is whether the correlation is direct, a marker for a less healthy diet, or something else. Large studies have not found a reduction in colorectal cancer among people eating a low-fat and/or a high-fiber diet, although postmenopausal women who ate a low-fat diet for eight years produced fewer polyps, suggesting that over time their cancer rate might decline.

Another theory is that folic acid (also known as folate, which is found in citrus and green vegetables as well as in multivitamins) may help to prevent polyps, while too much alcohol may encourage their growth. Analysis of the drinking habits of 16,000 participants in the Nurses' Health Study found that those women who drank more than two alcoholic drinks a day seemed to be at increased risk. Some studies also indicate that calcium and vitamin D may help protect against colon cancer. This theory is still being researched.

Data from the Nurses' Health Study also indicate that women who take more aspirin (four to six a week for 10 years) cut their rate of colorectal cancer in half. Nonsteroidal anti-inflammatory drugs (such as ibuprofen, acetaminophen,

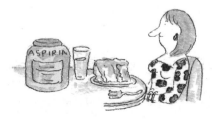

and naproxen sodium) are thought to have a similar effect. If you're considering taking a pain reliever for this purpose, talk to your doctor first to make sure such a strategy won't aggravate another condition, such as ongoing stomach problems.

Women (more than men) seem to be able to further lower their risk through exercise and by maintaining a healthy weight.

BLADDER CANCER

Men are twice as likely as women to get bladder cancer, and that may be why it can be initially misdiagnosed as a bladder infection, a fibroid, or another common problem. Caucasians are twice as likely to get bladder cancer as African-Americans and Hispanics; it's rare among Asians. If your symptoms don't go away with treatment, make sure you keep bringing them up to your doctor or consult a urologist. In the best case, bladder cancer is caught while it's still restricted to the lining of the bladder.

Who's at Higher Risk for Bladder Cancer?

Smokers and people whose work exposes them to a lot of carcinogens (especially those who work in the rubber industry or with chemicals or leather, as well as hairdressers, machinists, metal workers, printers, painters, textile workers, and truck drivers) are the most vulnerable. Others at risk include:

• Anyone with a personal or family history of bladder cancer

• People over 40 (risk increases with age)

• Caucasians

• People taking cyclophosphamide or arsenic to treat cancer or other diseases

• People with chronic bladder infections

Symptoms of Bladder Cancer

The symptoms below may be signs of something other than bladder cancer (such as a benign tumor or an infection) but should be checked out promptly by your internist or urologist.

• Blood but no pain when urinating (urine may appear slightly rusty to deep red)

• Pain during urination

• Frequent urination

• Frequent impulse to urinate without being able to do so

• Lower back pain

CANCER SUSPECTS

Q *I've heard that the chlorine in drinking water, as well as coffee, the artificial sweetener saccharin, and hair dye all cause bladder cancer. True?*

A All have been suspected and all have been widely studied, but none has been proven to cause bladder cancer in humans.

WHAT TO DO?

Q *What can I do to guard against bladder cancer?*

A While there is no specific screen for bladder cancer, symptoms of the disease (the presence of blood and/or cancer cells) can be detected through regular urine tests. Tumors can also be felt during abdominal, pelvic, or rectal examinations. So be sure to get regular medical exams.

To help guard against the disease, it's important to eat your share of fruits and vegetables. Studies indicate that people who eat these foods regularly are less likely to get bladder cancer. No specific supplement or nutrient has proven to be protective.

VULVAR CANCER

V ulvar cancer refers to the fairly rare malignancies of the external genitalia, including the pubic mound, the labia majora, the labia minora, the vaginal opening, the urethral opening, and the clitoris. The most common are caused by squamous cell carcinoma, which can occur on any surface or lining of a hollow organ in the body (such as your mouth, lungs, etc.) The two types of human papillomavirus (HPV) that are most responsible for cervical cancer cause about 40 percent of the cases of vulvar cancer. About 5 percent of vulvar cancers are caused by melanoma, a cancer that starts in the pigment-producing cells of the body. If caught early, about 90 percent of women survive these cancers.

Who's at Higher Risk for Vulvar Cancer?

Women with vulvar intraepithelial neoplasia (VIN), a precancerous area on the surface of the vulva typically diagnosed during a pelvic exam, are at risk for this disease. VIN can become full blown cancer but sometimes goes away on its own. It is believed to be associated with HPV and herpes simplex virus II, both of which are sexually transmitted diseases. Also at risk are:

• Women with multiple sexual partners

• Caucasian women (three times more likely to develop vulvar cancer than African-American women)

• Women with other reproductive system cancer

• Women with a history of HPV or genital warts

• Women with HIV

• Diabetic women and women who take drugs that suppress their immune systems

• Smokers

Symptoms of Vulvar Cancer

• Persistent itching of the vulvar area (the most common symptom)

• Pain or a burning sensation in the genital area

• Lumps or sores (white, red, dark, or raised) that appear on either the outer or inner lips of the vulva, as well as the clitoris or perineum (Symptoms are often mistaken for infections or other inflammations. If you're given a treatment to address these symptoms but they don't go away, be sure to follow up with your doctor.)

THE BEST PROTECTION

Q *What can be done to prevent vulvar cancer?*

A Since there is no specific screening test for vulvar cancer other than a pelvic exam, be sure to mention any changes or persistent symptoms (itching, burning, pain, lumps, sores) to your doctor during your annual visit. If you're given a treatment for these things and the problem doesn't go away, bring it up again. Regular physical exams and biopsies when necessary can help with early detection. If you have multiple sexual partners, use condoms and do whatever else you can to reduce your vulnerability to sexually transmitted diseases. And getting the HPV vaccine does offer protection against some causes of this cancer.

VAGINAL CANCER

Vaginal cancer, which refers to any of the cancers that start in the vagina, is rare. Most cancer found in the vagina actually starts elsewhere (in the uterus or cervix, for example) and eventually finds its way to the vagina. Some cases may be caused by human papillomavirus (HPV), a sexually transmitted disease. When vaginal cancer is caught early, the vast majority of women survive for more than five years.

Who's at Higher Risk for Vaginal Cancer?

• Women with HPV

• Cervical cancer survivors, as well as women diagnosed with precancerous conditions in the cervix

• Women whose mothers took diethylstilbestrol (DES) while pregnant with them

• Women who have had multiple sex partners or who became sexually active early

• Smokers

• African-American women

Symptoms of Vaginal Cancer

• Abnormal bleeding (heavy bleeding, spotting between periods, any bleeding after menopause)

• Pain or bleeding during or after intercourse

• Unusual vaginal discharge

• Pelvic pain

• A lump or mass in the vagina

• Painful or difficult urination

MELANOMA AND THE VAGINA

Q *I've heard that melanoma can start in the vagina. I thought it was caused by too much time in the sun.*

A Most of the time, malignant melanoma is a skin cancer related to excessive sun exposure, but it can develop in the vagina and other internal organs. When this occurs, it is usually not detected in its early stages and thus has been shown to have poor five-year survival rates.

HOW CAN I PROTECT MYSELF?

Q *Are there things I should be doing to protect myself against vaginal cancer?*

A While there is no specific screen for vaginal cancer, getting annual pelvic exams and regular Pap smears will help to ensure that precancerous conditions are found early. If you're starting to date again or have multiple sex partners, be sure to talk to your doctor about how best to protect yourself against HPV and HIV. The HPV vac-

cine offers protection against some causes of vaginal cancer.

CANCER AND MENOPAUSE

Dealing with cancer is stressful enough; adding menopause to the mix isn't anyone's idea of a blessing. Breast cancer survivors taking tamoxifen, raloxifene, and other anti-estrogen medications are among those most likely to have really bothersome hot flashes and vaginal dryness. The same is true of women who lose their ovaries as part of a cancer treatment. Women who have had radiation or surgery may have a harder time getting sexually aroused (for a variety of physical, psychological, or emotional reasons), and the loss of lubrication that comes with menopause doesn't help. If you're having mood or sleep or memory problems, it's often difficult to gauge how much is related to cancer treatment, menopause, aging, life in general, or all of the above.

The encouraging news is that there's more support and information than ever before, as well as more research. While most breast cancer survivors are discouraged from using hormone therapy, research has determined that antidepressants such as Effexor (venlafaxine) and Prozac (fluoxetine), as well as medications such as Neurontin (gabapentin), can help to reduce hot flashes. Also important is more research to see whether alternative treatments like soy and black cohosh are effective and safe. New treatments like Zestra genital massage oil and Eros, a handheld suction device, can help women who are recovering from cancer treatments feel more sexual.

Many chapters in this book include information specifically aimed at cancer survivors, and much of the general information for all midlife women—such as how to get a better night's sleep and wake up eager to face the day—is likely to help. While cancer survivors still have many unmet needs, at least they're not the forgotten women they once were.

CHAPTER 14

Diet and Exercise

Whether you've been a health nut or a coach potato, you're going to find menopause a challenge. You feel as if you gain weight just by *looking* at food . . . and where did all that flab come from? Perhaps you never had a belly before, and it's resisting your best efforts to flatten it out. You're too self-conscious to sign up at the gym, and as the pounds creep up, you want nothing more than a double date with Ben & Jerry. Well, don't give up. No matter how far you've strayed from a healthy lifestyle, you can come back. Start slowly, literally one step at a time. Walk around the block. Park a little farther away in the mall. Switch to low-fat dairy products. Cut out desserts. Choose whole-grain toast instead of pastry in the morning.

In this chapter, we'll tell you how you can maintain an energetic lifestyle to maintain healthy eating for many years to come. Don't habits and why exercise is no believe us? New research on longer optional. You need to longevity shows that the changes be active every day, not to turn yourself into a marathoner (although cal. There's no time to waste. if that's your goal, go for it). You need Put down the remote, get off to get on the right track now so that that couch . . . and get going.

DIET

If you're like most women, you've probably started and quit dozens of weight-loss plans over the years. So here's a new approach. Forget the "D" word. Instead, focus on permanent change. Promise yourself: This time, it's for keeps.

MORE THAN VANITY

Q *I've learned to live with being less than svelte. Why should I care about an extra 10 or 20 pounds?*

A Many of us have spent years trying to live up to an unreasonable Barbie doll ideal—basically a skinny body with big boobs. That body doesn't exist in nature without extensive help from plastic surgery and extreme dieting, and it's not what we're advocating here. We want you to get down to a healthy weight to lower your vulnerability to disease. Specifically, extra weight puts you at risk for type 2 diabetes, high blood pressure, heart disease, stroke, some types of cancer, sleep disorders, and osteoarthritis.

Nearly two-thirds of American women are overweight or obese. You don't want to be one of them if you plan on living a long and active life. But weight isn't the only risk factor. A sedentary lifestyle is equally unhealthy. That's why we want you to aim for both healthy eating and regular exercise habits.

If you have a lot of weight to lose, it can be discouraging to contemplate that dramatic loss all at once. Instead, pick an attainable intermediate goal of 5 or 10 pounds. Every 10 percent drop in weight (accompanied by an increase in physical activity) improves your overall health. A weight loss of 5 to 10 pounds can slow the development of osteoarthritis. Losing 5 to 10 percent of your total body weight can

When to See the Doctor

Your doctor can help you get started on a healthy weight-loss diet. You should also consider a complete physical if you're starting an exercise plan after a long period of inactivity. In addition, you should contact your doctor if you experience any of the following:

❖ A SUDDEN WEIGHT GAIN OR LOSS

❖ AN INABILITY TO LOSE WEIGHT DESPITE STICKING TO A DIET AND EXERCISE PLAN

❖ SEVERE PAIN IN FEET OR LEGS EXPERIENCED AFTER EXERCISING BUT UNRELIEVED BY REST

What Can Happen

✤ Most women's metabolism slows down at midlife, so it's easier to gain and harder to lose weight.

✤ Your tried-and-true quick weight loss tricks won't work the way they used to.

✤ When you gain weight, you may find that fat goes to unexpected parts of your body like your neck or your belly.

✤ Your tolerance for alcohol and caffeine may decline.

✤ If you start exercising too vigorously after years of inactivity, you may experience unexpected aches and pains.

raise the level of HDL (good) cholesterol in your blood, and for every two pounds you lose, the LDL (bad) cholesterol level goes down 1 percent. A weight loss of 20 pounds may reduce LDL levels by 15 percent, reduce triglyceride levels by 30 percent, increase HDL by 8 percent, and cut total cholesterol by 10 percent.

So get started now, and remember that major lifestyle changes can be self-reinforcing. The more success you have, the more you're inspired to keep going.

STARTING OUT

Q *I'm an expert on diets. I've tried a million over the years, but I always gain the weight back. Is there a trick to keeping weight off? And what's the best way to start?*

A Here's the trick: Eat less and exercise more. That's easy to say and very difficult to put into practice . . . which is why many dieters not only gain back what they lose but can even end up heavier than they were when they started. One of the best sources of information on successful dieting is the National Weight Control Registry, which tracks about 4,500 people who have maintained a 30-pound weight loss for at least a year. These successful dieters have certain behaviors in common: a low-fat, high-carbohydrate diet; eating breakfast almost every day; frequently checking with the scale; and a high level of physical activity (from 60 to 90 minutes a day). The dieters ate from 1,300 to 1,500 calories a day, with less than 25 percent of those calories coming from fat. They went to fast-food restaurants about once a week and ate four to five times a day. By the way, "high carbs" doesn't translate into tons of bread and pasta. These dieters tended to get their carbs from beans and many different kinds of vegetables.

Take cheer that many of these people struggled for years to lose weight. Ninety percent said they had failed to drop pounds in the past. Most had weight problems when they were young: 46 percent were overweight by age 11, a quarter became overweight between 12 and 18, and 28 percent gained the excess weight as adults. Family history also seems to count. Forty-six percent had at least one overweight parent, and 27 percent said both parents were overweight. The mean weight loss was 66 pounds.

So how should you get started? A good first step is to analyze what you eat now. Keep a rigorous diary for a week— and we mean rigorous. (For sources of accurate calorie counts, see Appendix II.) Write down everything, then add up the calories. You may find that a lot of small transgressions are turning into a big weight gain. For example, just one four-inch-diameter doughnut during coffee breaks five days a week could mean a gain of about 20 pounds a year, so

---

OBESITY-RELATED DISEASES

If you're overweight or obese, you're at increased risk for:

◆ Type 2 diabetes

◆ Cardiovascular disease

◆ Stroke

◆ Hypertension

◆ High cholesterol

◆ Congestive heart failure

◆ Osteoarthritis

◆ Gout

◆ Fatty liver disease

◆ Sleep apnea and other breathing problems

◆ Kidney stones

◆ Stress urinary incontinence

◆ Cancer of the endometrium, breast, kidney, colon and rectum, esophagus, and gallbladder

---

you would lose weight just by cutting that out.

Your food diary should provide some other clues as well. Are you a midnight snacker? Are you tired and susceptible to temptation in the late afternoon? Are you gorging on comfort food when you're feeling low? If you see a pattern, you can plan for it. Fight calorie-rich late-night binges with a scheduled healthy snack like an apple or a couple of rice cakes before bed. Don't turn to food for emotional comfort; instead, call a friend or take a walk around the block.

Another tip from successful dieters: Don't try to lose all the weight at once. Make changes that you can live with and then stick to them. If you do, the pounds will disappear and stay off.

BMI BLUES

Q *I know I'm over my ideal weight, but how can I tell how much I need to lose? My doctor referred to a BMI chart, but it confuses me. The range seems so great.*

A The body mass index (BMI) table provides a ratio of height to weight. The range of what's considered healthy, overweight, and obese allows for differences in your natural frame. Depending on your stature, a BMI of 18.5 could be healthy; so could 24.9. But anything over 29 is obese. Generally, overweight means you're at least 10 percent above the ideal weight

The Body Mass Index

In the lab, researchers can use CT scans, in which a computer translates X-ray images, to measure abdominal fat. Scientists also use magnetic resonance imaging (MRI) and electrical impedance, in which electrodes attached to the body estimate the percentage of water (the higher the water, the higher the fat). But unless you volunteer for a research study, your best tool is the BMI table. Check out where you stand.

	HEALTHY WEIGHT						OVERWEIGHT					OBESE		
BMI	19	20	21	22	23	24	25	26	27	28	29	30	35	40
Height (inches)	Weight (pounds)													
58	91	96	100	105	110	115	119	124	129	134	138	143	167	191
59	94	99	104	109	114	119	124	128	133	138	143	148	173	198
60	97	102	107	112	118	123	128	133	138	143	148	153	179	204
61	100	106	111	116	122	127	132	137	143	148	153	158	185	211
62	104	109	115	120	126	131	136	142	147	153	158	164	191	218
63	107	113	118	124	130	135	141	146	152	158	163	169	197	225
64	110	116	122	128	134	140	145	151	157	163	169	174	204	232
65	114	120	126	132	138	144	150	156	162	168	174	180	210	240
66	118	124	130	136	142	148	155	161	167	173	179	186	216	247
67	121	127	134	140	146	153	159	166	172	178	185	191	223	255
68	125	131	138	144	151	158	164	171	177	184	190	197	230	262
69	128	135	142	149	155	162	169	176	182	189	196	203	236	270
70	132	139	146	153	160	167	174	181	188	195	202	207	243	278
71	136	143	150	157	165	172	179	186	193	200	208	215	250	286
72	140	147	154	162	169	177	184	191	199	206	213	221	258	294
73	144	151	159	166	174	182	189	197	204	212	219	227	265	302
74	148	155	163	171	179	186	194	202	210	218	225	233	272	311
75	152	160	168	176	184	192	200	208	216	224	232	240	279	319
76	156	164	172	180	189	197	205	213	221	230	238	246	287	328

for your height; obese is defined as at least 30 percent over the ideal weight. But BMI is only part of the story. Another important gauge, especially at midlife, is your waist size, a measure of abdominal fat. If it's more than 35 inches (40 inches for a man), you're at increased risk of health problems.

GOOD FATS, BAD FATS

Q *I used to think fat was bad. Now I'm reading that some fats are good. Why is that? And how can I tell the difference?*

A You're right, all fats are not created equal. In general, you should keep your total fat intake to between 20 and 35 percent of calories with as much as possible coming from good fats. Here's the difference:

BAD FATS. Basically, these are saturated fats and trans fats. They raise the LDL (bad) cholesterol in your blood, which increases your risk of heart disease. (For a more detailed explanation of how cholesterol works in your body, see Chapter 12.) Saturated fat is in food from animals, such as beef, veal, pork, lamb, butter, cream, whole milk, and cheese. It's also in plant-based foods, like coconut and palm oil, that are used in commercial baked goods and snack foods. Processed foods are generally high in saturated fats. Trans fats are created during the manufacture of cooking oil, shortening, and margarine. That's why you'll find them in commercial cakes, cookies, and crackers. These fats raise your bad cholesterol *and* lower your HDL (good) cholesterol, which makes them doubly bad. You can now find the amount of saturated and trans fats right on the label of food products, so you have no excuse.

GOOD FATS. Monounsaturated and polyunsaturated fats don't raise your LDL cholesterol but can raise your HDL cholesterol. Monounsaturated fats are found in some oils (olive and peanut) and avocados. Polyunsaturated fats are in many nuts and seeds, including safflower, sesame, and sunflower. Eat and enjoy.

DRUG THERAPY

Q *I just don't have the discipline to diet. Can't I take a pill to keep me from eating so much?*

A The simplest way to lose weight is to eat less and exercise more, but some people may indeed need extra help, especially if they're obese or have other complications. Medications are currently prescribed for people who have either a BMI higher than 30 or a BMI higher than 27 with two or more obesity-related conditions, such as high blood pressure or diabetes. The FDA has approved two types of drugs to treat long-term obesity. One type suppresses your appetite by restricting your ability to pick up the brain chemicals serotonin and norepinephrine, which regulate satiety. Meridia (sibutramine) is one of these drugs, which are classified as sympathomimetic because their actions mimic the responses of the sympathetic nervous system. Lipase inhibitors, the other class of anti-obesity medications, stop the action of lipases, the enzymes that break down fat, and prevent about a third of the fat you eat from being absorbed by your body. Xenical (orlistat) is a lipase inhibitor that has been approved by the FDA for use by obese adolescents as well as adults. Other drugs that work in different ways are in the research pipeline.

In addition to these medications designed specifically for obesity, other drugs may cause you to lose weight. For example, bupropion (brand names Wellbutrin and Zyban) is an antidepressant and antismoking drug that can result in some weight loss. These are all options that you need to discuss with your doctor. Any medication has side effects, so you have to balance the potential benefits against the risks.

You may be tempted to try over-the-counter diet medications. Be extremely cautious. Many contain ingredients that can be dangerous or, at best, ineffective. As always, talk to your doctor about anything you're thinking about taking—even if you can buy it without a prescription.

From the Past

Body image issues are nothing new. In the 19th century, women were expected to have a figure that defied biology—well-developed bosoms and hips and a tiny waist created by torturously tight corsets. No wonder they needed fainting couches! Fortunately, a matronly look was no disgrace as a woman aged, and the voluminous fashions of the time hid what we might consider figure flaws. Slim female bodies became the ideal in the first decades of the 20th century, around the same time that women earned the right to vote, became more educated, and started entering the workforce in larger numbers.

BAD FOR BELLY FAT

Q *Do certain foods, like beer and white bread, make you put on abdominal weight more quickly than other foods?*

A Nutrition scientists say there's no good evidence to support that claim. No controlled trials have shown that people who like beer or bread or other refined carbs gain more weight than they would if they consumed the same amount of calories in other foods. The problem is that it's easy to drink too much beer or eat too much bread. If a typical 12-ounce can of beer contains 150 to 200 calories and you drink three

◼ WHAT YOU NEED EVERY DAY ◼

Calories are units of energy, and how many you need each day depends on your age, height, and level of physical activity. Middle-aged and older adults usually need fewer calories than younger people do. That's why you may be gaining weight even if you've been eating exactly the same things for years. In general, nutrition scientists say that women and older adults should take in about 1,600 calories a day to maintain their weight. If you want to lose, you have to eat fewer calories. A pound is about 3,500 calories, so if you eat 500 calories less than you need each day, you will lose a pound a week.

The Department of Agriculture's food pyramid is a great resource for planning a healthy daily menu. Go to www.mypyramid.gov and plug in your age and activity level. You'll get an individualized plan with links to a printable version and a customized food diary.

In general, you should aim for less than 10 percent of total calories from saturated fat and no more than 30 percent from total fat. Here are some other guidelines:

◆ **Cholesterol:** less than 300 milligrams a day

◆ **Fiber:** 25 to 30 grams a day

◆ **Protein:** 10 to 35 percent of daily calories

◆ **Carbohydrates:** 45 to 65 percent of daily calories

◆ **Sodium:** no more than 2,400 milligrams per day

of them, you've just added 450 to 600 calories to your diet for the day. Similarly, it's easy to load up on calories by eating chocolate, potato chips, cookies, and other refined carbs. It's much harder to pack in as many calories eating broccoli, even if you knock down a whole plateful. It really comes down to a question of calories and the caloric density of foods.

But moving beyond the question of whether calories make you gain more weight, do they go preferentially to your belly? Again, the answer is no. For genetic reasons, bodies tend to accumulate fat in different areas, leading to an apple shape in some people and a pear shape in others. No matter which type you are, an excess of calories will be distributed among different fat depots. So, yes, excess beer and bread can add fat to your belly, but not faster than other foods of equal caloric density.

Now that we've shot down a myth, we'll give you some reasons to avoid too many foods composed of refined carbs. These foods tend to be nutritional lightweights, short on health-giving vitamins, minerals, and fiber. And because they're highly refined—hence already processed—your body doesn't have to process them much itself. As a result, they enter the bloodstream quickly (assuming you're not eating enough fiber at the same time to slow absorption). The more refined carbs you eat, the greater the spikes of blood sugar you will experience. Your body then needs to produce more insulin to help store the glucose in the form of glycogen in your muscles and liver. The amplified insulin response helps drive down blood sugar quickly, which in turn can lead to cravings for more. In addition, the more frequently you challenge your body with these insulin spikes over the years, the more likely you are to develop insulin resistance, a first step on the path to type 2 diabetes. One solution: Eat a lot of fiber and a little bit of fat at the same meal. Fiber and fat slow the absorption of glucose into the bloodstream.

BELLY BLOAT

Q *I've always had a fairly flat tummy, even after three pregnancies. Why am I developing a jelly belly now?*

A Our guess is that the scale has been creeping up a bit over the years. Since your metabolism slows down as you get older, you'll gain weight if you don't cut calories. No wonder women add an average of a pound a year during perimenopause. Many women say the extra weight is landing in places that are new for them—like the tummy. Part of

"APPLE" VS. "PEAR"

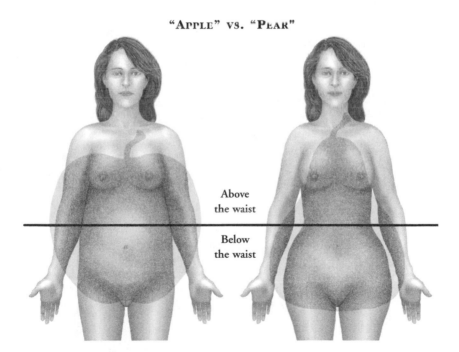

Above the waist

Below the waist

THE SHAPE YOU'RE IN
Are you heavier in your middle or in your hips? Where your fat is stored depends largely on genetics, but you can lower your risk of disease by getting rid of abdominal fat. This kind of fat is generally the first to melt away when you lose weight.

BLOATED PORTIONS

Remember when a muffin used to fit in the palm of your hand? Today they're so big that you need two hands to hold one! And restaurant portions seem to have been blown up as well.

Many nutritionists say expanded portion size is a major factor in the current obesity epidemic. When we supersized Big Macs, we supersized America. The problem is so acute that you might have a hard time remembering what a normal portion looks like. We don't expect you to carry a scale or measuring cup with you, but visualizing "official" serving sizes can help. Below are some examples of how the USDA defines a serving of various foods.

1 Serving Looks Like . . .

GRAIN PRODUCTS

1 cup of cereal flakes = fist

 1 pancake = compact disc

½ cup of cooked rice, pasta, or potato = ½ baseball

 1 slice of bread = bar of soap

1 piece of cornbread = bar of soap

1 Serving Looks Like . . .

VEGETABLES AND FRUIT

1 cup of salad greens or 1 medium fruit = baseball

½ cup of fresh fruit = ½ baseball

 ¼ cup of raisins = large egg

 1 baked potato = fist

1 Serving Looks Like . . .

DAIRY AND CHEESE

 1½ oz. cheese = 4 stacked dice or 2 cheese slices

½ cup of ice cream = ½ baseball

FATS

1 tsp. margarine or spreads = 1 die

1 Serving Looks Like . . .

MEAT AND ALTERNATIVES

3 oz. meat, fish, or poultry = deck of cards

3 oz. grilled /baked fish = checkbook

 2 tbsp. peanut butter = Ping-Pong ball

the explanation is that after menopause women tend to accumulate fat where men do—in the neck, chin, and abdominal areas—perhaps because of the shifting estrogen-androgen ratio. Your genes also help determine where fat accumulates on your body, as does your activity level. Even if you haven't gained weight, the flabbiness could come from lack of exercise. As we get older, we tend to be more sedentary, which means more fat and less muscle. Changes in skin tone that come with the loss of estrogen also make your abdominal area seem looser and flabbier.

You can improve much of this by watching what you eat and exercising more. One recent study of 164 overweight and obese women in Minnesota suggested that lifting weights may be one of the best ways to beat belly fat. Women who did supervised weight training for two years had only a 7 percent increase in intra-abdominal fat, compared to 21 percent for women who were just given exercise advice.

Fighting the belly bloat is not just vanity. Some of the weight you may gain at menopause will be stored as subcutaneous fat in the thighs, abdomen, or elsewhere. And some will be stored as visceral fat, close to vital organs in your abdominal area. Subcutaneous and visceral fat cells differ not only in their location, but also in the danger they pose to your health. Laboratory studies of visceral fat cells have found that they're more active than subcutaneous fat cells. How this difference plays out in your body is still not clear, but there is an association between high levels of visceral fat and disease risk. Fatty acids and triglycerides very quickly move in and out of visceral fat cells, which are like short-term storehouses for fats. So if you're consuming excess calories, some of them will certainly be stored in visceral fat. On the other hand, this is the first place you'll lose weight when you start to slim down, no matter where your long-term fat depots are.

To be clear, abdominal fat puts you at higher risk for high cholesterol, high blood pressure, and insulin resistance, which can lead to type 2 diabetes. In fact, researchers have found that women who have apple-shaped bodies are more vulnerable to these diseases than women with pear-shaped bodies—even if they weigh the same.

FATTY FOODS AND ESTROGEN

Q *Can you increase estrogen levels in your body by eating food with a lot of fat?*

A Studies are inconclusive on this, but most endocrinologists don't think a fatty diet affects estrogen levels in any significant way. What we can say for sure is that peripheral fat cells in your body convert cholesterol to steroid hormones, including estrogen. The more body fat you have, the more estrogen. This means that obesity—and not the fat in your diet—increases estrogen levels.

EGG EATERS

Q *Although I love eggs, I only eat egg substitutes or egg whites because my cholesterol is on the high side. Is there any benefit to eating real eggs?*

A Eggs are high in protein and low in fat, but you should still limit your intake. In one recent study of the relationship between eye health and nutrition, participants were instructed to eat an egg every day for three months. All the test subjects had a low cholesterol count at the beginning of the study, but by the end almost everyone's numbers were worse. About 15 percent of the participants had to quit the study early because their cholesterol levels rose so steeply that they qualified for a prescription for statins after only a month or two.

If you do decide to eat real eggs on occasion, look for omega-3 eggs, which are produced by chickens that have been fed flaxseed. Not only do they have three or more times the "good" omega-3 fatty acids found in regular eggs, but they also tend to be lower in cholesterol.

While we're on the subject of eggs, we should mention that low-cholesterol eggs are now available in some parts of the country. These eggs are touted to have half the cholesterol of regular eggs, and as they become more widely available, you may be able to increase your egg intake. A couple of eggs a week is fine, according to the latest nutritional thinking. But be careful. The average restaurant-made omelet these days can contain three or four eggs. Before you start eating more eggs of any kind, talk to your doctor about their likely impact on your cholesterol count.

VITAMINS FOR MENOPAUSE?

Q *When I was pregnant, I took prenatal vitamins. Now that I'm going through menopause, do I need to start taking vitamins again?*

A A multivitamin tablet is a good idea at any age. A few years ago, a panel of 19 leading health and nutrition experts combed the scientific literature and concluded that a multivitamin could help adults enhance their immune systems and reduce their risks of chronic diseases such as osteoporosis, heart disease, and colon cancer. In elderly people, multivitamins lowered the risk of infectious disease. The panel found no evidence that one brand is better than another.

Although multivitamins can meet most of your vitamin and mineral needs, they don't give you your recommended daily amount of calcium (at least 1,200 milligrams a day for postmenopausal women). A quick look at calcium supplements will tell you why. They're huge pills. For this reason, most multivitamins include only about 100 milligrams of calcium.

And what about vitamin D, which your body needs in order to absorb calcium? The recommended daily amount for women until the age of 70 is 400 international units (IUs). You generally get 200 from most multivitamins and should be able to get the rest from food and sunshine. Beyond that, there may be specific reasons for taking other supplements, but this would be on a case-by-case basis, not a blanket recommendation. If you're taking cholesterol-lowering statins, for example, it's a good idea to take CoQ-10 because statins deplete this critical antioxidant.

PROTECTING BONE HEALTH

Q *What's the healthiest way to control my weight and still keep my bones healthy?*

A Extreme dieting depletes the body's nutritional stores and takes its toll on bones. The way to keep weight down and also be good to your bones is to exercise at least 30 minutes a day and, if you can't get adequate calcium and vitamin D through food, to take supplements. Foods with high levels of calcium include milk, some leafy green vegetables, soybeans, yogurt, and cheese. (For more details, see Chapter 10.) Vitamin D is produced in the skin through exposure to the sun and is also found in fortified milk and other foods. The National Osteoporosis Foundation recommends an intake of at least 1,200 milligrams of calcium from foods or supplements and 400 to 800 international units (IUs) of vitamin D—again from foods or supplements. Other experts recommend 1,000 IUs a day. A consensus seems to be coalescing around 800 to 1,000 IUs.

LOW-CARB DIETS AND BONES

Q *A low-carb diet helps me lose weight, but I've heard that it might also increase my risk for osteoporosis. Is this true?*

A There's no need to worry if you follow a low-carbohydrate diet for a few months. But if you're on that regimen for the long term, you may well increase your risk of osteoporosis. Low-carb, high-protein diets can cause problems because the high quantities of animal protein may increase the acidity of your blood, which in turn accelerates bone loss. If you're on a low-carb diet, osteoporosis specialists recommend vegetable-based proteins such as soy products and nuts, which have less effect on acid balance. Another risk of low-carb diets is that eliminating fruit also cuts out many minerals that are required for optimal bone health.

What About Dairy Products?

Q *Is there a connection between weight loss and how many dairy products you eat? Can I lose more weight if I increase my intake?*

A The jury is still out on this, although you've probably seen plenty of TV and magazine ads promoting the connection. A number of studies (some paid for by the dairy industry) indicate that milk products may help, but most nutritionists and dietitians aren't convinced. In any case, dairy products will never be a cure-all for fat. You can't simply add low-fat milk or yogurt to your current diet without reducing calories and expect to lose weight. Study participants who benefited from dairy also reduced their caloric intake by 500 calories a day. What's more, the effects were seen with approximately three servings of dairy a day, not single servings, and only certain types of dairy—namely, milk, yogurt, and perhaps some kinds of cheese—appear to be useful. Eating ice cream, cottage cheese, or cream cheese didn't help. Two final caveats: None of the studies specifically looked at menopausal women, and, as we all know, it gets harder to lose weight as you age. Also, the participants in these studies were seriously overweight or obese to start with. There is no evidence that dairy has any special weight-loss effects in women who are just 5 or 10 pounds over their ideal weight.

Dairy products can be part of any balanced weight-loss program. The USDA recommendation is three servings a day. That's important to remember, because women who are dieting tend to reduce their dairy consumption. And dairy products are an excellent source of calcium, essential to bone health.

Vegetarians and Menopause

Q *I've read that vegetarians go into menopause sooner than meat eaters. Is this true?*

A It's unlikely, especially if the rationale is that they're not getting enough protein. In the industrialized world, most people get adequate protein even if they're vegetarians. It is possible that women in poor countries who are restricted to a limited vegetarian diet might see some difference, but there's no clear evidence of this.

Eating lots of vegetables might even delay the transition. A Japanese study (which wasn't looking at vegetarianism per se) found that later onset of menopause was associated with higher consumption of green and yellow vegetables. In another study done by the University

A Better Way

We all love whipped cream and butter. In an alternate universe, they're health foods.
But while you're still here on Earth, you should avoid these and other diet busters. Here's how to
get similar taste in recipes with fewer calories and less cholesterol:

INGREDIENT	RECOMMENDATION
Cream cheese	Use nonfat or low-fat versions.
Eggs	In baking or cooking, use 2 egg whites and ¼ cup of cholesterol-free egg substitute instead of 1 egg, or 3 egg whites and 1 yolk instead of 2 whole eggs.
Sour cream	Blend 1 cup low-fat, unsalted cottage cheese with 1 tablespoon of nonfat milk and 2 tablespoons of lemon juice. Another choice: plain, nonfat yogurt.
Butter	Use margarine that lists liquid vegetable oil as the first ingredient on the nutrition label. In cooking, use spray oil. You can also dip bread in olive oil.
Chocolate	Use 3 tablespoons of cocoa instead of 1 ounce of baking chocolate. To replace the fat in chocolate, use 1 tablespoon or less of vegetable oil.

of Aberdeen, higher meat consumption was associated with earlier natural menopause in a group of women between the ages of 45 and 49.

So vegetarians should relax and concentrate on eating a healthy diet. On the other hand, if you're a frequent meat eater and you're also worried about cholesterol, you might want to cut down on fatty meats. Even if this doesn't delay menopause, it should improve your overall health.

WATER, WATER, EVERYWHERE

Q *For years, I've heard that you're supposed to drink eight glasses of water a day. Now that I'm older, I already have to go to the bathroom constantly. Is all that water really necessary?*

A Don't sweat this one. An Institute of Medicine report in 2004 dismissed the idea that there is some particular number of glasses of water one should drink every day. The reason is simple. The report said people meet their hydration needs by drinking all kinds of beverages, including coffee and soft drinks. Even the water in solid foods—like fruits and vegetables—adds to your fluid intake. The vast majority of healthy people drink plenty of liquids.

How much does that mean we actually consume? Actually, it's a lot more than the equivalent of eight eight-ounce glasses a day. The Institute of Medicine panel found that most women consume 91 ounces of water a day, the equivalent of 11.4 glasses, with 80 percent coming from beverages and the other 20 percent

What to Tell Your Daughter

The obesity epidemic is affecting children as well as adults. In the past two decades, the proportion of overweight children aged 6 to 11 has more than doubled; among 12-to-19-year-olds, the number has tripled. Fat kids are likely to stay fat; about half of obese adolescents become obese adults. And people who grow up fat are even more at risk for diseases like diabetes and atherosclerosis that are associated with obesity. Vigilance can't stop at the door of adulthood. Women who gain more than 20 pounds between the age of 18 and midlife double their risk of breast cancer after menopause. The message for your daughter is clear: Eat wisely, exercise daily, live well.

from food. Men average even more—125 ounces a day.

We all have different fluid requirements, and your needs may change depending on what you're doing and where you are. You may need more if you're physically active, if the temperature is above 80 degrees, if the humidity is low, or if you're at a higher elevation. In the last two cases, you'll lose more water to perspiration. Dark, strong-smelling urine is a signal that you need to drink more. Chronic constipation is another. Usually, thirst will make you drink enough.

MIXED DRINKS

Q *I'm getting such mixed signals on alcohol. Drinking red wine is supposed to be good for your heart, but I also hear that alcohol is bad for your bones. And does it raise or lower your breast cancer risk?*

A Alcohol plays a kind of Jekyll-and-Hyde role in your diet. Researchers describe what they call a J-shaped risk curve for alcohol consumption. With moderate drinking, mortality falls, basically because of the reduction in heart attack deaths. But as you drink more, total mortality rises, with an increase in deaths from cancer, liver disease, and accidents.

Alcohol helps to reduce heart attack deaths because it raises the level of HDL (good) cholesterol in your blood and also makes your blood less likely to form unwanted clots. Too much alcohol, however, raises blood pressure. And years of heavy drinking increase the risk of heart problems. The key is to drink in moderation. What does that mean? For a man, it's two drinks a day; for women, just one. A drink is defined as 12 ounces of beer, 5 ounces of wine, or 1.5 ounces of distilled spirits. Remember, moderate consumption for men is *twice* what it is for women. According to the National Institute on Alcohol Abuse and Alcoholism, when alcohol enters a woman's bloodstream, it typically reaches a higher level than a man's, even if both are drinking the same amount. Alcohol mixes with water in the body, and because women's bodies generally have less water than men's, the alcohol is less diluted. That's why women become more impaired by alcohol and are more vulnerable to alcohol-related illness.

As far as cancer is concerned, an analysis of 156 studies on a total of 116,702 subjects found that risks of many cancers increased with increasing alcohol consumption, especially cancers of the mouth, esophagus, and larynx. There was less of a correlation with cancers of the colon, rectum, liver, and breast. Although breast cancer risk does not increase as much as the others, the effect kicks in at lower levels. Just one drink a day can raise the risk by 10 percent. At two drinks a day, the risk increases to 20 to 25 percent; at 3.5 drinks, by 55 percent. And it continues to rise as you drink more. At 100 grams of alcohol a day (seven drinks), the risk for breast cancer is 2.4 times higher than if you drank no alcohol.

On bone health, the evidence is mixed. The one thing that's absolutely clear is that chronic alcohol abuse is associated with low bone density and high risk of fracture. More than two drinks a day interferes with calcium metabolism. Alcoholics also have high levels of cortisol, which have been linked to decreased bone formation and increased bone resorption. Alcohol has a direct toxic effect on the cells that build bone while stimulating the cells that break it down. H. Wayne Sampson, professor of human anatomy at the Texas A&M Health Science Center College of Medicine, has found that in young rats alcohol lowers bone mineral density and that the effects are not completely reversible as the rats age. However, *moderate* alcohol consumption in menopausal women may actually have a modest protective effect on bone. The Nurses' Health Study, after controlling for age, menopause status, BMI, estrogen levels, smoking status, physical activity, calcium and vitamin D intake, protein, and caffeine, found that postmenopausal women who consumed a drink a day had higher bone density than nondrinking women did. Why would this be true? According to the National Institutes of Health, it has to do with estrogen. In postmenopausal women, alcohol increases the conversion of testosterone into bone-protective estradiol, the most potent form of estrogen.

The advice that experts usually give is that if you don't drink, don't start. If you do drink, moderation is critical.

BERRY GOOD NEWS

Q *I keep hearing that berries are a "superfood." Is that true?*

A Antioxidants in blue, deep red, and purple berries cut the level of LDL cholesterol in your blood, reducing your risk of cardiovascular disease and stroke. The USDA's Human Nutrition Research Center says blueberries rank at the top of 40 fruits and vegetables studied for their antioxidant activity. Why is that so important? Antioxidants neutralize the damaging metabolism by-products called free radicals.

RECITES

Okay. You've heard the evidence, and you're ready to change your eating habits. In the course of preparing this book, we looked through dozens of diet guides and cookbooks. The one we liked best as a starting point is free if you access it online and costs only $4 if you want a copy already printed out. It's called *Keep the Beat: Heart Healthy Recipes from the National Heart, Lung and Blood Institute*. In addition to recipes, it contains information for designing your own diet plan. Below are a few of our favorite recipes. For more, check out www.nhlbi.nih.gov/health/public/heart/other/ktb_recipebk/.

Bean and Macaroni Soup

2 16-ounce cans Great Northern beans
1 tablespoon olive oil
½ pound fresh mushrooms, sliced
1 cup coarsely chopped onion
2 cups sliced carrots
1 cup coarsely chopped celery
1 clove garlic, minced

3 cups peeled and cut-up fresh tomatoes
   (or 1½ pounds canned, whole, cut up)*
1 teaspoon dried sage
1 teaspoon dried thyme
½ teaspoon dried oregano
freshly ground black pepper to taste
1 bay leaf, crumbled
4 cups uncooked elbow macaroni

1. Drain beans and reserve liquid. Rinse beans.

2. Heat oil in a six-quart kettle. Add mushrooms, onion, carrots, celery, and garlic. Sauté for 5 minutes.

3. Add tomatoes, sage, thyme, oregano, pepper, and bay leaf. Cover and cook over medium heat for 20 minutes.

4. Cook macaroni according to package directions, using unsalted water. Drain when cooked. Do not overcook.

5. Combine reserved bean liquid with water to make 4 cups.

6. Add liquid, beans, and cooked macaroni to vegetable mixture.

7. Bring to boil. Cover and simmer until soup is thoroughly heated. Stir occasionally.

* If you're using canned tomatoes, the sodium content will be higher. Look for canned tomatoes with no added salt to keep sodium lower.

YIELD: 16 servings ◆ SERVING SIZE: 1 cup

EACH SERVING PROVIDES:
CALORIES: 158
TOTAL FAT: 1 gram
SATURATED FAT: less than 1 gram
CHOLESTEROL: 0 milligrams
SODIUM: 154 milligrams
TOTAL FIBER: 5 milligrams
PROTEIN: 8 milligrams
CARBOHYDRATES: 29 grams
POTASSIUM: 524 milligrams

Gazpacho

3 medium tomatoes, peeled and chopped

½ cup seeded and chopped cucumber

½ cup cored and chopped green pepper

2 green onions, sliced

2 cups low-sodium vegetable juice cocktail

1 tablespoon lemon juice

½ teaspoon dried basil

¼ teaspoon hot pepper sauce

1 clove garlic, minced

1. In a large mixing bowl, combine all ingredients.

2. Cover and chill in refrigerator for several hours.

YIELD: 4 servings ◆
SERVING SIZE: 1¼ cups

EACH SERVING PROVIDES:

CALORIES: 52

TOTAL FAT: less than 1 gram

SATURATED FAT: less than 1 gram

CHOLESTEROL: 0 milligrams

SODIUM: 41 milligrams

TOTAL FIBER: 2 grams

PROTEIN: 2 grams

CARBOHYDRATES: 12 grams

POTASSIUM: 514 milligrams

Barbecued Chicken

8 pieces of chicken (about 3 pounds: breasts, drumsticks, and/or thighs), skin and fat removed

1 large onion, thinly sliced

3 tablespoons vinegar

3 tablespoons Worcestershire sauce

2 tablespoons brown sugar

Black pepper to taste

1 tablespoon hot pepper flakes

1 tablespoon chili powder

1 cup chicken stock or broth, fat skimmed from top

1. Preheat oven to 350°F. Place chicken in a 13-inch by 9-inch by 2-inch pan. Arrange onions over top.

2. Mix together vinegar, Worcestershire sauce, brown sugar, pepper, hot pepper flakes, chili powder, and stock. Pour mixture over chicken and bake for 1 hour or until done. While cooking, baste occasionally.

YIELD: 8 servings ◆ SERVING SIZE: 1 chicken part with sauce

EACH SERVING PROVIDES:

CALORIES: 176

TOTAL FAT: 6 grams

SATURATED FAT: 2 grams

CHOLESTEROL: 68 milligrams

SODIUM: 240 milligrams

TOTAL FIBER: 1 gram

PROTEIN: 24 grams

CARBOHYDRATES: 7 grams

POTASSIUM: 360 milligrams

Bavarian Beef

1¼ pounds lean beef stew meat, trimmed
    of fat and cut into 1-inch pieces
1 tablespoon vegetable oil
1 large onion, thinly sliced
1½ cups water
¾ teaspoon caraway seeds
½ teaspoon salt

⅛ teaspoon black pepper
1 bay leaf
¼ cup white vinegar
1 tablespoon sugar
½ small head red cabbage,
    cut into 4 wedges
¼ cup crushed gingersnaps

1. Brown meat in oil in a heavy skillet. Remove meat and sauté onion in the same pan until golden. Return meat to skillet. Add water, caraway seeds, salt, pepper, and bay leaf. Bring to boil. Reduce heat, cover, and simmer for 1¼ hours.

2. Add vinegar and sugar. Stir. Place cabbage on top of meat. Cover and simmer for an added 45 minutes.

3. Remove meat and cabbage, arrange on a platter, and keep warm.

4. Strain drippings from skillet and skim off fat. Add enough water to drippings to yield 1 cup of liquid.

5. Return to skillet with crushed gingersnaps. Cook and stir until thickened and mixture boils. Pour over meat and vegetables, and serve.

YIELD: 5 servings ◆ SERVING SIZE: 5 oz.

EACH SERVING PROVIDES:
CALORIES: 218
TOTAL FAT: 7 grams
SATURATED FAT: 2 grams
CHOLESTEROL: 60 milligrams
SODIUM: 323 milligrams
TOTAL FIBER: 2 grams
PROTEIN: 24 grams
CARBOHYDRATES: 14 grams
POTASSIUM: 509 milligrams

Bay Scallop Kebabs

3 medium green peppers,
    cut into 1½-inch squares
1½ pounds fresh bay scallops
1 pint cherry tomatoes
¼ cup dry white wine

¼ cup vegetable oil
3 tablespoons lemon juice
Dash garlic powder
Black pepper to taste
4 skewers

1. Parboil green peppers for 2 minutes.

2. Alternately thread peppers, scallops, and tomatoes on skewers.

3. Combine wine, oil, and lemon juice. Season with garlic powder and black pepper.

4. Brush kebabs with wine/oil/lemon mixture, then place on grill or under broiler.

5. Grill for 15 minutes, turning and basting frequently.

YIELD: 4 servings ◆ SERVING SIZE: 1 kebab (6 oz.)

EACH SERVING PROVIDES:

CALORIES: 224

TOTAL FAT: 6 grams

SATURATED FAT: 1 gram

CHOLESTEROL: 43 milligrams

SODIUM: 355 milligrams

TOTAL FIBER: 3 grams

PROTEIN: 30 grams

CARBOHYDRATES: 13 grams

POTASSIUM: 993 milligrams

Classic Macaroni and Cheese

2 cups uncooked macaroni

Nonstick cooking spray, as needed

½ cup chopped onion

½ cup evaporated skim milk

1 medium egg, beaten

¼ teaspoon black pepper

1¼ cups (4 oz.) finely shredded
    low-fat sharp Cheddar cheese

1. Cook macaroni according to package directions, using unsalted water. Drain and set aside.

2. Preheat oven to 350°F. Spray a casserole dish with nonstick cooking spray.

3. Lightly spray a saucepan with nonstick cooking spray. Add onion to saucepan and sauté for about 3 minutes.

4. Combine macaroni, onion, and rest of the ingredients in a bowl. Mix thoroughly.

5. Transfer mixture to casserole dish.

6. Bake for 25 minutes or until bubbly. Let stand for 10 minutes before serving.

YIELD: 8 servings ◆ SERVING SIZE: ½ cup

EACH SERVING PROVIDES:

CALORIES: 200

TOTAL FAT: 4 grams

SATURATED FAT: 2 grams

CHOLESTEROL: 34 milligrams

SODIUM: 120 milligrams

TOTAL FIBER: 1 gram

PROTEIN: 11 grams

CARBOHYDRATES: 29 grams

POTASSIUM: 119 milligrams

Zucchini Lasagna

Nonstick cooking spray, as needed

¾ cup grated part-skim mozzarella cheese

¼ cup grated Parmesan cheese

1½ cups fat-free cottage cheese*

1½ cups no-salt-added tomato sauce

2 teaspoons dried basil

2 teaspoons dried oregano

¼ cup chopped onion

1 clove garlic

⅛ teaspoon black pepper

½ pound lasagna noodles, cooked in
    unsalted water

1½ cups sliced raw zucchini

(continued on page 398)

1. Preheat oven to 350°F. Lightly spray a 9- by 13-inch baking dish with vegetable oil spray.

2. In a small bowl, combine ⅛ cup mozzarella and 1 tablespoon Parmesan cheese. Set aside.

3. In a medium bowl, combine remaining mozzarella and Parmesan cheese with all of the cottage cheese. Mix well and set aside.

4. Combine tomato sauce with the next five ingredients. Spread a thin layer of tomato sauce in bottom of baking dish. Add a third of the noodles in a single layer. Spread half of the cottage cheese mixture on top. Add a layer of zucchini.

5. Repeat layering. Add a thin coating of sauce. Top with noodles, sauce, and reserved cheese mixture. Cover with aluminum foil.

6. Bake for 30 to 40 minutes. Cool for 10 to 15 minutes.

* Use unsalted cottage cheese to reduce the sodium content. New sodium content for each serving is 196 grams.

YIELD: 6 servings ◆ SERVING SIZE: 1 piece

EACH SERVING PROVIDES:

CALORIES: 276

TOTAL FAT: 5 grams

SATURATED FAT: 2 grams

CHOLESTEROL: 11 milligrams

SODIUM: 380 milligrams

TOTAL FIBER: 5 grams

PROTEIN: 19 grams

CARBOHYDRATES: 41 grams

POTASSIUM: 561 milligrams

Banana Mousse

2 tablespoons low-fat milk

4 teaspoons sugar

1 teaspoon vanilla

1 medium banana, cut into quarters

1 cup plain low-fat yogurt

8 ¼-inch slices banana

1. Place milk, sugar, vanilla, and banana in blender. Process for 15 seconds at high speed until smooth.

2. Pour mixture into small bowl and fold in yogurt. Chill.

3. Spoon into four dessert dishes and garnish each with two banana slices before serving.

YIELD: 4 servings ◆ SERVING SIZE: ½ cup

EACH SERVING PROVIDES:

CALORIES: 94

TOTAL FAT: 1 gram

SATURATED FAT: 1 milligram

CHOLESTEROL: 4 milligrams

SODIUM: 47 milligrams

TOTAL FIBER: 1 gram

PROTEIN: 1 gram

CARBOHYDRATES: 18 grams

POTASSIUM: 297 milligrams

EXERCISE

First, a confession. Neither of us would ever qualify as a jock. But we do try to stay as active as we can, especially now that we're at midlife. We've tried everything— walking, running, swimming, biking, yoga, Pilates, workouts at the gym, video workouts—and we've come to the conclusion that any activity helps as long as you do something regularly. In this section, we give you a little background on activities that might work for you and a set of simple exercises to get even the most out-of-shape reader on the road to health.

First Steps

If you notice that you're winded after climbing a flight of stairs or even walking around the block, your body is telling you that it's time to shape up. This is a message you shouldn't ignore. The value of exercise is probably the most consistent finding in the reams of medical research published every year. If you're inspired to give fitness another shot, here's some advice from the experts on how to start an exercise program and, more important, how to stay the course.

FOCUS ON GOALS. Think about what you want to accomplish. Your goal might be something as specific as an upcoming hiking vacation or as general as being able to play ball with your children or grandchildren. Having a meaningful goal in mind will keep you going when you hit the inevitable rough spots.

RESEARCH YOUR CHOICES. One good place to start is the website of the American College of Sports Medicine at www.acsm.org. The site contains lots of information on different types of exer-cises as well as topics like how to pick a personal trainer. After you zero in on what might work for you, check out fitness options in your community, such as joining a gym, walking with a friend around the high school track, or signing up for classes at the Y. At this stage, you might also consult your doctor. If you haven't been active in a while, you probably need a checkup to make sure you're ready to start training.

CREATE A SUPPORT SYSTEM. Get your partner or spouse on board. Try to enlist a friend to exercise with you. The social surround of exercise seems to matter more to women than to men. You'll keep each other going on those days when working out seems like too much trouble.

BE PREPARED. If you're going to start a walking program, for example, buy comfortable and supportive shoes. If a gym workout is on your agenda, schedule it for the period of your day when you have the most control over your time. For many people, that's early morning—

before the day's craziness has gotten in the way. Other good bets are "transition" times: at lunch or on your way home. Keep your gym bag in your car so you're ready whenever the urge hits you.

DON'T OVERREACH AT THE START. You may be dreaming of a triathalon, but for now, focus on the next couple of months and exercising for a specific number of days a week. You might try 15 minutes at first and then add more minutes as you progress. The important thing in the beginning is to make exercise as much a part of your routine as brushing your teeth. Research shows that it takes about eight weeks to establish this kind of habit. It's a lot easier to concentrate on that specific, short-term goal than to imagine what it will take to get you in shape to run 26-plus miles. A good rule for avoiding injuries is to increase your workout by around 10 percent a week.

VARY YOUR WORKOUT. Ultimately, you want to work up to a regimen that includes exercises that increase cardiorespiratory endurance, muscular fitness, and flexibility. All three types of activities are important. Cardiorespiratory activities could include something as simple as 30 minutes of brisk walking. Muscular fitness is especially important for women because it helps to maintain bone strength, especially after menopause. Working with free weights or using resistance bands builds muscles and strengthens bone. Muscle cells also burn more calories than fat cells do—a boost to dieting. Flexibility and stretching exercises keep you limber and help to prevent injury.

KEEP A JOURNAL. You won't see overnight change in your body, but marking down everything you're doing can give you a sense of accomplishment in the meantime. Even something as simple as putting check marks on your calendar works to reinforce the message that you're making progress.

ANTICIPATE RELAPSE. No matter how great a start you get, you'll fall off at some point—perhaps because of a crush of projects at work, illness, or some other personal issue. Don't let it escalate. Make a plan with your friend to get back to the routine on a specific day and stick to that. Researchers tell us that getting back into the zone isn't easy if you've been away for more than two weeks, but that's no excuse for letting a couple of weeks turn into four and then eight.

HAVE FUN. The main reason most exercise plans fail is because they're boring. If you're on the treadmill or the stair machine, listen to music on your iPod. When you're walking or running with a friend, think of it as a social activity as well as exercise. If you're feeling ambitious, take up a sport like tennis or skiing or biking. After a while, exercise becomes an accepted part of your life and you'll wonder what you ever did without it.

JOINING A GYM

Q *I have friends who work out at three different gyms near me and say good things about each. How can I tell which is right for me?*

A Since there are more than 26,000 health clubs in the United States with more than 41 million members, your options are many—maybe too many! But positive word of mouth from your friends is a good place to start. Take the time to test-drive each recommended gym. Many gyms give members free passes for friends; some clubs will let you join for a week or a month as a trial membership. In any case, ask for a tour and keep your eyes open. Ask to see group classes. Are they well organized? Is the changing area clean? Watch for adequate lighting and ventilation. Is there enough parking? Is the gym convenient? Does it offer a prescreening to determine your fitness level? Do staff members have appropriate certification and training? Is there a grace period during which you can cancel your membership? Are all the fees for services posted?

One warning: If the sales manager or membership coordinator who shows you around pressures you to sign a contract, move on to the next facility.

STRENGTH OR FLEXIBILITY?

Q *I'm confused by all the different possibilities: yoga, weight training, swimming, running. What do I really need to do in order to get my body in shape?*

A A good exercise program has three major components: cardiorespiratory endurance, muscular fitness, and flexibility. You need to include all three if you want to really get in shape—both inside and outside. Cardiorespiratory endurance is the capability to perform high-intensity exercise using large muscle groups for an extended period. Activities like jogging or brisk walking build up your cardiorespiratory endurance and lower your risk of heart disease. Muscular fitness involves both muscle strength and endurance. You don't need to look like a weight lifter to be muscularly fit. Generally, toned muscles will boost your muscle mass, which means a higher metabolic rate since muscle burns more calories an hour than fat does. A higher muscle mass also reduces your vulnerability to osteoporosis. You can use free weights, weight-lifting machines, or even cans of soup to build up your muscles. The important thing is to start slowly and increase the weight gradually so you don't overload your muscles and injure yourself. Finally, flexibility exercises are especially critical as you get older; you should be doing them every day. You don't need any special equipment—just enough space to stretch muscle groups. Activities like yoga, Pilates, and tai chi are great for building both flexibility and strength. Many women also say they're stress busters.

How do you know what specific exercises you should be doing? It really depends on your current fitness level. We'll give you some sample exercises at

DO PEDOMETERS WORK?

Not all pedometers are equally accurate, but using one can be a good way to keep track of your activity level and encourage you to push it up a notch. Pedometers track movements that cause your hips to move up and down (like walking and running). Each of these movements is recorded as a step. Some models also calculate distance and calories expended. Walking too slow lowers the level of accuracy. For best results, wear the pedometer on your waist parallel to your right knee. The American College of Sports Medicine says the most accurate brands are Yamax, Kenz, New Lifestyles, and Walk4Life. In general, they work best for tracking steps and are less effective at tracking distance and calories. A good goal is 10,000 steps a day, but don't try to reach that level your first day if you've been inactive. Work up to it gradually.

The ACSM suggests this simple test of a pedometer's accuracy:

1. Put on the pedometer and find a space where you can walk at your typical pace.

2. Reset the pedometer to zero.

3. Walk 20 steps.

4. Carefully open the pedometer (too much jiggling can add steps).

5. Ratings:

Perfect = 20 steps

Good = 19 to 21 steps

Acceptable = 18 to 22 steps

Unacceptable = less than 17 or more than 23 steps

the end of this chapter, but if you're really serious about this, you might invest in a session with a well-qualified personal trainer who can individualize a program for you. Also, recreation departments in many communities offer low-cost, professionally taught exercise classes that are geared to people of different ages and abilities.

PICKING A TRAINER

Q *How do I know that a personal trainer is qualified and not just a glorified gym rat?*

A The American College of Sports Medicine maintains a list of ACSM-certified professionals on its website, www.acsm.org. Look for the Pro Finder link. If you're a gym member, watch trainers in action who have clients of your age and general physical activity level. If you're interested in hiring a particular trainer you've seen outside of the gym, ask for a resumé and references from current clients and find out if he or she has a certification from ACSM or another nationally recognized organization such as the American Council on Exercise (www.acefitness.org). Also make sure the trainer is certified in CPR and has professional liability insurance. Ask about educational background; many trainers have a college degree in exercise science or physical education. You need to discuss your goals with your trainer and see if your needs mesh with his or her ideas. If you have a particular physical problem, ask about the trainer's experience with bad backs or weak knees or whatever your problem is. You don't want the trainer to mollycoddle you, but you do want to make sure you'll get a workout appropriate for your physical condition. Finally, be sure you understand the fee schedule and cancellation penalties.

DOES HOUSEWORK COUNT?

Q *I've never belonged to a gym, but I live in a three-story house and I do all the cleaning—vacuuming, mopping floors, laundry, changing beds, dusting. I feel pretty fit. Could my housecleaning be the reason?*

A We're in awe—and not just because your cleaning routine puts us to shame. Yes, housework counts as physical activity, especially when you're running up and down stairs all day. If you're making beds, mopping, vacuuming, and all the rest, you're probably expending plenty of calories and building muscles in your arms and legs. But you might still want to consider strength-training exercises for your bones. You're also missing the pleasure physical activity can bring. Try signing up for a yoga class, or just take a brisk walk every day with a friend. In the meantime, the chart in the next column will give you some idea of how many calories a healthy woman weighing between 120 and 150 pounds burns doing daily activities.

ACTIVITY	CALORIES PER HOUR
Walking up and down stairs	150
Raking leaves	300
Washing windows or floors	150
Washing dishes, ironing clothes	100
General cleaning, vacuuming, mopping	200
Mowing lawn (manual mower)	400
Mowing lawn (self-propelled mower)	200
Washing, waxing car	300

WORKOUT STYLE

Q *Do I need to spend a fortune on special work-out clothes, or can I just wear any old pair of sweats?*

A Some women find that more attractive clothes make them feel confident in the gym, but a glam look is no necessity. You should wear easy-fitting clothing that lets you move freely—a style that comes in all price ranges. Just make sure that what you're wearing is safe; pants that are too long can get caught in equipment and cause an accident. You might also want to invest in clothes made of wicking fabrics that take moisture away from your body. Wicking underwear and T-shirts can make your workout more comfortable by eliminating chafing from sweaty clothes sticking to your body. If you're going to spend money on one item, we suggest a really supportive bra—look for "no jiggle" models.

IF THE SHOE FITS

Q *I'm ready to start training and I went to my local shoe store to buy some running shoes. The choices were mind-boggling!*

A Unless you're planning on participating in a sport two or three times a week, you can rule out shoes designed for specific games like basketball. Instead, if your workout includes lots of brisk walking or running, look for shoes that have comfortable soft uppers plus good shock absorption, cushioning, flexibility, and traction. Try on shoes after a workout or at the end of the day when your feet are at their largest. Wear athletic socks—not panty hose. In well-fitting shoes, you should be able to wiggle all your toes. Try to run a few steps to see how the shoes will feel in action. Your heels should not slip when you move. Finally, if you're really working out regularly, you'll need to replace your shoes every six months or so.

HOW MUCH IS ENOUGH?

Q *How much time do I have to spend exercising every day?*

A In general, you should aim for 30 to 60 minutes of physical activity *every* day. This doesn't mean you have to go to the gym and sweat on the treadmill for an hour. In fact, research shows that most people are more likely to adhere to a fitness routine if they vary their activities: a brisk walk one day, a game of ten-nis another, and perhaps an afternoon cleaning out the attic. Everything counts. You can even turn the most routine movements into physical training. Increase the number of steps you take each day by getting off the bus a stop or two early. Use stairs instead of the escalator. Carrying groceries out to the car instead of using the cart builds upper body strength. You can improve your flexibility the same way. When you're brushing your teeth, stretch out your calf muscles by putting one leg behind the other (don't bend your knee). Invest in a set of small hand-sized dumbbells and keep them in the family room so you can lift during your favorite TV programs.

WATER POWER

Q *Everyone at my gym carries a bottle of water around. I just drink from the fountain before I start and after I finish. Am I doing something wrong?*

A If you feel okay, that's fine. The need to rehydrate *constantly* is a myth that has been around athletic circles for years; in fact, recent research has shown that too much water can be dangerous—at least for endurance athletes. One other point: You may see oxygenated water advertised as an energy booster. No high-quality studies back up this claim. So save your money and drink from the fountain or your own water bottle if you feel thirsty.

WARMING UP AND COOLING DOWN

Trainers generally recommend both warming up and cooling down to prevent injuries. You can warm up your muscles by something as simple as walking to the gym instead of driving or by starting your exercise routine slowly for the first 5 or 10 minutes and then ratcheting up the intensity. A common warm-up is to stretch the muscles in your shoulders, back, arms, and legs through a series of exercises. Similar exercises also help after you finish your workout. Here are some examples from the American Academy of Orthopaedic Surgeons (www.aaos.org):

For shoulders. While standing or sitting, interlace your fingers. With palms facing up, push your arms slightly back and up. Hold for 15 seconds. (Figure 1) With your arms overhead, hold the elbow of one arm with your other hand. Gently pull the elbow behind your arm. Hold for 15 seconds. Stretch both arms. (Figure 2) Gently pull your elbow across your chest toward your opposite shoulder. Hold for 10 seconds. Repeat with the other elbow. (Figure 3)

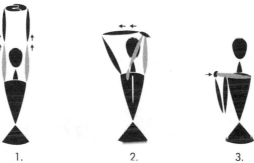

1.   2.   3.

For knee and calf. Hold the top of your left foot with your right hand and gently pull it toward your buttocks. Hold for 30 seconds and repeat with the other leg. (Figure 1) Standing close to a wall or other solid support, lean on your forearms with your head resting on your hands. Bend one leg and place it on the ground in front of you with the other leg straight behind. Slowly move your hips forward while keeping your back flat. Hold for 15 to 30 seconds. Do not bounce. (Figure 2)

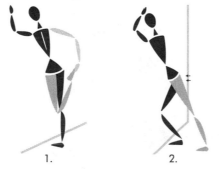

1.   2.

For hip and groin. Sit with the bottoms of your feet touching. Hold your feet with your hands while slowly pushing down on your knees with your elbows. Hold for 5 to 8 seconds. (Figure 1) Place one leg forward while your other leg is resting on the floor. Without changing the position of your knee on the floor or the forward leg, sit into your forward hip. Hold for 30 seconds. (Figure 2)

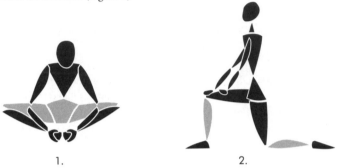

1.   2.

For lower back. Lie down on your back. Pull your left leg toward your chest while keeping the back of your head on the floor. Hold for 30 seconds. Repeat with your right leg.

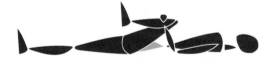

For hamstring. Sit down and straighten your left leg. The sole of your right foot should be next to the inside of your straightened leg. Lean forward and try to touch your foot with your fingers. (Reach only as far as you can while keeping your leg straight.) Keep your left foot upright with your ankle and toes relaxed. Hold for 30 seconds. Repeat with right leg.

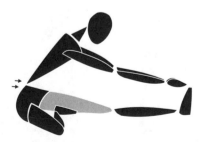

Easy Beginnings

Just to get you going, we've included these exercises from the National Institute on Aging. They're designed especially for older people, so they should qualify as a gentle start for someone at midlife. There's nothing overly strenuous here, but they do cover the different categories of exercise. You can access the whole booklet, which contains more exercises, at www.nia.nih.gov/HealthInformation/Publications/ExerciseGuide/. By the way, if you're just starting to work out, you can begin with weights of a pound or two. Add more as you get stronger.

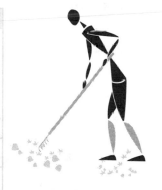

Endurance Activities

Endurance activities increase your heart rate and breathing for an extended period. You don't have to go to the gym to do this, as you can see below. Build up endurance gradually, starting out with as little as five minutes at a time if that's what you need to do. Your goal is 30 minutes of endurance exercise on most days of the week.

MODERATE	VIGOROUS
Swimming	Climbing stairs or hills
Bicycling	Shoveling snow
Cycling on a stationary bicycle	Brisk bicycling up hills
Gardening (mowing, raking)	Tennis (singles)
Walking briskly on a level surface	Swimming laps
Mopping or scrubbing floor	Cross-country skiing
Golf, without a cart	Downhill skiing
Tennis (doubles)	Hiking
Volleyball	Jogging
Rowing	
Dancing	

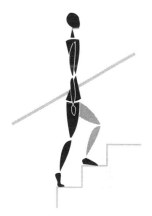

Strength Exercises

Arm Raise

This exercise strengthens your shoulder muscles.

1. Sit in an armless chair with your back supported by the back of the chair.

2. Keep your feet flat on the floor, shoulder-width apart.

3. Hold the hand weights straight down at your sides, with your palms facing inward.

4. Raise both arms out to the side, shoulder height.

5. Hold the position for 1 second.

6. Slowly lower your arms to your sides. Pause.

7. Repeat 8 to 15 times.

8. Rest; then do another set of 8 to 15 repetitions.

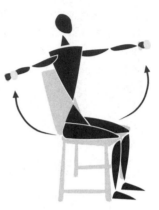

Chair Stands

As you become stronger, try to do this exercise without using your hands. The goal is to strengthen the muscles in your abdomen and thighs.

1. Place a pillow on the back of a chair.

2. Sit toward the front of the chair, knees bent and feet flat on the floor.

3. Lean back against the pillow, keeping your back and shoulders straight.

4. Raise your upper body forward until you're sitting upright, using your hands as little as possible (or not at all, if you can).

5. Slowly stand up, again using your hands as little as possible.

6. Slowly sit back down. Pause.

7. Repeat 8 to 15 times.

8. Rest; then do another set of 8 to 15 repetitions.

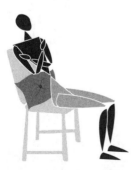
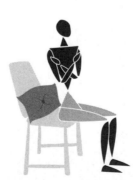
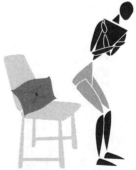

Biceps Curl

Do this to improve the strength of your upper-arm muscles.

1. Sit in an armless chair with your back supported by the back of the chair and your feet flat on the floor shoulder-width apart.

2. Hold the hand weights straight down at your sides, with your palms facing inward.

3. Slowly bend one elbow, lifting the weight toward your chest. (Rotate your palm to face your shoulder while lifting the weight.)

4. Hold this position for 1 second.

5. Slowly lower your arm to the starting position. Pause.

6. Repeat with your other arm.

7. Alternate arms until you've completed 8 to 15 repetitions with each arm.

8. Rest; then do another set of 8 to 15 alternating repetitions.

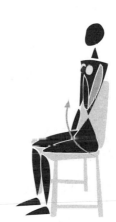

Plantar Flexion

This exercise may look familiar; It's one that we included in Chapter 10. It's also part of the National Institute on Aging program because it's a great way to strengthen your ankle and calf muscles. Use ankle weights if you're ready for them.

1. Stand straight with your feet flat on the floor. Hold on to a chair or table for balance.

2. Slowly stand on tiptoe, as high as possible.

3. Hold this position for 1 second.

4. Slowly lower your heels all the way back down. Pause.

5. Do the exercise 8 to 15 times.

6. Rest; then do another set of 8 to 15 repetitions.

Variation: As you become stronger, do the exercise standing on one leg only, alternating legs for a total of 8 to 15 times on each leg. Rest; then do another set of 8 to 15 alternating repetitions.

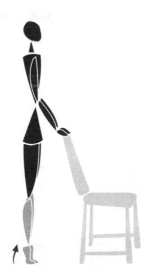

Triceps Extension

We included a version of this exercise in our chapter on hot flashes. As we mentioned, there's no point in wearing sleeveless tops under your suits if you're embarrassed about your arms. This exercise strengthens the muscles in the backs of your upper arms. Keep supporting your arm with your hand throughout the exercise. (If your shoulders aren't flexible enough to do this exercise, see the "Dip" exercise below.)

1. Sit in a chair with your back supported by the back of the chair.

2. Keep your feet flat on the floor, shoulder-width apart.

3. Hold a weight in your left hand. Raise your left arm straight toward the ceiling, palm facing in.

4. Support your left arm, below the elbow, with your right hand.

5. Slowly bend your left arm, bringing the hand weight toward your left shoulder.

6. Slowly straighten your left arm toward the ceiling.

7. Hold this position for 1 second.

8. Slowly bend your left arm toward your shoulder again. Pause.

9. Repeat the bending and straightening until you've completed the exercise 8 to 15 times.

10. Repeat 8 to 15 times with your right arm.

11. Rest; then do another set of 8 to 15 repetitions.

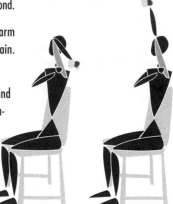

Alternative "Dip" Exercise for Back of Upper Arm

This pushing motion will strengthen your arm muscles even if you aren't yet able to lift yourself up off of the chair. Don't use your legs or feet for assistance, or use them as little as possible.

1. Sit in a chair with armrests.

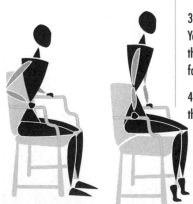

2. Lean slightly forward, keeping your back and shoulders straight.

3. Grasp the arms of the chair. Your hands should be level with the trunk of your body, or slightly farther forward.

4. Tuck your feet slightly under the chair, heels off the ground and weight on the toes and balls of your feet.

5. Slowly push your body off the chair, using your arms (not your legs).

6. Slowly lower your back down to the starting position. Pause.

7. Repeat 8 to 15 times.

8. Rest; then do another set of 8 to 15 repetitions.

Knee Flexion

If you're ready, use ankle weights when you do this exercise, which strengthens the muscles in the backs of your thighs.

1. Stand straight, holding on to a chair or table for balance.

2. Slowly bend your right knee as far as possible. Don't move your upper leg at all.

3. Hold this position for 1 second.

4. Slowly lower your right foot all the way back down. Pause.

5. Repeat with your left leg.

6. Alternate legs until you've completed 8 to 15 repetitions with each leg.

7. Rest; then do another set of 8 to 15 alternating repetitions.

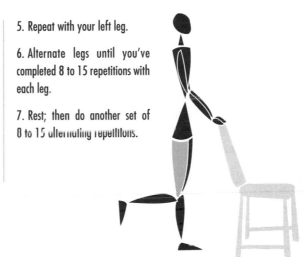

Hip Flexion

Again, use ankle weights when you're ready. This exercise strengthens your thigh and hip muscles.

1. Stand straight behind or to the side of a chair or table, holding on for balance.

2. Slowly bend your right knee toward your chest, without bending your waist or twisting your hips.

3. Hold this position for 1 second.

4. Slowly lower your right leg all the way down. Pause.

5. Repeat with your left leg.

6. Alternate legs until you've completed 0 to 15 repetitions with each leg.

7. Rest; then do another set of 8 to 15 alternating repetitions.

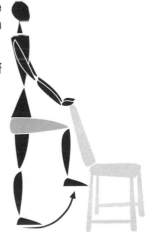

Shoulder Flexion

Do this exercise to strengthen your shoulder muscles.

1. Sit in an armless chair with your back supported by the back of the chair.

2. Keep your feet flat on the floor, shoulder-width apart.

3. Hold the hand weights straight down at your sides, with your palms facing inward.

4. Raise both arms to shoulder height in front of you, keeping them straight and rotating your wrists so that your palms face upward.

5. Hold this position for 1 second.

6. Slowly lower your arms to your sides. Pause.

7. Repeat 8 to 15 times.

8. Rest; then do another set of 8 to 15 repetitions.

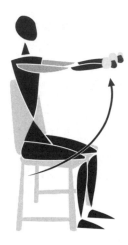

Knee Extension

This is another exercise where you can use ankle weights when you're ready. It strengthens the muscles in the front of your thigh and around your shin.

1. Sit in a chair with only your toes and the balls of your feet resting on the floor. Place a rolled towel under your knees, if needed, to lift your feet. Rest your hands on your thighs or on the sides of the chair.

2. Slowly extend your left leg as straight as possible in front of you.

3. Flex your left foot so that your toes point toward your head.

4. Hold this position for 1 to 2 seconds.

5. Slowly lower your left leg back down. Pause.

6. Alternate legs until you've completed 8 to 15 repetitions with each leg.

7. Rest; then do another set of 8 to 15 alternating repetitions.

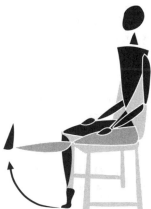

Hip Extension

These movements will strengthen your buttocks and lower-back muscles. Use ankle weights if you're ready.

1. Stand 12 to 18 inches from a chair or table, feet slightly apart.

2. Bend forward at the hips at about a 45-degree angle; hold on to the chair or table for balance.

3. Slowly lift your right leg straight backwards without bending your knee, pointing your toes, or bending your upper body any farther forward.

4. Hold this position for 1 second.

5. Slowly lower your right leg. Pause.

6. Repeat with your left leg.

7. Alternate legs until you've completed 8 to 15 repetitions with each leg.

8. Rest; then do another set of 8 to 15 alternating repetitions.

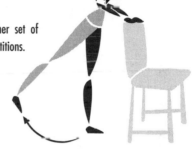

Side Leg Raise

This exercise works the muscles at the sides of your hips and thighs. When you're ready, add ankle weights.

1. Stand straight, directly behind a chair or table, with your feet slightly apart.

2. Hold on to the chair or table for balance.

3. Slowly lift your right leg 6 to 12 inches out to the side. Keep your back and both legs straight. Don't point your toes outward; keep them facing forward.

4. Hold this position for 1 second.

5. Slowly lower your right leg. Pause.

6. Repeat with your left leg.

7. Alternate legs until you've completed 8 to 15 repetitions with each leg.

8. Rest; then do another set of 8 to 15 alternating repetitions.

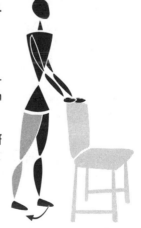

Examples of Strength/Balance Exercises

Plantar Flexion

Plantar flexion is already included in your strength exercises. Add modifications as you progress. Hold on to a chair or table with one hand, then one fingertip, then no hands; then do the exercise with your eyes closed, if steady.

1. Stand straight; hold on to a chair or table for balance.

2. Slowly stand on tiptoe, as high as possible.

3. Hold this position for 1 second.

4. Slowly lower your heels all the way back down. Pause.

5. Repeat 8 to 15 times.

6. Rest; then do another set of 8 to 15 repetitions.

Do modifications to your ability.

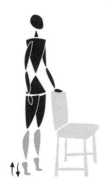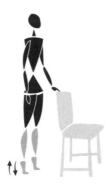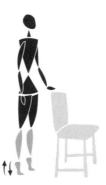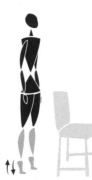

Knee Flexion

Do knee flexions as part of your regularly scheduled strength exercises, and add modifications as you progress. Hold on to a chair or table with one hand, then one fingertip, then no hands; then do the exercise with your eyes closed, if steady.

1. Stand straight; hold on to a chair or table for balance.

2. Slowly bend your right knee as far as possible, so that your right foot lifts up behind you.

3. Hold this position for 1 second.

4. Slowly lower your right foot all the way back down. Pause.

5. Repeat with your left leg.

6. Alternate legs until you've completed 8 to 15 repetitions with each leg.

7. Rest; then do another set of 8 to 15 alternating repetitions.

Do modifications to your ability.

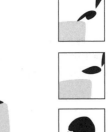

Hip Flexion

Do hip flexions as part of your regularly scheduled strength exercises, and add modifications as you progress. Hold on to a chair or table with one hand, then one fingertip, then no hands; then do the exercise with your eyes closed, if steady.

1. Stand straight; hold on to a chair or table for balance.

2. Slowly bend your right knee toward your chest, without bending your waist or twisting your hips.

3. Hold the position for 1 second.

4. Slowly lower your right leg all the way down. Pause.

5. Repeat with your left leg.

6. Alternate legs until you've completed 8 to 15 repetitions with each leg.

7. Rest; then do another set of 8 to 15 alternating repetitions.

Do modifications to your ability.

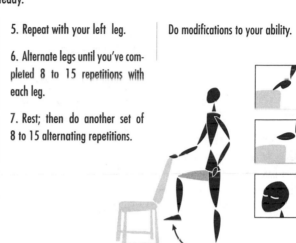

Hip Extension

Do hip extensions as part of your regularly scheduled strength exercises, and add modifications as you progress. Hold on to a chair or table with one hand, then one fingertip, then no hands; then do the exercise with your eyes closed, if steady.

1. Stand 12 to 18 inches from a chair or table, with your feet slightly apart.

2. Bend forward at the hips at about a 45-degree angle; hold on to the chair or table for balance.

3. Slowly lift your right leg straight backwards without bending your knee, pointing your toes, or bending your upper body any farther forward.

4. Hold this position for 1 second.

5. Slowly lower your right leg. Pause.

6. Repeat with your left leg.

7. Alternate legs until you've completed 8 to 15 repetitions with each leg.

8. Rest; then do another set of 8 to 15 alternating repetitions.

Do modifications to your ability.

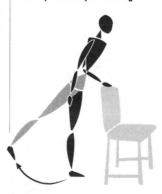

Side Leg Raise

Do leg raises as part of your regularly scheduled strength exercises, and add modifications as you progress. Hold on to a chair or table with one hand, then one fingertip, then no hands; then do the exercise with your eyes closed, if steady.

1. Stand straight, directly behind a chair or table, with your feet slightly apart.

2. Hold on to the chair or table for balance.

3. Slowly lift your right leg 6 to 12 inches out to the side. Keep your back and both legs straight. Don't point your toes outward; keep them facing forward.

4. Hold this position for 1 second.

5. Slowly lower your right leg all the way down. Pause.

6. Repeat with your left leg.

7. Alternate legs until you've completed 8 to 15 repetitions with each leg.

8. Rest; then do another set of 8 to 15 alternating repetitions.

Do modifications to your ability.

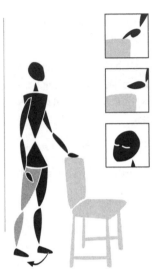

"Anytime, Anywhere" Balance Exercises

These types of exercises also improve your balance. You can do them almost anytime, anywhere, and as often as you like, as long as you have something sturdy nearby to hold on to if you become unsteady.

Examples:

• Walk heel-to-toe. Position your heel just in front of the toes of the opposite foot each time you take a step. Your heel and toes should touch or almost touch. (See illustration.)

• Stand on one foot (for instance, while waiting in line at the grocery store or at the bus stop). Alternate feet.

• Stand up and sit down without using your hands.

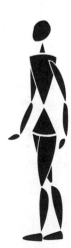

Stretching Exercises

Hamstrings Stretch

This exercise stretches the muscles in the backs of your thighs.

1. Sit sideways on a bench or other hard surface (such as two chairs placed side by side).

2. Keep your left leg stretched out straight on the surface, toes pointing up.

3. Keep your right leg off the surface, with your foot flat on the floor.

4. Straighten your back.

5. If you feel a stretch at this point, hold the position for 10 to 30 seconds.

6. If you don't feel a stretch, lean forward from your hips (not your waist) until you feel stretching in your left leg, keeping your back and shoulders straight. Omit this step if you've had a hip replacement, unless your surgeon/therapist approves.

7. Hold this position for 10 to 30 seconds.

8. Repeat with your right leg.

9. Repeat 3 to 5 times on each side.

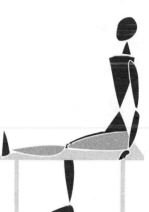

Alternative Hamstrings Stretch

This is another way to stretch the muscles in the backs of your thighs.

1. Stand behind a chair, holding on to the back with both hands.

2. Bend forward from your hips (not your waist), keeping your back and shoulders straight at all times.

3. When your upper body is parallel to the floor, hold the position for 10 to 30 seconds. You should feel a stretch in the backs of your thighs.

4. Repeat 3 to 5 times.

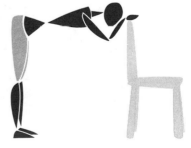

Ankle Stretch

Here's how to stretch your front ankle muscles.

1. Remove your shoes. Sit toward the front edge of a chair and lean back, using a pillow to support your back.

2. Stretch your legs out in front of you.

3. With your heels still on the floor, bend your ankles to point your feet toward you.

4. Bend your ankles so that your feet point away from you.

5. If you don't feel the stretch, repeat with your feet slightly off the floor.

6. Hold this position for 1 second.

7. Repeat 3 to 5 times.

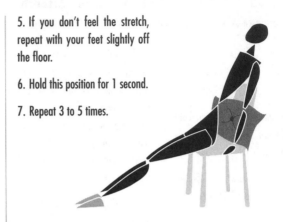

Calf Stretch

You can stretch your calves with knee straight and knee bent.

1. Stand with your hands against a wall, with your arms outstretched and elbows straight.

2. Keeping your left knee slightly bent and the toes of your right foot slightly turned inward, step back 1 to 2 feet with your right leg, keeping your right foot flat on the floor. You should feel a stretch in your calf muscle, but you shouldn't feel uncomfortable. If you don't feel a stretch, move your foot farther back until you do.

3. Hold this position for 10 to 30 seconds.

4. Bend the knee of your right leg, keeping your heel and foot flat on the floor.

5. Hold this position for another 10 to 30 seconds.

6. Repeat with your left leg.

7. Repeat 3 to 5 times for each leg.

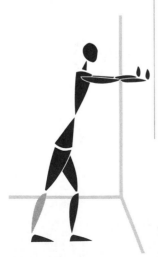

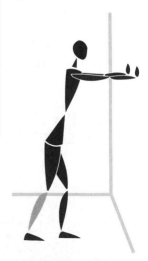

Triceps Stretch

Use a towel to stretch the muscles in the backs of your upper arms.

1. Hold one end of a towel in your left hand.

2. Raise and bend your left arm to drape the towel down your back. Keep your left arm in this position, and continue holding on to the towel

3. Reach behind your lower back and grasp the bottom end of the towel with your right hand.

4. Climb your right hand progressively higher up the towel, which also pulls your left arm down. Continue until your hands touch,

or as close to that as you can comfortably go.

5. Reverse positions.

6. Repeat each position 3 to 5 times.

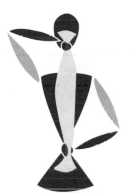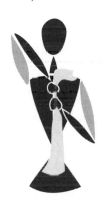

Wrist Stretch

This exercise stretches your wrist muscles.

1. Place your hands together in a praying position.

2. Slowly raise your elbows so your arms are parallel to the floor, keeping your hands flat against each other.

3. Hold this position for 10 to 30 seconds.

4. Repeat 3 to 5 times.

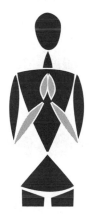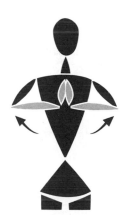

Quadriceps Stretch

Do this exercise to stretch the muscles in front of your thighs.

1. Lie on your left side on the floor. Your hips should be lined up so that one is directly above the other one.

2. Rest your head on a pillow or your hand.

3. Bend your right knee.

4. Reach back and grab the heel of your right foot. If you can't reach your heel with your hand, loop a belt over your foot and hold the belt ends.

5. Gently pull your right leg until the front of your thigh stretches.

6. Hold this position for 10 to 30 seconds.

7. Reverse position and repeat.

8. Repeat 3 to 5 times on each side. If the back of your thigh cramps during this exercise, stretch your leg and try again, more slowly.

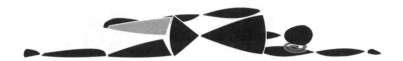

Double Hip Rotation

Don't do this exercise, which stretches the outer muscles of your hips and thighs, if you've had a hip replacement—unless your surgeon approves.

1. Lie on the floor on your back, knees bent and feet flat on the floor.

2. Keep your shoulders on the floor at all times.

3. Keeping your knees bent and together, gently lower your legs to one side as far as possible without forcing them.

4. Hold this position for 10 to 30 seconds.

5. Return to the original position.

6. Repeat toward the other side.

7. Repeat 3 to 5 times on each side.

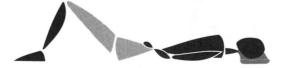

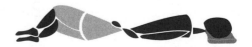

Single Hip Rotation

Don't do this exercise, which stretches the muscles of your pelvis and inner thighs, if you've had a hip replacement—unless your surgeon approves.

1. Lie on your back on the floor, knees bent and feet flat on the floor.

2. Keep your shoulders on the floor throughout the exercise.

3. Lower your right knee slowly to the side, keeping your left leg and your pelvis in place.

4. Hold this position for 10 to 30 seconds.

5. Bring your right knee back up slowly.

6. Repeat with your left knee.

7. Repeat 3 to 5 times on each side.

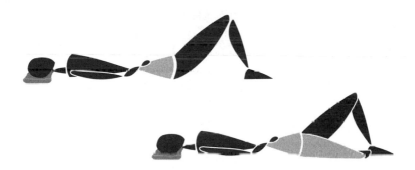

Neck Rotation

Do this exercise to stretch your neck muscles.

1. Lie on the floor with a phone book or other thick book under your head.

2. Slowly turn your head from side to side, holding your position each time for 10 to 30 seconds on each side. Your head should not be tipped forward or backward, but should be in a comfortable position. You can keep your knees bent to keep your back comfortable during this exercise.

3. Repeat 3 to 5 times.

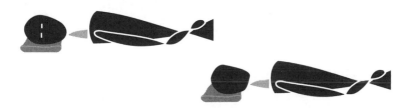

Shoulder Rotation

Here's a stretching exercise for your shoulders.

1. Lie flat on the floor with a pillow under your head and your legs straight. If your back bothers you, place a rolled towel under your knees.

2. Stretch your arms straight out to the side. Your shoulders and upper arms will remain flat on the floor throughout this exercise.

3. Bend your elbows so that your hands are pointing toward the ceiling. Let your arms slowly roll backwards from the elbow. Stop when you feel a stretch or slight discomfort, and stop immediately if you feel a pinching sensation or a sharp pain.

4. Hold this position for 10 to 30 seconds.

5. Slowly raise your arms, still bent at the elbow, to point toward the ceiling again. Then let your arms slowly roll forward, remaining bent at the elbow, to point toward your hips. Stop when you feel a stretch or slight discomfort.

6. Hold this position for 10 to 30 seconds.

7. Alternate pointing above your head, then toward the ceiling, then toward your hips. Begin and end with pointing-above-head position.

8. Repeat 3 to 5 times.

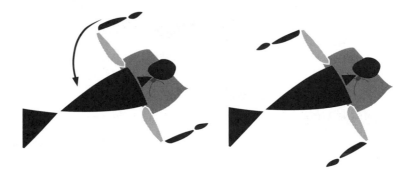

CHAPTER 15

Looking Good

Who is that strange woman in the mirror? She's got dark pouches under her eyes, lines around her mouth, and a long, dark hair sprouting from her chin. You know you're not 25 anymore, but it's discouraging when these external signs of aging begin to show up in your 30s or 40s. Even if you've been a regular at the gym and are meticulous about watching your weight, your skin and hair will start to change as you get older. Your skin loses elasticity and becomes prone to wrinkling. Your hair may be thinner on the top of your head and more plentiful in places where you don't want it . . . like on your face. Your nails may become more brittle.

These changes aren't life-threatening, but they certainly can be demoralizing. Sure, inner beauty is great, but we all want to shine on the outside, too. Besides, in our youth-obsessed culture, looking your age can be a distinct disadvantage at work and even in social interactions. No woman wants to be at a party and suddenly feel she looks like the oldest person in the room (even if her chronological age tops the rest of the crowd).

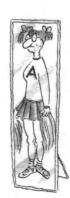

And very few of us want (or can afford) cosmetic surgery to fix every imperfection. By understanding why your appearance is changing and what you can do—short of invasive surgery—you can look better and feel better about yourself as the years go by.

SKIN

Often, the earliest signs of aging are fine lines around your eyes or pale tan spots on your hands. It can be a shock when these first appear, because you might only be in your late 30s or early 40s. The rate at which your skin ages depends on two things: your genes and your lifestyle. You can't do anything about your genes, but you can look younger for longer by avoiding sun damage, not smoking, and maintaining a steady weight. If you're generally healthy, it shows in your skin. Drink plenty of water and get enough sleep. Eating right and exercising also give your skin a more youthful glow.

Skin is actually your largest organ, weighing about nine pounds in total. Your eyelids have the thinnest skin, while the soles of your feet have the thickest.

What Can Happen

❖ Fine lines around the eyes and mouth

❖ Generally drier skin

❖ Some loss of skin elasticity

❖ Flat brown spots on hands and face

❖ A few dark hairs on chin or upper lip

❖ Some hair loss from scalp, arms, legs, and pubic area

❖ Graying hair

Below is a description of your skin's three layers and what they do for you.

EPIDERMIS: the outermost layer of skin, about as thick as a piece of paper.

The epidermis keeps germs out and fluids in. It has four layers of cells that are constantly flaking off and being renewed, so that every 28 days it has a completely new set of cells. The stratum corneum contains keratinocytes, cells that produce a tough protein to form a flexible shield. The bottom layer contains melanocytes, which produce melanin, the pigment that gives skin its color. If you're out in the sun a lot, you produce more melanin; that's why you tan or get freckles. The epidermis also contains Langerhans cells, part of your immune system. They help ward off infection.

DERMIS: the middle layer of skin, thicker than the epidermis and containing collagen, blood and lymph vessels, nerves, hair follicles, and sweat and oil glands.

The blood vessels in the dermis expand and contract to maintain constant body temperature. These are the blood vessels that spring into action when you get a hot flash. The dermis nourishes the epidermis. Collagen and another molecule, elastin, help skin stay firm when stretched. As you get older, some of the elastin fibers disappear, causing wrinkles. The dermis also contains white blood cells that catch any germs that might have slipped through the epidermis.

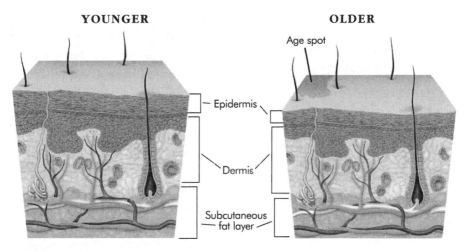

YOUNGER   **OLDER**

Age spot

— Epidermis

Dermis

Subcutaneous
— fat layer —

UNDER THE SKIN

As you get older, your skin loses elasticity and the fatty layer shrinks.

SUBCUTANEOUS TISSUE: the bottom layer of skin, consisting mainly of connective tissue, sweat glands, blood vessels, and cells that store fat.

This layer helps keep you warm and shields you from injury.

SMILE LINES

Q *I have lines around my eyes and mouth, and I can see that these are the parts of my face that fold when I smile. Has too much laughter made me wrinkled?*

A Remember when you were little and your mother told you not to make weird faces because your features might freeze that way? Well, she was actually sort of right. Repeated movements of skin and facial muscles —like smiling or frowning—do begin to make permanent lines as you get older because your skin is thinner and

less elastic. Young skin bounces back from movement, like a rubber band, but older skin doesn't. It's more like tissue paper; the creases settle in. Another thing that happens as you get older is that your skin cells don't turn over as rapidly as they did when you were young. You may find that it takes longer for injuries to heal. When you were a kid, a cut was gone in less than a week. Now it could be around for a month. The fatty layer under your skin also gets thinner. You might think this is a good thing, but it isn't when it makes you look older. For example, you may be able to see the veins on the backs of your hands. Your skin also produces less oil and loses its ability to retain moisture. All of these changes are reasons to treat your skin more gently now. In other words, keep smiling but use lots of moisturizer and sunscreen.

═ YOUR PLACE IN THE SUN: ═ A GLOSSARY

Sun damage or photo-aging: makes the skin look leathery, accelerates the wrinkling process.

Sun exposure: breaks down collagen and elastin, which support the epidermis, causes skin to sag.

Sunburn: leads to inflammation that damages collagen and elastin.

SUN DAMAGE

Q *I'm in my mid-40s and have been a beach lover since I was in my teens. I feel like I'm suddenly looking much older than friends my age. I suspect I know the answer, but could it be all those summers in the sun? And what can I do about it now?*

A You didn't see the changes in your skin until recently, but the effects of sun exposure have been accumulating under the surface of your skin for decades. Longtime sun exposure can make you look 5 or even 10 years older than you are. You may also be noticing small brown or tan spots (known as sun spots or age spots) on your hands and face—or any part of your body that has seen a lot of sun. Just compare your hands to your bottom. Assuming you're not a nudist, you'll be able to see the damage up close and personal.

You suspected that all that fun in the sun made you look older, but you know what you have to do now. Always, always, always (even on cloudy days, when 80 percent of the sun's rays still reach the ground) use a sunscreen that protects against ultraviolet A (UVA) rays, the cause of most skin aging, and ultraviolet B (UVB), which is most likely the culprit behind skin cancers (although there is some dispute about that among scientists). Check your sunscreen, and while you're at it, be sure it has the highest SPF (sun protection factor) you can find, since only the most diligent among us apply sunscreen as thickly and frequently as scientists do in the lab, where the numbers are created. Look for products that contain micronized zinc oxide or titanium oxide, which provide a physical barrier to sun exposure. And be sure to reapply often if you're swimming or sweating a lot.

You might also consider clothes and hats designed to block out sun. Stores specializing in equipment for hikers carry these, and some are relatively fashionable and okay for the beach. Finally, if you love that tanned look but want to avoid further damage, check out self-tanners. These products can be tricky to master at first without getting orange streaks all over, but once you get the hang of them, no one will be able to tell whether your healthy glow comes from the beach or a bottle.

When to See the Doctor

If you notice any of these changes, you should make an appointment for a checkup:

❖ A NEW SPOT ON YOUR SKIN THAT IS RAISED, IS MORE THAN ONE COLOR, OR HAS AN IRREGULAR SHAPE

❖ ANY OLD SPOTS OR MOLES THAT APPEAR TO BE CHANGING

❖ SUDDEN, EXTENSIVE HAIR GROWTH ON YOUR FACE OR CHEST

❖ PATCHY HAIR LOSS ON YOUR SCALP

SMOKING

Q *My sister is five years younger than me and a smoker. Now we're both in our 40s, and she looks 10 years older. I think smoking is to blame. Am I right?*

A Smokers' skin generally does age faster than nonsmokers' skin, and women are more vulnerable than men because our skin is thinner. Nicotine and other chemicals in cigarettes decrease blood flow, preventing oxygen and essential nutrients from reaching the skin. Some dermatologists think the damage comes not only from chemicals in the cigarettes, but also from the constant exposure to heat.

Every cigarette you smoke hurts your skin; you can even see facial changes in young women who have been smoking for only 10 years. A 2002 study found that smokers as young as 20 may have wrinkles that are visible under a microscope. By the time a woman hits her late 30s or early 40s, she often develops a characteristic pattern of wrinkles called "smoker's face." The main damage is around the eyes, mouth, and cheeks. Wrinkles around the eyes come from squinting to keep smoke out. Lines above the lip result from dragging on cigarettes. Wrinkles in the middle of the cheek develop after repeated inhaling and exhaling. You may also see skin discoloration on the fingers that hold cigarettes. Overall, the skin of a longtime smoker's face is often slightly yellowed or sallow. Skin around the eyes may be paler than the rest of the face—probably because of constricted blood flow. Stopping smoking helps, even when you're older. People who have smoked for years or smoked heavily when they were young show fewer wrinkles and better skin tone after they quit.

You probably know that smoking causes lung cancer, but it's also associated with skin cancer and an increased risk of death from melanoma, the most dangerous kind.

What to Tell Your Daughter

*H*ere's another great opportunity to be a positive role model. Stress the importance of starting good skin care habits at an early age. Remind your daughter to use sunscreen. Some dermatologists think that children may get 80 percent of their total lifetime sun exposure before they're 18. Sun damage accumulates throughout your lifetime, and severe sunburns early in life are a specific risk factor for melanoma, the deadliest form of skin cancer, as well as a major source of premature skin aging. That's also true of smoking, which causes wrinkles and makes you look old before your time.

DRIED OUT

Q *My skin feels dry and itchy all over. I've never had this problem before. Is this just aging, or could it be something serious?*

A Very dry skin could be a sign of an underactive thyroid. If you're also feeling unusually tired and have gained a few pounds, check with your doctor. (For more on thyroid disease, see Chapter 7.) Other disorders that can cause dry skin include diabetes and kidney disease. In any case, dry skin is much more common as you get older, because of both aging and sun damage.

If you're not already moisturizing your face morning and night, it's time to start. If your skin is especially dry, try cream moisturizers, rather than lotions. The alcohol in lotions makes them easier to pour and apply, but it can dry out your skin. Stay away from expensive department store brands; you're mostly paying for marketing. Dermatologists will tell you that the more moderately priced brands you buy in the drugstore may even be better than the pricey ones. You can use them on any part of your body that needs help: face, arms, legs, even the soles of your feet. The best time to apply moisturizers is after your bath or shower, when your skin is still slightly damp. A good lotion or cream will help seal in the moisture. You should be using lukewarm rather than very hot water, which can be drying. Also, stick to super-fatted soaps (like Dove) or gentle cleansing bars. Pat your skin dry with a towel; don't rub it. For your face, look for tinted moisturizers with SPF; that way, you need only one product to soothe your skin, help prevent further damage, and even out blotchy areas. You might also try using a humidifier at home or leaving a pan of water on top of the radiator to keep the air moist.

HOPE IN A JAR

Q *There must be a thousand anti-wrinkle creams on the market. Do they work? Or do I have to go under the knife to get help?*

FIRST AID FOR YOUR SKIN

What can creams and lotions do for you? It depends on the problem.

General dryness and loss of elasticity. Moisturize, moisturize, moisturize. If you're just starting to see wrinkles, the most effective products are very aggressive hydrating creams. Look for those containing ceramides, triglycerides, or cholesterol. Products with retinol could stimulate cell growth, which should help as well.

Age spots. Also called sun spots or liver spots, these are flat areas of brown skin on the face, neck, chest, and tops of the hands or forearms. If you have a lot of them, you should check with a dermatologist because they may indicate that you've had considerable sun damage and therefore are at higher risk for skin cancer. Nonprescription products that may help the problem contain the bleaching agent hydroquinone. Combining a bleaching agent with an exfoliant, retinol creams, or glycolic acid creams and lotions can accelerate the fading you get from bleaching. But you need to use a good sunscreen as well; otherwise, any bleaching will be wiped away by a few strong rays. If there's no improvement in a few months, see a physician. A dermatologist can prescribe more powerful bleaching agents or administer peels and other treatments.

Fine lines and puffiness around eyes. Wrinkles anywhere look better if the skin is moisturized. Again, the most expensive moisturizer is not necessarily the most effective. Retinols and alpha hydroxy acids such as glycolic acid smooth skin as well. Many products are sold specifically as eye cream. Whether you really need them is debatable. Doctors say that products for the face are generally mild, and you should try those first for lines around the eyes before you invest in another jar or tube.

Puffy eyes are harder to fix. If the problem is allergies or lack of sleep, you need to take antihistamines or get more rest. Traditional cures like cucumber slices, tea bags, or astringent gels can also help if the puffiness is just temporary. But in many cases the cause is herniated fat pads above or beneath the eyes. Then you really need to see a doctor for surgery to remove the pads. Nothing sold in a drug or department store is likely to be of much help.

Laugh lines and lines around lips. Dermatologists aren't very impressed with any of the products that are sold over the counter. If you're really troubled by lines like these, see a doctor. Possible treatments include injectable fillers and resurfacing.

A The answer really depends on what you expect from them. Nothing you can buy over the counter will give you the results you get from prescription products or procedures that

only a doctor can perform. (In any case, if you have concerns about a new dark spot or rough patch on your skin, it's a good idea to see a dermatologist to rule out skin cancer.) Also, no cosmetic product can erase the damage caused by the two biggest enemies of healthy skin: sun exposure and smoking. If you've been bad, you're paying for it now.

The cosmetics industry has spawned a gigantic new category of products called cosmeceuticals, which purport to erase aging without a scalpel or needle. These products fall into a regulatory gray area: they're neither drugs nor cosmetics, and you have no guarantee that they'll do what they claim to do. You can purchase cosmeceuticals in chic department stores, where they may cost a week's salary, or in your local drugstore, where they're a lot more reasonable. Dermatologists say there's no connection between effectiveness and price, so you're better off going with cheaper products from well-known manufacturers like Oil of Olay, Aveeno, Neutrogena, or Eucerin.

Collagen Creams

Q *I see lots of products advertised that contain collagen. I know you lose collagen as you age. Would these creams help?*

A You do lose collagen as you age, but you won't get it back by smearing it on your face. Collagen isn't absorbed through the skin, and those creams don't make your body produce more. If your skin looks better, it's because the cream you're using is working as a moisturizer. Bottom line: Don't waste your money on collagen.

Retinoids

You've probably heard a lot about these vitamin A–based drugs. They're not exactly the fountain of youth, but they are promising. Tretinoin, marketed as Renova and Retin-A, was first used to treat acne in the 1970s. Researchers found that it also fades actinic keratosis spots (precursors to skin cancer) and speeds skin cell turnover. And then, in 1996, the FDA approved Renova to treat wrinkles. Tretinoin works by increasing new collagen production and stimulating the growth of new blood vessels in the skin. It also fades age spots and softens patches of rough skin. You'll see some changes in a few months, but it can take up to a year to get the full benefit. There is a downside, however. Tretinoin can cause skin irritation, and you'll need to wear a sunscreen (which you should be using anyway) because it increases your skin's sensitivity to sunlight. And if you stop using it, the benefits go away. Prices vary from $40 to more than $90, depending on where you buy it.

Adult Acne

Q *This doesn't seem fair, but I'm still seeing some blackheads as I enter perimenopause. I know teenage acne is hormonal. Is that true now as well?*

A Women whose breakouts are associated with their menstrual cycle usually find that they get pimples or blackheads about two to seven days before the start of their period. That problem tends to go away after menopause, so you can look forward to some relief! However, you may still break out occasionally during the transition. Fluctuating hormones could indeed be the problem. Although doctors don't really understand what causes acne, they do know that an increase in androgens (male sex hormones) is an important factor. And, as you know, you do experience a change in the estrogen-androgen ratio during the menopause transition. In studies, women who had acne have higher levels of circulating androgens than women without acne. Similarly, women who had acne during adolescence also often get it again at midlife. Other possible causes: greasy makeup, medications (such as lithium for bipolar disorder or barbiturates used to control seizures) and even resting your cheek on your hand (a source of bacteria). Contrary to myth, chocolate, fried foods, and dirty skin do *not* cause acne. Neither does stress, but it can aggravate acne, so try to relax more.

If pimples are really troubling you, try over-the-counter acne medications containing benzoyl peroxide, resorcinol, salicylic acid, or sulfur. These break down blackheads and whiteheads and reduce oil production in your skin. But don't slather them on as you might have done when you were a teenager. Put the medication just on the spot—not on the

HORMONE THERAPY AND WRINKLES

Most of the controversy over hormone therapy at menopause has centered on the risks of cancer and heart disease. But many women who use estrogen say they like it because it makes them look younger. What's the science behind their claims? Estrogen therapy does not alter the effects of genetic aging, and it can't reverse the damage from sun exposure or smoking. It has no effect on the risk of skin cancer. But clinical trials have shown that systemic estrogen may have some benefits for skin. It appears to limit collagen loss, maintain skin thickness, improve firmness and elasticity, and decrease wrinkle depth and pore size. Researchers say the data aren't convincing enough to recommend taking estrogen for this reason alone and it's not FDA approved for this purpose. Research is ongoing.

area around it. Your skin is drier now, so you need to be careful. You should look for products made for adults, including some specifically formulated for menopausal women.

If you're still not getting relief, see a dermatologist for antibiotics or other prescription medication. Oral contraceptives and menopausal hormone therapy may also help. (For more on using these medications, see Chapter 2.)

In the meantime, wash your face gently; don't scrub or rub it. That will only exacerbate the problem.

MAKEUP TIPS

If you're still using makeup products you chose in your 20s, you're way overdue for a change. Here's some advice from a friend of ours, Laura Snavely, a makeup artist for Bobbi Brown.

◆ Slather on moisturizer and use eye cream if you need it. To even out skin tone, use a tinted moisturizer or a hydrating foundation. Skin loses moisture because of hormonal changes. Look for moisturizers and foundation that contain sunscreen (which you should always use).

◆ Wear mostly matte eyeshadows. White, bone, and shell are colors that will make your eyes appear bigger and more open.

◆ Line your lids. You don't want a thick slash . . . just definition. Gel liner and damp shadow liner work wonders when applied "tight" into the lash line. Softly smudge the line with a Q-tip or smudge brush for a softer look.

◆ If your lids are starting to droop, don't use liner or mascara on the lower edge. Use white eyeshadow under the arch of your brow to draw the eye up. Use a blush color (pale pink, apricot) that will brighten your face. Dark, intense blushes will make the skin look "saggy." Bronzers should be used to give skin warmth and evenness. They shouldn't make the skin look "dirty."

◆ A lighter lip color is more youthful. You can still use an intense color—just avoid heavy hues, especially dark browns. Use liner to prevent seepage and keep lipstick on your lips.

◆ Pick out a feature that you particularly like, such as your eyes, and make that your focal point. Keep everything else soft.

◆ Skin needs to be beautiful from the inside out. Eat right, drink water, exercise, and have a good attitude!

PILLOW TALK

Q *This may sound weird, but I'm convinced that the way I sleep has left its mark on my face. I'm a side sleeper, and when I lie on the pillow, my cheek pushes the skin above my lip a little. Now I have a line there. Is there a connection?*

A There certainly could be a connection. Resting your face on the pillow the same way for years can lead to wrinkles. Early on, you may see these lines only when you wake up in the morning. They disappear as the day goes on. But as you get older, the lines become permanent. According to the American Academy of Dermatology, people who sleep on their back don't get these wrinkles. Women tend to sleep on their sides and get characteristic lines on their chins and cheeks. Men are more likely to sleep with their heads pressed against the pillow and get lines on their foreheads. You might consider changing your sleep position to keep wrinkles to a minimum.

SHINGLES

Q *I have a sharp, burning pain in the skin on one side of my back. There's also a cluster of blisters in this area. Does this have anything to do with menopause?*

A You could have shingles, a viral infection of the nerves that causes just this kind of blistering rash. The virus that's attacking you is called varicella-zoster, and it's the same one that brings on chicken pox. If you had the disease as a child, the virus remains dormant in your spinal cord for the rest of your life. Sometimes the virus wakes up again, usually in people over 60 or those with a weakened immune system. The first symptoms are the kind of pain you describe, followed by a blistering rash. The blisters form along nerve pathways, often along the ribs or on the face, and they last several weeks. The pain may persist for months. Sometimes, the affected area becomes overly sensitive, so that anything that touches it (clothes, sheets) brings on excruciating pain. This is caused by nerve damage.

If you think you have shingles, see your doctor immediately. Early treatment shortens the amount of time you have to suffer. Your doctor may prescribe an antiviral drug or a painkiller to make you more comfortable.

ROSACEA

Q *I've noticed tiny red pimples on my chin, but nowhere else. They seem to come out when I'm drinking something hot or during a hot flash. What's happening?*

A It sounds like you might be suffering from rosacea, a skin condition characterized by redness and pimples that usually affects only the face—especially the forehead, nose, cheeks, and chin. It's more common in women than in men, particularly during menopause. Typically, a person with rosacea will have fair rather than darker skin. People who blush frequently are more likely to get it. No one really knows what causes rosacea, but scientists think it could result from abnormalities of small blood vessels, sun damage to connective tissue, or an abnormal inflammatory response. Many people report specific triggers for flare-ups such as spicy foods, alcohol, or hot beverages. Women who develop rosacea for the first time at menopause often say it's triggered by hot flashes. The eyes and eyelids can also become inflamed, and rosacea sufferers report redness, dryness, and itching (a feeling like sand in the eyes). You should see your dermatologist; while there's no cure for rosacea, you can control it with a topical or oral antibiotic. Keep a written record to see if you can identify your triggers and avoid them. You should also be scrupulous about wearing sunscreen and avoid irritating cosmetics.

Could It Be Cancer?

Skin cancer is becoming a serious public health problem as baby boomers get older. Most of us spent lots of time in the sun when we were young. In the 1950s and '60s, many people believed that looking tan was a sign of health—even for kids. Although some people used sunscreen, it wasn't as popular or as effective as today's products. That's why you should be familiar with the warning signs of skin cancer and get an annual checkup by a dermatologist, especially if you're fair-skinned and burn easily.

Several kinds of lesions appear on sun-exposed skin. Some are potentially dangerous; others are not.

Noncancerous

FRECKLES indicate significant sun exposure. They're more common in fair-skinned people and tend to be small. Any freckle that seems unusual—in size, shape, or color—should be examined by a doctor.

MOLES (technically called nevi) are extremely common and mostly benign. However, any mole can change and become malignant, so your doctor should examine each one carefully.

ACTINIC KERATOSIS is a precancerous skin condition that looks like a scaly pink or reddish brown rough patch on sun-exposed areas of skin such as the arms, the backs of the hands, or the face. Fair-skinned people are more vulnerable than those with darker skin. These patches aren't dangerous in themselves and can be easily removed by cryosurgery, prescription creams, patches, laser resurfacing, or chemical peels. It's important to get them treated, because the FDA estimates that almost half of all skin cancer cases began as actinic keratosis spots.

Cancerous

BASAL CELL CARCINOMAS are the most common form of skin cancer, responsible for about 80 percent of all cases. Often, these growths take the form of a pearly bump, a white or yellowish scar, or a scaly red patch in an area of the skin that has been exposed to sun. Many have

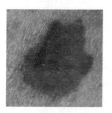

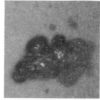

A **Asymmetry** (one half unlike the other half).

B **Scalloped** or poorly circumscribed border.

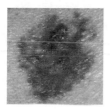

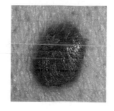

C **Color** varies from one area to another and can include shades of tan and brown, black, white, red, or blue.

D **Diameter** larger than six millimeters as a rule (diameter of pencil eraser).

DANGER SIGNS IN PIGMENTED LESIONS OF THE SKIN

very faint blood vessels on the skin surface. These cancers come from the lower layer of the epidermis (the basal layer). Malignant cells destroy surrounding tissue and ultimately form a painless bump that can become an open sore with a hard edge. Basal cell carcinomas grow very slowly and do not develop into the more serious melanomas.

SQUAMOUS CELL CARCINOMAS can be flaky and scaly like actinic keratosis but are thicker. These malignant growths, about 16 percent of skin cancers, start in the middle layer of the epidermis. They

usually affect only the immediate surrounding area of the skin but eventually can grow and form a raised patch with a rough surface ranging in size from a pea to a walnut. Squamous cell carcinomas are more common in men than in women and generally aren't fatal unless they spread to the lymph nodes or vital organs.

MELANOMA is a cancer that originates in melanocytes, cells deep in the epidermis or in moles. Although melanoma accounts for only 4 percent of skin cancer cases, it's responsible for more than

How to Examine Yourself for Skin Cancer

Check yourself regularly and see a dermatologist annually.

1. Examine your body front and back in front of the mirror. Raise your arms and look at both right and left sides.

2. Use a mirror to look at your scalp face, ear, neck, and shoulder area.

3. Carefully look at your forearms, palms of hands, and between your fingers.

4. Examine your feet; look at the backs of your legs, the soles of your feet, and between your toes.

75 percent of all deaths caused by skin cancer. Unless it's diagnosed early, it spreads to lymph nodes and internal organs, particularly the lungs and the liver. The incidence of melanoma has risen dramatically in recent years, and researchers suspect that sun exposure is the reason. However, melanoma can develop anywhere on your body, even in places like your vagina and the soles of your feet that get no sun exposure. Blondes, redheads, and other fair-skinned people have a higher risk of melanoma than people with darker skin. However, darker-skinned people can get melanoma, too. Your risk is greater if your parent, child, or sibling has had melanoma. (See Appendix I.)

Odd-Looking Moles

Q *When should you worry about a mole? I've always had one on the side of my neck, but now another has cropped up and its shape is odd. It looks sort of like a raisin.*

A You need to have a dermatologist look at it right away. Melanoma, the deadliest form of skin cancer, can make its appearance in a mole that shows up in adulthood or a mole that has changed shape. Moles that you've had from birth (called congenital nevi) or that appeared soon afterwards are often removed because they're more likely to develop into melanoma than moles acquired after you're a year and a half old. Removing a mole is a simple procedure usually done in a doctor's office. The mole is sent to a lab to be examined for any cancerous cells.

Nail Health

Q *Now that I'm older, my nails look terrible. They break easily and have ridges. What does this mean?*

A Nails are living tissue, just like skin. In fact, they're composed primarily of the skin protein keratin. As your skin gets drier with age, your nails do, too. But that doesn't mean you have to resign yourself to a lifetime of ugly nails. You just need to treat them with more kindness and gentleness. Don't overuse products like nail polish, nail hardeners, and polish remover. Keep

What Your Nails Say About You

Nails that break easily or are discolored could signal a medical problem or be a sign that your body lacks essential vitamins and nutrients. Your nails could also be damaged by the kind of cleaning fluid you use, false fingernails, or even gardening without gloves. The table below is meant as a guideline; only your doctor or health-care provider can make an accurate diagnosis.

WHAT THE NAIL LOOKS LIKE	WHAT IT MIGHT MEAN
Nail is white	Liver disease
Nail is half pink, half white	Kidney disease
Nail bed is red	Heart conditions
Yellowing and thickened nail that is slow-growing	Lung disease
Pale nail beds	Anemia
Yellowish nails with a slight blush about the base	Diabetes

your nails clean and dry; this prevents bacteria from collecting under the nails. Don't remove your cuticles, because that makes it easier for infection to develop. When you rub lotion on your hands, be sure you get it in the area around the nails. Avoid harsh chemicals; they can damage your nails. Many women say rubbing cuticle oil into your nails at bedtime helps make them much less brittle.

VARICOSE VEINS

Q *I've noticed enlarged dark blue veins poking out on my calves. It's a relatively new problem. Does it have any connection to menopause?*

A Not to menopause specifically, but varicose veins are related to aging. When the valves that push blood through your vascular system don't close properly and some blood pools in your legs, the normally elastic walls of the veins get stretched out, making them widen, bulge, and twist. Women are more likely than men to get varicose veins, possibly because estrogen makes vein walls relax and stretch. Pregnancy or medications containing hormones may bring on varicose veins or make the problem worse. Heredity is also a major risk factor. If your mother or grandmother had varicose veins, you are more likely to have them as well. Other risk factors include age, obesity, and jobs that require standing for long periods of time.

Varicose veins aren't just unsightly; they can also cause swelling, burning, and aching in the affected area. Pain can get worse if a distended vein pushes

TREATMENTS FOR VARICOSE VEINS

A varicose vein specialist offers a number of procedures to help eliminate those unsightly bulges. Here's a rundown:

Stripping. Usually reserved for larger veins, this procedure is generally done by a vascular surgeon in a hospital. The vein is tied off or completely removed.

Sclerotherapy. Medication is injected into small and medium-size veins to irritate and then collapse them. Scar tissue forms and closes down the veins. Nearby veins take up the blood flow. The scar tissue is eventually absorbed by the body. This procedure is usually performed in a doctor's office without an anesthetic. It may take more than one treatment to make the veins invisible, but you can return to your regular activities right away. Sometimes, doctors use ultrasound to guide them in this procedure. One drawback: New veins that grow afterwards may also become varicose veins. Other side effects may include a slight swelling, bruising, redness, and itching at the site of the injection.

Phlebectomy. In this procedure, an enlarged vein is removed through tiny incisions along its length. It can be used for both varicose and spider veins. It takes place in a doctor's office under local anesthesia. Afterwards, you'll need to wear a bandage or a compression stocking for a short time.

Electrodesiccation. An electrical current is used to seal off enlarged veins.

Laser surgery. Lasers used to be effective only on smaller, superficial veins, but new technology has enabled doctors to use them on larger veins as well. In laser therapy, the doctor uses ultrasound to guide a laser fiber into the vein through a needle inserted near the patient's knee. The laser pulses destroy visible veins so they fade and then disappear. It can take two to five treatments, depending on the size and density of the veins. After the procedure, you will need to wear thigh-high compression stockings for a week.

against a nerve. You may also be more vulnerable to leg wounds, blood clots, and phlebitis, an inflammation of a vein.

If you have varicose veins, you may also notice their smaller cousins: spider veins. These are distillations of small blood vessels near the surface of the skin. They can appear anywhere, but they usually show up on your legs or face.

Fortunately, there's help for both conditions. The first step would be simple measures such as compression stockings that brace the vein walls from outside and often may be enough to relieve discomfort. If you're overweight, losing a few pounds may help, as may exercises like walking and bicycling. You should also try to keep your feet up whenever possible.

If these measures don't work, consider talking to your doctor about procedures to fix the veins. The cost of these various treatments depends on whether they're performed in a doctor's office or a hospital and whether or not you need an anesthetic. Ask your primary care physician to recommend a clinic or specialist. Don't just go to one of the "vein treatment clinics" you see advertised in the newspaper.

BREASTS

When we were young teenagers, we couldn't wait for them to grow. Later on, they were symbols of sexual desirability. Some of us nursed children. And now . . . what happens to our breasts after menopause? Are we doomed to sagging and bagging? Not necessarily. Lots of factors affect how our breasts appear and feel over time, including childbirth, breast-feeding, age, gravity, and weight gain and loss. And, of course, hormones, specifically the amount of estrogen and progesterone in our bodies. Estrogen got our breasts growing in the first place, way back when.

Glandular tissue grows during puberty in response to increased production of estrogen and progesterone. At the same time, estrogen prompts the fat and fibrous tissues in your breasts to become more elastic. When your hormone levels rise during a menstrual cycle, the breast tissue swells and the milk glands and ducts enlarge. They also retain more water. So it's not surprising that as estrogen levels fall, the process goes into reverse, and there is a corresponding decrease in the glandular tissue of the

---

WHAT'S INSIDE

Your breasts are composed of three types of tissue:

◆ Glandular tissue includes the lobules (the bulbous-shaped milk glands) and the ducts (the passages that connect the lobules to the nipple).

◆ A layer of fat cushions the breast glands and is found throughout the breast. Fat gives breasts their soft, squishy feel.

◆ Fibrous connective tissue supports and suspends the lobules and the ducts. Fibrous strands known as Cooper's ligaments hold breast tissue to the chest wall.

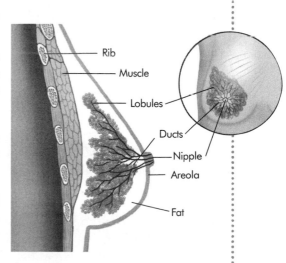

Rib

Muscle

Lobules

Ducts

Nipple

Areola

Fat

breasts. Fat usually takes its place. The connective tissues often become weaker and less elastic. Nipples may become smaller and less erect. Depending on weight gain and the amount of fat in the breasts, they may get bigger or smaller as you get older. They may also change in shape and appear to sag more than before. The silver lining to this change is that most women's breasts become less dense over time, making it easier for radiologists to detect abnormalities and early signs of breast cancer.

IS BIGGER BETTER?

Q *I've heard that my breasts could get bigger after menopause. That sounds like a good thing!*

A Usually, it's not. Bigger breasts after menopause are generally a sign that you're gaining weight. Bigger breasts can also cause back pain. You should be watching your weight and making sure you're exercising, especially your upper body. The better your muscles, the less you'll sag no matter what your bra size.

SHRINKING ON ONE SIDE

Q *I'm 55 and just noticed that one of my breasts seems to be shrinking. Is this part of postmenopause?*

A You should get that promptly checked out by a doctor. While it's not unusual for both breasts to become less dense over time, it's unusual

to experience a change in one but not the other. Sometimes this is due to a growth within the breast that causes the tissue to contract, making the overall breast look smaller.

HORMONE THERAPY AND BREASTS

Q *If I start taking hormones, will my breasts look the way they did when I was younger?*

A If your breasts were sagging before you reached menopause, hormone therapy won't reverse things. Hormones can make the breasts denser, but no knowledgeable health professional would recommend hormone therapy primarily for breast enhancement. Combination therapy (estrogen and a progestogen), which may be recommended for women who still have a uterus and are troubled by severe hot flashes, has been shown to increase the risk of breast cancer after five years. Estrogen-only therapy has not been shown to increase breast cancer risk, but estrogen can feed some types of breast tumors.

BUST BOOSTERS

Q *What can I do to make my breasts look better?*

A Because the fat content of your breasts increases as you get older, exercise and weight loss are a good place to start. Getting your pectoral muscles toned can make your breasts

YOUR BREAST CHOICE

Did you know that a really well-fitting bra can make you look 10 pounds sleeker? And that most women are wearing the wrong size bra? Breast sizes, shapes, and density change over time, and if you're not occasionally making adjustments, you're probably not maximizing your assets.

How do you go about putting your best breast forward?

◆ Start by getting a professional bra fitting, at least once every couple of years. A well-trained and experienced bra saleswoman will give you objective advice on what size, style, and brand will work best for you. Don't be afraid to mention your price limit.

◆ Remember that old ditty "Do your boobs hang low, do they wobble to and fro?" Low-hanging breasts make you look heavier than you are (especially when you're also thickening around the middle). Tightening your bra straps probably won't fix the problem. The band that runs under your breasts and the cut of the cup actually provide most of your uplift.

◆ When a bra fits properly, the front band should line up with the band in back or be slightly below it. If the back is higher than the front, your bra doesn't fit properly or has stretched out. The front part of the band should lie flat and snug against the breastplate but shouldn't be tight.

◆ You've got a good fit if your entire breast is inside the cup (this doesn't apply to push-up or demi bras). If the top edge of the bra is pressing down into breast flesh and making it bulge out, the bra doesn't fit.

◆ A new bra should fit snugly on the loosest eye. As the bra stretches out, you can move the hook up to the other eyes. If your bra fits on the tightest hook when you buy it, it will be too loose-fitting within a month or two. If the band is too tight, an inexpensive solution may be an extender.

◆ Research indicates that the wrong bra is responsible for a lot of back and shoulder pain. Bra straps that are too narrow can cause damage to the cervical nerve, which can cause headaches as well as neck, shoulder, arm, and hand pain.

◆ If your breasts have visible stretch marks, that's a sign that your breast tissue is breaking down because you're not providing enough support during the day or when you're exercising.

◆ Perimenopausal breasts can be super sensitive because of fluctuating hormone levels. As a result, an underwire bra may not be your best choice right now. The top of the wire usually hits at a particularly sensitive spot.

◆ If your postmenopausal breasts are not as dense as they used to be, you may need to switch to a different bra. Lingerie departments have a variety of enhancers, pads, and specially designed bras to fix whatever problem you have.

look more compact and less flabby. Weight training is a particularly effective way to do this.

You should also consider getting your next bra professionally fitted. Seek out a lingerie shop or department with a fitter who really knows her business. What worked when you were 30 may not be doing you any good now. Getting a bra that really fits and provides good support can make you look a lot thinner and younger. Take this opportunity to get rid of all those stretched-out, ill-fitting bras that you've stuffed in your lingerie drawer.

HAIR

Many women have a love-hate relationship with their hair. It's too curly, too straight, too thick, too thin, a blah color . . . the list of flaws can be long. But at midlife you might come up with some new concerns. Basically, it boils down to this: too much or too little. More specifically, you might have too much hair where you don't want it and too little where you do want it.

CHIN WHISKERS

Q *I'm 46 and still getting regular periods, but I'm starting to see a few long, dark hairs on my chin and upper lip. Is this hormone-related?*

A Hormones do affect hair growth, but so does genetics. Hair growth on your face might indicate an excess of male hormones, but it could also be hereditary, especially if you're of Mediterranean origin.

Look carefully at your face, and you'll see that you have two kinds of hair: vellus, which is fine and colorless, and terminal, which is coarse, dark, and sometimes curly. In women, vellus hair normally covers the face, chest, and back and gives the impression of hairlessness, although you do actually have hair almost everywhere on your body. (The only hairless parts are the soles of your feet, the palms of your hands, and your lips.) Terminal hair grows on your scalp, in your pubic area, and in your armpits. The hair on your lower arms and legs is a mixture of terminal and vellus hair.

What you may be noticing now is that hair that was once soft and fine is growing in coarse and darker. If it's just a few hairs, it could be a sign that your hormones are fluctuating even though you're still menstruating. Your hair follicles are sensitive to hormones, and a slight imbalance between androgens and estrogen may have caused some vellus hairs to change into terminal hairs. Once that happens, they usually don't change back.

Many women find that while they have a few stray dark hairs around the time of the menopause transition, this problem doesn't get much worse and can be easily fixed by tweezing. You may also notice that the hair on your legs, lower arms, and pubic area is somewhat sparser.

Women who experience more extensive facial hair growth in a pattern common to men (on the chin, lips, and cheeks) may be suffering from a serious hormone imbalance and need to be checked out by an endocrinologist. If this new hair growth had happened when you were younger and your periods suddenly became irregular at the same time, one possibility might be polycystic ovary syndrome (PCOS), a condition in which the ovaries produce excessive amounts of androgens.

In any case, you should have your doctor look over this new hair growth for a more objective opinion of its severity.

HAIR REMOVAL

Q *I've always heard that tweezing makes hair grow back darker. Is that true? Are there methods of hair removal that would be more effective (and less tedious) than tweezing?*

A Tweezing generally doesn't make hair grow back darker, and it's a perfectly adequate method of hair removal if you have only a few stray hairs on your chin. However, it can be tedious and time-consuming if you have a lot of ground to cover. To make it easier, invest in good tweezers and a high-magnification mirror. Tweezing is easiest after a hot shower or bath. If the growth is a little heavier, you might try other temporary methods. (Shaving is effective on your legs, but not a good choice for your face.)

In addition to plucking, your options include waxing, bleaching, and chemical depilatories. Waxing keeps hair at bay four to six weeks. Plucking, bleaching, and depilatories last about two to three weeks or less. Each method has pros and cons. Waxing removes hair quickly and smoothly but can be painful and expensive if you get it done in a salon. You also run the risk of damaging your hair shafts and getting ingrown hairs. Bleaching is pretty easy, but it can burn and sting if you leave it on too long. Be sure to use a product made especially for the face, not the arms or legs. It's a good option if your hair color contrasts with your skin color. The day before, test a patch on your inner wrist to make sure you don't get redness or swelling. You should do a patch test with depilatories as well. These products, which come in aerosol, lotion, cream, and roll-on preparations, contain a chemical that dissolves the surface of the hair, separating it from the skin. Read instructions very carefully; leaving a depilatory on too long can irritate your skin. Also, make sure you get a preparation made specifically for the part of your body you're targeting. A product aimed at hair on your legs could well be too strong for your face. In any case, you shouldn't use depilatories around your eyes or on inflamed or broken skin.

For longer-term hair removal, you can hit hair follicles with the more expensive options of lasers or electrolysis. Lasers work best when you're attacking dark hair on pale skin; however, some newer methods target other skin and hair combinations. It usually takes several treatments to get at hair in different stages of growth. Electrolysis also takes several treatments and can be painful; if your technician isn't properly trained, you could get an infection from an unsterile needle or even scarring. And both of these procedures can be costly. For either, be sure to check the credentials of the operator. Most states require people to be specially licensed to perform these procedures. If you can, get a recommendation from a dermatologist or your physician.

You may have seen ads for face creams and moisturizers that claim to slow hair growth. Try these products and see if you notice a difference. They may not actually slow growth but rather make it less obvious. That could be enough for you. If it isn't, you might ask your doctor about prescription medications to slow hair growth. One of the newest is Vaniqa (eflornithine HCl). After about eight weeks, you may find that you need to tweeze or wax less frequently.

HAIR LOSS

Q *I've always had thin hair, but now that I've passed menopause it's really bad. I'm worried I might actually become bald. Is this possible?*

A After menopause, changes in the level of androgens (male hormones) can affect your hair growth. Many women find that the hair on their scalp starts to thin, though in a different pattern than that experienced by men. While men's hairlines recede, women's don't. Instead, their hair generally gets thinner all over the scalp. Although this thinning is common after menopause, you should still ask your doctor about it. Changing hormone levels aren't the only reason your hair might be getting thinner. In some cases, it could be styling treatments or twisting and pulling of the hair. Also, certain medications and skin diseases can cause hair loss. Thyroid disease can also cause hair loss.

THE BALD TRUTH

Q *Don't tell me I have to live with being bald. Isn't there something I can do?*

A You might be surprised that some women don't care about losing their locks! But if you're concerned about your appearance or if the hair loss is progressing, talk to your doctor about minoxidil, which is used on the scalp to help hair loss. You apply it to your scalp twice a day, and it takes about four months to see results. Tests show that minoxidil may make hair grow in about 20 to 25 percent of women; in others, it slows or stops hair loss. This drug is pricey, however, and the benefits stop when you stop using it.

Consider a new style, such as a layered cut, which can help hide thinning hair. You should be extra careful about how you handle your hair now; avoid any styles that pull, like ponytails or braids. Try shampooing your hair less often—a daily shampoo is not necessary—and use gentler products and a cream rinse or conditioner. Wet hair is more fragile, so don't rub it roughly with a towel and avoid vigorous combing or brushing. Use wide-toothed combs and smooth-tipped brushes.

LESS DOWN THERE

Q *I used to tease my poor husband about his thinning scalp—until one day I noticed that my pubic hair seems to be thinning out as well. Please tell me it's my imagination.*

A You might as well look at this from a positive point of view. You'll need fewer bikini waxes in the future. Pubic hair does thin out as we age, and over time you'll have a lot less. Hormone therapy—estrogen, progestogens, or testosterone—won't bring it back. And don't even think about using Rogaine down there.

PATCHWORK SCALP

Q *At my last appointment, my hairdresser told me there are quarter-size bald patches on my scalp. She said she can comb my hair over them so they don't show. Why is this happening? Will they go away?*

A Your problem sounds like alopecia areata, an autoimmune disorder that causes hair loss in small, round patches. In other words, your immune system is attacking the roots of your hair. Scientists don't really understand why this happens. People with alopecia areata have a higher risk of other autoimmune diseases, like thyroid disease, as well as eczema, asthma, and nasal allergies. Family members are also more likely to have these conditions.

The good news is that your hair will probably grow back, although it might fall out again later. The course of alopecia areata varies widely among individuals. Some people experience it only once; others have repeated episodes.

If the condition doesn't go away, ask your doctor about possible treatments. Corticosteroids that suppress the immune system may help in certain circumstances. Minoxidil, used to treat baldness, may promote hair growth. Another possibility is anthralin, a tar-like substance that changes immune function in the affected areas when it's applied for 20 to 60 minutes a day and then washed off. Your doctor might suggest a combination of treatments.

SHAPERS AND SLIMMERS

If you ever doubted whether Mother Nature has a sense of humor, look at what she's doing to your body. You're fighting back—exercising more and trying to eat smarter—but your favorite pair of slacks is still too tight. What's the solution, short of a surgery? Check out the growing number of products that offer a little help where you need it. NYDJ's Tummy Tuck jeans, a soft denim-and-lycra combination, include a stomach flattening panel in front and a derriere lifter in back. You can probably buy them a size or two smaller than your normal jeans, and the label sewn onto the back pocket does *not* say "tummy tuck." (That would have been a deal breaker!) Bathing suits also come with tummy panels or are made of special fabrics created to make you look noticeably thinner (Miraclesuit and Carol Wior's Slimsuits, among them). And in the foundation world, more and more products are being designed to be both comfortable and slimming. We like the Spanx line. It includes "power panties" and footless panty hose, which give a smooth, slim line under tight slacks and skirts, without wedgies, strangulating leg bands, or visible panty lines. They also make shirts, slacks, and skirts with built-in tummy panels. A less expensive control panty by the same manufacturer is sold at Target under the brand name Assets.

Endnote

Every major transition in life is a beginning and an end. Menopause is no exception. If you're like most women, you've probably spent much of your life up to this point focusing on the people who need you: your spouse or partner, your children, your aging parents, your friends, your coworkers. Meanwhile, you have a list of things you want to accomplish for yourself. Maybe you want to learn another language, see the Greek islands, get a degree, or just have enough time to get more exercise. Whatever your goal, chances are you've put it off until tomorrow. What have we learned from writing this book? Tomorrow is here.

Researching this book has given us the push we desperately needed. We wanted to live healthier lives, but we were procrastinators. Now we understand what constitutes a normal menopause and when to seek help. We know lots of effective ways to deal with hot flashes, vaginal dryness, moodiness, and irritability, and we know when hormone therapy makes sense. We know that it's really important to watch your weight and to get all three types of exercise (aerobics, weight lifting, and flexibility).

We know what to eat and what to avoid—and that we need to watch how many cocktails we drink. We're trying to be better about scheduling our annual physical, our pelvic exam, our mammograms and colonoscopies and bone mineral density tests. We know the warning signs of many more cancers as well as heart disease. We've learned that we need to see the dentist, the dermatologist, and the eye doctor more often. We know we're supposed to get more sleep, reduce our stress, become more social, and challenge our brains. All these things could make a big difference in how we feel as we make the transition through menopause and move into the rest of our lives.

How have we used this new knowledge? Since we started researching this book, we've changed in so many ways—some small, some profound. We know we have to mention anything that worries us to our doctor, even if we're embarrassed or it makes us feel like hypochondriacs. We're running a lot more errands on foot, and we're walking up the escalator instead of just riding along. We go to the gym, and we've put a set of hand weights in our offices, right next to the moisturizer and artificial tears. We dragged ourselves to a really good lingerie shop and had ourselves properly fitted for new bras (we were both wearing the wrong size). We had our makeup updated. We're eating better—more salads, more vegetables and fruit, less junk. We make sure we get our calcium and vitamin D, and more skim milk than coffee in our mugs. We're making more time for our friends and welcoming new challenges that will keep our minds sharp. We recognize that our days in miniskirts are over, and we're just fine with that. We've learned to embrace the joys of this new phase. We're savvier, more confident, and ready to take on anything.

Of course, we're not perfect. Some days we end up with nothing but good intentions (we meant to get to the gym, we really didn't mean to eat that bag of Cheetos, we knew we shouldn't have slurped down that second frosty cosmopolitan). But the next day we start again and try a little harder. And we can honestly say that we've got more energy and are more upbeat than when we started this project. In other words, we've found the "menopausal zest" we've heard so much about.

Tomorrow is here—and it looks pretty good to us.

APPENDICES

Appendix I: Charts, Graphs, and Sources

Throughout the book, we've tried not to bog you down with too many charts and technical terms. In Appendix I, you'll find some very useful information, organized by chapter and theme, which you may want to turn to if a subject interests you in a particular way. (You may have noticed references to these charts and graphs in the text.) You'll also find some of our sources listed here.

CHAPTER 1: WHAT'S HAPPENING?

Recommended Screening Schedule for Women at Average Risk			
SCREENING TEST	AGES 40 TO 49	AGES 50 TO 64	AGES 65 AND ABOVE
General health Full checkup, including height and weight	Discuss schedule with your doctor or nurse.	Discuss schedule with your doctor or nurse.	Discuss schedule with your doctor or nurse.
Thyroid test (TSH)	Every 5 years.	Every 5 years.	Every 5 years.
Heart health Blood pressure test	At least every 2 years.	At least every 2 years.	At least every 2 years.
Cholesterol test	Depending on results, discuss with your doctor or nurse.	Depending on results, discuss with your doctor or nurse.	Depending on results, discuss with your doctor or nurse.
Bone health Bone mineral density test	Discuss with your doctor or nurse.	Discuss with your doctor or nurse.	Be tested at least once. Talk to your doctor or nurse about repeat tests.
Diabetes Blood sugar test	Start at age 45, then every 3 years.	Every 3 years.	Every 3 years.
Breast health Mammogram	Every 1 to 2 years. Discuss with your doctor or nurse	Every 1 to 2 years. Discuss with your doctor or nurse	Every 1 to 2 years. Discuss with your doctor or nurse.
Reproductive health Pap test and pelvic exam	Ideally, every year.	Ideally, every year.	Discuss with your doctor or nurse.
Chlamydia test	If you are at high risk for chlamydia or other STDs, you may need this test.	If you are at high risk for chlamydia or other STDs, you may need this test.	If you are at high risk for chlamydia or other STDs, you may need this test.
Tests for sexually transmitted diseases (STDs)	Both partners should be tested for STDs (including HIV) before initiating sexual intercourse.	Both partners should be tested for STDs (including HIV) before initiating sexual intercourse.	Both partners should be tested for STDs (including HIV) before initiating sexual intercourse.

Screening Test	Ages 40 to 49	Ages 50 to 64	Ages 65 and Above
Colorectal health Fecal occult blood test		Yearly.	Yearly.
Flexible sigmoidoscopy (preferred with fecal occult blood test)		Every 5 years (if not having a colonoscopy).	Every 5 years (if not having a colonoscopy).
Double contrast barium enema (DCBE)		Every 5 to 10 years (if not having a colonoscopy or sigmoidoscopy).	Every 5 to 10 years (if not having a colonoscopy or sigmoidoscopy).
Colonoscopy		Every 10 years.	Every 10 years.
Rectal exam	Discuss with your doctor or nurse.	Every 5 to 10 years with each screening (sigmoidoscopy, colonoscopy, or DCBE).	Every 5 to 10 years with each screening (sigmoidoscopy, colonoscopy, or DCBE).
Eye and ear health Eye exam	Every 2 to 4 years or more often if you have vision problems.	Every 2 to 4 years; yearly after 60.	Yearly.
Hearing test	Every 10 years.	Discuss with your doctor or nurse.	Discuss with your doctor or nurse.
Skin health Mole exam	Monthly self-exam; by a doctor every year.	Monthly self-exam; by a doctor every year.	Monthly self-exam; by a doctor every year.
Oral health Dental exam	One to two times every year.	One to two times every year.	One to two times every year.
Immunizations Influenza vaccine	Discuss with your doctor or nurse.	Yearly.	Yearly.
Pneumococcal vaccine			One time only.
Tetanus-diphtheria booster vaccine	Every 10 years.	Every 10 years.	Every 10 years.

Source: National Women's Health Information Center.

Pregnancy Risks for Older Mothers

As you age, the risks of pregnancy increase for you and your baby.

BABY/PREGNANCY	MOTHER
Miscarriage	Diabetes
Stillbirth	Hypertension and preeclampsia
Birth defects	Heart disease
Preterm labor and delivery	Kidney problems
Low birth weight (less than 5½ lbs.)	Abruptio placentae; placenta previa
Ectopic pregnancy	Cesarean section
	Cancer
	Maternal death

Risk of Having a Live Baby with Any Chromosomal Problem

AGE	BIRTHS PER 1,000
20	1.9
25	2.1
30	2.6
35	5.2
40	15.2
45	47.6

Source: American College of Obstetricians and Gynecologists.

Maternal Age and Down Syndrome

Down syndrome is a genetic disorder characterized by mental retardation, abnormal facial development, and heart problems. It is caused by the presence of an extra chromosome. The odds that a woman will have a baby with Down's increases very rapidly after age 40.

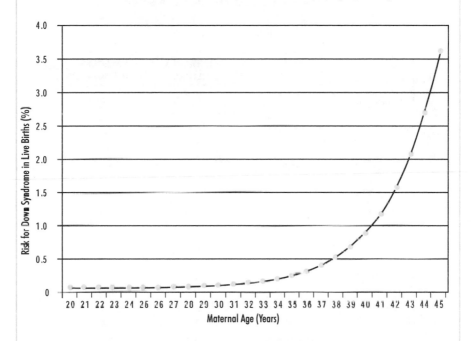

Source: H.S. Cuckle, N.J. Wald, and S.G. Thompson, "Estimating a woman's risk of having a pregnancy associated with Down syndrome using her age and serum alpha-fetoprotein level," *British Journal of Obstetrics and Gynaecology* (1987), 94.

Page Notes

Page 7: Stages of Reproductive Aging Workshop (STRAW) model, *Menopause* (2001).

Page 8: Graph, Life Expectancy vs. Age of Menopause, M.R. Soules et al., *Journal of the American Geriatric Society* (1982), 30.

Page 23: Chart, Risk of Miscarriage, American Society for Reproductive Medicine.

CHAPTER 2: THE HORMONE QUESTION

Profile of Women's Health Initiative Participants

The women who took part in this study represented a range of races, ages, and health problems. Compare them with yourself to help determine how these results are relevant to you.

		ESTROGEN ALONE	ESTROGEN PLUS PROGESTIN
Participants		10,739	16,608
Race	Caucasian	75%	84%
	African-American	15	7
	Hispanic	6	5
Average age		*64*	*63*
	50 to 59	31%	33%
	60 to 69	45	45
	70 to 79	24	23
Hormone use	Ever	35%	20%
	At enrollment	13	6
BMI	Normal	21%	31%
	Overweight	35	35
	Obese	45	34
Smoking	Ever	38%	40%
	At enrollment	10	11
Treated for high blood pressure		48%	36%

Source: National Heart, Lung and Blood Institute.

Results from the Women's Health Initiative by Age Group

In the WHI, younger women who took estrogen and a progestin
generally had fewer problems than older women did.

| | AGES 50 TO 59 | | AGES 60 TO 69 | | AGES 70 TO 79 | |
| | (NUMBER OF CASES PER 10,000 WOMEN PER YEAR) | | | | | |
	Estrogen plus Progestin	Placebo	Estrogen plus Progestin	Placebo	Estrogen plus Progestin	Placebo
Coronary heart disease	22	17	35	34	78	55
Stroke	14	10	32	23	61	48
Venous thromboembolism	19	8	35	19	62	27
Breast cancer	31	26	44	36	54	41
Colorectal cancer	4	5	10	19	14	28
Hip fracture	1	3	9	11	33	48

In the estrogen-alone arm of the study, younger women
also did better than older women.

| | AGES 50 TO 59 | | AGES 60 TO 69 | | AGES 70 TO 79 | |
| | (NUMBER OF CASES PER 10,000 WOMEN PER YEAR) | | | | | |
	Estrogen	Placebo	Estrogen	Placebo	Estrogen	Placebo
Coronary heart disease	17	27	57	61	96	86
Stroke	16	16	49	30	71	57
Venous thromboembolism	15	13	31	23	40	28
Breast cancer	21	29	26	36	32	34
Colorectal cancer	7	12	16	19	32	15
Hip fracture	4	1	4	11	32	52

Estrogen-Progestogen Products

These products are available in the United States and Canada for postmenopausal use.

(E = estrogen; P = progestogen)

COMPOSITION	PRODUCT NAME	DAILY DOSAGES
Oral Continuous-Cyclic (or Sequential) Regimen Conjugated estrogens (E) + medroxyprogesterone acetate (P) (E alone for days 1–14, followed by E+P on days 15–28)	Premphase*	0.625 milligram E + 5.0 milligrams P (2 tablets: E and E+P)
Oral Continuous Combined Regimen Conjugated estrogens (E) + medroxyprogesterone acetate (P)	Prempro*	0.625 milligram E or 5.0 milligrams P (1 tablet); 0.3 or 0.45 milligram E + 1.5 milligrams P (1 tablet); 0.45 milligram E + 1.5 milligrams P (1 tablet)
	Premplus**	0.625 milligram E + 2.5 or 5.0 milligrams P (2 tablets: E+P)
Ethinyl estradiol (E) + norethindrone acetate (P)	Femhrt* FemHRT**	5.0 micrograms E + 1.0 milligram P (1 tablet)
17-beta estradiol (E) + norethindrone acetate (P)	Activella*	1.0 milligram E + 0.5 milligram P (1 tablet)
17-beta estradiol (CE) + drospirenone (P)	Angelig*	1.0 milligram E + 0.5 milligram P
Oral Intermittent Combined Regimen 17-beta estradiol (E) + norgestimate (P) (E alone for 3 days, followed by E+P for 3 days, repeated continuously)	Prefest*	1.0 milligram E + 0.09 milligram P (2 tablets: E and E+P)
Transdermal Continuous Combined Regimen 17-beta estradiol (E) + norethindrone acetate (P)	CombiPatch* Estalis**	0.05 milligram E + 0.14 milligram P (9 cm² patch, twice/week); 0.05 milligram E + 0.25 milligram P (16 cm² patch, once/week)
17-beta estradiol (E) + levonorgestrel (P)	Climara Pro*	0.045 milligram E + 0.015 milligram P (22 cm² patch, once/week)

*Available only in the United States.
**Available only in Canada.

Source: North American Menopause Society.

Oral Estrogen Products

These products are available in the United States and Canada for postmenopausal use.

COMPOSITION	PRODUCT NAME	AVAILABLE DOSAGES (MILLIGRAMS)
Conjugated estrogens (formerly conjugated equine estrogens)	Premarin	0.3, 0.45*, 0.625, 0.9, 1.25
Synthetic conjugated estrogens, A	Cenestin*	0.3, 0.45, 0.625, 0.9, 1.25
	Congest**	0.3, 0.625, 0.9, 1.25, 2.5
	C.E.S.**	0.3, 0.625, 0.9, 1.25
	PMS-Conjugated**	0.3, 0.625, 0.9, 1.25
Synthetic conjugated estrogens, B	Enjuvia*	0.625, 1.25
Esterified estrogens	Menest*	0.3, 0.625, 0.9, 1.25
17-beta estradiol, micronized	Estrace	0.5, 1.0, 2.0
	Various generics	0.5, 1.0, 2.0
Estradiol acetate	Femtrace*	0.45, 0.9, 1.8
Estropipate (formerly piperazine estrone sulfate	Ortho-Est*	0.625 (0.75 estropipate, calculated as sodium estrone sulfate 0.625), 1.25 (1.5), 2.5 (3.0)
	Ogen**	0.625 (0.75), 1.25 (1.5), 2.5 (3.0)
	Various generics	0.625 (0.75), 1.25 (3.0)

*Available only in the United States.
**Available only in Canada.

Source: North American Menopause Society.

Transdermal and Topical Estrogen Products

These products are available in the United States and Canada for postmenopausal use.

COMPOSITION	PRODUCT NAME	DELIVERY RATE (MILLIGRAMS PER DAY)	DOSING
17-beta estradiol matrix patch	Alora*	0.025, 0.05, 0.075, 0.1	Twice weekly
	Climara	0.025, 0.375*, 0.05, 0.075, 0.1	Once weekly
	Esclim*	0.025, 0.0375, 0.05, 0.075, 0.1	Twice weekly
	Estradot**	0.025, 0.0375, 0.05, 0.075, 0.1	Twice weekly
	Menostar*	0.014	Once weekly
	Oesclim**	0.05, 0.1	Twice weekly
	Vivelle	0.025, 0.0375, 0.05, 0.075, 0.1	Twice weekly
	Vivelle-Dot*	0.025, 0.0375, 0.05, 0.075, 0.1	Twice weekly
	Various generics	0.05, 0.1	Once or twice weekly
17-beta estradiol reservoir patch	Estraderm	0.05, 0.1	Twice weekly (patch cannot be cut)
17-beta estradiol transdermal gel	EstroGel 0.06%* Estrogel 0.06%**	0.035	Daily application; 1 metered pump delivers 1.25 grams of gel containing 0.75 milligrams of 17-beta estradiol
17-beta estradiol topical emulsion	Estrasorb**	0.05	Daily application of two packets (1.74 grams/packet)

*Available only in the United States.
**Available only in Canada.

Source: North American Menopause Society.

Progestogens Used for Estrogen-Progestogen Therapy

These products are available in the United States and Canada for postmenopausal use.
Note: Progestogens include natural progesterone and synthetic progestin.

COMPOSITION	PRODUCT NAME	AVAILABLE DOSAGES
Oral tablet: progestin Medroxyprogesterone acetate	Provera, various generics	2.5, 5, 10 milligrams
Norethindrone (formerly norethisterone)	Micronor, Nor-Q.D.,* various generics	0.35 milligram
Norethindrone acetate	Aygestin,* various generics	5 milligrams
Norgestrel	Ovrette*	0.075 milligram
Megestrol acetate	Megace	20,* 40 milligrams
Oral capsule: progesterone Progesterone, micronized	Prometrium	100, 200* milligrams (in peanut oil)
Intrauterine system: progestin Levonorgestrel intrauterine system	Mirena	20 micrograms (daily approximate release rate); 52-milligram intrauterine system has five-year use.
Vaginal gel: progesterone Progesterone	Prochieve 4%	45 milligrams/applicator

*Available only in the United States.

Source: North American Menopause Society.

Vaginal Estrogen

These products are available in the United States and Canada
for the treatment of postmenopausal vaginal dryness.

COMPOSITION	PRODUCT NAME	DOSING
Vaginal creams 17-beta estradiol	Estrace Vaginal Cream*	Initial: 2 to 4 grams daily for 1 to 2 weeks Maintenance: 1 gram daily (0.1 milligram active ingredients/gram)
Conjugated estrogens (formerly conjugated equine estrogens)	Premarin Vaginal Cream	0.5 to 2 grams daily (0.625 milligram active ingredients/gram)
Vaginal rings 17-beta estradiol	Estring	Device containing 2 milligrams releases 7.5 micrograms daily for 90 days (local levels)
Estradiol acetate	Femring*	Device containing 12.4 milligrams or 24.8 milligrams estradiol acetate releases 0.05 milligram daily or 0.10 milligram daily estradiol for 90 days (systemic levels)
Vaginal tablet Estradiol hemihydrate	Vagifem	Initial: 1 tablet daily for 2 weeks Maintenance: 1 tablet twice/week (tablet containing 25.8 micrograms of estradiol hemihydrate equivalent to 25 micrograms of estradiol)

*Available only in the United States.
**Available only in Canada.

Source: North American Menopause Society.

Page Note

Page 33: Chart, Overall Results of the Women's Health Initiative, National Heart,
Lung and Blood Institute.

CHAPTER 3: HOT FLASHES

Medicine Chest: Hot Flashes

The North American Menopause Society reviewed research on treatments for hot flashes and came up with recommendations based on the best available evidence. They concluded that women should start by making lifestyle changes such as losing weight, getting regular exercise, lowering room temperatures, and stopping smoking. If those don't work, other remedies are available.

ALTERNATIVE REMEDIES

TYPE OF DRUG	DOES IT WORK?	POSSIBLE SIDE EFFECTS
Soy and red clover From plants with hormonal and nonhormonal properties	Mixed results.	For soy, minimal in dosages of 40 to 80 milligrams daily; long-term safety of red clover unclear.
Black cohosh From an herb; often sold as Remifemin	Mixed results; use recommended by NAMS for less than six months.	Stomach upset; effects of long-term use unknown. Should not be used by women with breast cancer. There is some evidence that it may cause liver damage.
Vitamin E	No proven benefit.	Women with vitamin K deficiency may have uterine bleeding with high doses. Studies indicate that 400 international units a day and above slightly increase risk of dying from all causes.
Magnet therapy	No proven benefit.	Unknown. Not recommended by NAMS for hot flash relief.

PRESCRIPTION HORMONES

TYPE OF DRUG	DOES IT WORK?	POSSIBLE SIDE EFFECTS
Progestogen alone	Proven effective but primary use is for endometrial protection from unopposed estrogen.	Side effects the same as for progestogen used with estrogen. Appears to increase breast cancer risk. NAMS says it's an option.

PRESCRIPTION HORMONES *(coninued)*		
TYPE OF DRUG	**DOES IT WORK?**	**POSSIBLE SIDE EFFECTS**
Estrogen and estrogen-progestogen therapy Estrogen alone for women without a uterus; a progestogen added for women with a uterus.	Proven effective in many clinical trials; may take 4 weeks or more to feel full effect.	Estrogen-progestogen therapy linked to increased risk for coronary heart disease, breast cancer, blood clots, stroke, and dementia, especially in older women. Side effects of estrogen therapy alone include breast tenderness, uterine bleeding, nausea, abdominal bloating, fluid retention, headache, dizziness, and hair loss. With progestogen added, adverse effects include mood changes and more uterine bleeding than with estrogen alone. Should not be used by women with a history of hormone-sensitive cancer, liver disease, blood clotting disorders, and cardiovascular disease. Recommended by NAMS for moderate to severe hot flashes in smallest effective dose for shortest possible time consistent with treatment goals.
Medroxprogesterone acetate (MPA) A progestin.	Proven effective in clinical trials.	Weight gain, uterine bleeding, amenorrhea, nervousness. Should not be used by women with a history of hormone-sensitive cancer, liver disease, blood clotting disorders, or cardiovascular disease.
Megestrol acetate A progestin.	Proven effective in a clinical trial; full effect takes up to 4 weeks.	Increased appetite, possible exacerbation of existing diabetes, risk of blood clots. Women on tamoxifen may experience increase in hot flashes before decrease. No long-term data on safety for women with breast cancer.
Oral contraceptives Estrogen and a progestin.	Proven effective in a randomized study.	Nausea, vomiting, abdominal bloating, breakthrough uterine bleeding, change in menstrual flow, edema, skin discoloration, migraine. Should not be used by women with a history of blood clots, cardiovascular disease, migraines, hormone-sensitive cancers, jaundice, or liver disease. NAMS supports the use of low-dose oral contraceptives by nonsmoking perimenopausal women with no risk factors who need hot flash relief and birth control.
Estrogen-androgen therapy Esterified estrogens and methyltestosterone.	No clinical data.	Same as for estrogen along with additional side effects from androgen: hair loss, acne, deepening of the voice, hirsutism. Long-term effects in women unknown.

OTHER PRESCRIPTION MEDICATIONS

Type of Drug	Does It Work?	Possible Side Effects
Effexor (venlafaxine) An antidepressant (serotonin and norepinephrine reuptake inhibitor, or SNRI).	Proven in clinical trial; full effect within 2 weeks.	Sleepiness, dizziness, constipation, sexual dysfunction. Should not be used with MAOIs. Recommended by NAMS at dosages of 37.5 to 75 milligrams daily for women with hot flashes who can't use hormone therapy, including women with breast cancer.
Paxil (paroxetine) An antidepressant (selective serotonin reuptake inhibitor, or SSRI).	Proven in clinical trial.	Muscle weakness, sweating, nausea, decreased appetite, insomnia, sleepiness, dizziness. Should not be used with MAOIs, thioridazine. Caution if taken with Coumadin (warfarin). Recommended by NAMS at dosages of 12.5 to 25 milligrams daily for women with hot flashes who can't use hormone therapy, including women with breast cancer.
Prozac (fluoxetine) An antidepressant (selective serotonin reuptake inhibitor, or SSRI).	Proven in clinical trial but not as great a reduction as Effexor.	Weakness, sweating, nausea, decreased appetite, insomnia, sleepiness, dizziness. Should not be used with MAOIs, thioridazine. Recommended by NAMS at dosage of 20 milligrams daily for women with hot flashes who can't use hormone therapy, including women with breast cancer.
Neurontin (gabapentin) An anticonvulsant.	Proven in clinical trial.	Sleepiness, dizziness, problems with coordination, fatigue, vision problems.
Catapres (clonidine) An antihypertensive.	Proven in clinical trials.	Dry mouth, dizziness, drowsiness, constipation, sedation. Should not be used by women with sinus node function impairment. Possible heart arrhythmias at high doses.

MAOI = monoamine oxidase inhibitor

CHAPTER 4: SLEEP

Page Notes:

Page 83: Chart, "Foods That Can Keep You Up," National Sleep Foundation and Center for Science in the Public Interest.

Pages 88–89: Sleepiness Diary, National Sleep Foundation (Sleepiness Scale, C. Maldonado, A. Bentley, and D. Mitchell, in *Sleep* (2003), 27.

CHAPTER 5: SEX

Medicine Chest: Sexual Dysfunction

At the time of this writing, no drugs have been approved by the FDA to treat women with sexual dysfunction. However, some medications approved by the FDA for other purposes have been used over the last 50 years to treat women's sexual complaints, with mixed results. Keep in mind that when it comes to the placebo effect, sexual problems are particularly vulnerable. Talk to your doctor before starting any of these.

NONPRESCRIPTION	DOES IT WORK?	POSSIBLE SIDE EFFECTS
ArginMax A nonprescription dietary supplement that combines the amino acid L-arginine with three herbs long thought to improve sexuality (Korean ginseng, gingko, and damiana), together with 14 vitamins and minerals. The ingredients are standardized, and the amounts of active ingredients are specified.	Effective in one double-blind placebo-controlled clinical study. A subgroup of women nearing menopause reported a 91% improvement in the frequency of intercourse, compared with a 20% increase in the placebo group.	Consult your physician if you're receiving chemotherapy, antibiotics, or medications for diabetes, blood pressure, clotting, migraine, or cardiovascular problems. Women with a history of cancer, heart disease, stroke, migraines, renal failure, liver failure, or severe allergies, as well as those who are pregnant or nursing, should also talk to their doctor before starting this supplement.
Zestra A genital massage oil made of borage seeds and evening primrose oil.	Effective in one small randomized clinical trial involving 20 women. All subjects reported improvement in arousal, desire, genital sensation, and ability to reach orgasm.	Three of the 20 women complained that, while using Zestra, they felt mild genital burning that lasted 5 to 30 minutes. In each case, this burning occurred only the first five times they used it.
L-arginine An amino acid that increases the amount of nitric oxide in the blood, which has a role in improving sexual functioning. Found naturally in nuts, meat, and dairy products and as a dietary supplement.	There is preliminary evidence that it improves genital blood flow and engorgement. More studies are needed to determine what dose is safe and effective for women.	Women with asthma, diabetes, or liver or kidney problems, as well as those taking anticoagulant or antiplatelet medications, should consult their doctor before using. Can cause severe allergy reactions (anaphylaxis) if injected or asthma symptoms if inhaled. Stomach distress also reported.

NONPRESCRIPTION	DOES IT WORK?	POSSIBLE SIDE EFFECTS
Asian ginseng (*Panax ginseng*) An herbal tonic. Active ingredient: ginsenoside.	Research indicates that ginsenoside boosts nitric oxide, which has a role in improving sexual functioning. Significant quality-control issues exist; some products contain no ginsenoside.	Contradictory evidence related to cancer growth; may have estrogenic effect. Reported side effects include increased uterine bleeding, headaches, depression, anxiety, insomnia, and worsened menopausal symptoms. Women with cardiovascular disease, high or low blood pressure, or diabetes should consult a doctor before using. Can elevate blood pressure and reduce glucose levels. Should not be taken with anticoagulants, ma huang, ephedrine, guarana, other stimulants, steroids, or antipsychotic drugs.
Ginkgo biloba An herb.	Mixed results. Studies that exhibited effectiveness had no control group	Ginkgo is an anticoagulant and should not be used with similar medications, blood thinners, or medication for blood pressure. Increased risk of uncontrolled bleeding if used with other botanicals, including feverfew, garlic, ginseng, dong quai, and red clover. General side effects include headaches, nausea, diarrhea, dizziness, weakness, heart palpitations, and skin rashes.
Damiana (*Turnera aphrodisiaca, Turnera diffusa*) Dried leaves of a small bush that grows in the southwestern U.S., Mexico, and Central America.	Small studies indicate that damiana has a modest ability to dilate blood vessels.	Consult your doctor before using if you have a history of breast cancer, schizophrenia, mania, diabetes, or Parkinson's disease.
DHEA (dehydroepiandrosterone) Made in your body by the adrenal glands; an estrogen and androgen precursor. Some "natural" DHEA products are derived from wild yams.	Mixed results for treatment of low sex drive or vaginal pain. Current thinking is that DHEA made from wild yams cannot be converted to DHEA in the body.	No studies on the long-term safety of DHEA have been conducted; theoretically, it should have the same risks as estrogen and testosterone. As with all hormones, start with a low dose; as little as 5 to 10 milligrams may be effective.

NONPRESCRIPTION	DOES IT WORK?	POSSIBLE SIDE EFFECTS
Yohimbe Bark of a West African tree. May also refer to yohimbine hydrochloride, a chemically similar prescription medication. Active ingredient: yohimbine.	Yohimbine hydrochloride has been approved by the FDA to treat erectile dysfunction; there is a theory that it might help with female desire issues, but research to date consists of a few poor-quality studies. The National Institutes of Health and the FDA both say there is not enough data on natural yohimbine to determine its safety or effectiveness.	The effective dose is slightly lower than the toxic dose. Serious side effects include renal failure, seizures, and death; especially dangerous when taken in high doses with red wine, cheese, or liver (all products containing tyramine) or with nasal decongestants or diet aids containing phenylpropanolamine. Anyone with low blood pressure, diabetes, or heart, liver, or kidney disease should also avoid this supplement. Can cause anxiety, panic attacks, and increased heart rate.

PRESCRIPTION HORMONES	DOES IT WORK?	POSSIBLE SIDE EFFECTS
Estratest and Estratest-HS (half-strength) Oral medication made of a combination of esterified estrogen with methyltestosterone, a synthetic version of testosterone. Not approved by the FDA (may be prescribed while lingering in the equivalent of regulatory limbo).	Mixed results.	Estrogen may increase likelihood of stroke, blood clots, and heart disease in some women. Possible side effects include breast tenderness and uterine bleeding. More than doubled the risk of breast cancer in older women (most of whom were longtime hormone therapy users) compared to those who had never used hormone therapy. Testosterone can cause acne as well as masculinizing traits such as excessive facial hair and receding hairline. Long-term effects on cardiovascular system unknown. Women with an intact uterus will need to add a progestogen to reduce risk of endometrial cancer.

Prescription Hormones	Does It Work?	Possible Side Effects
Depo-Testadiol (generic name: testosterone cypionate/estradiol cypionate) Injectable testosterone made by Pharmacia & Upjohn. Dosage: testosterone, 50 milligrams; estradiol, 2 milligrams per milliliter.	Developed for men; used off-label for women. Good-quality research indicates that testosterone improves sexual functioning in some women, but optimal dosage and long-term safety remain unclear.	Testosterone can cause acne and unwanted hair. Little is known about its long-term effects on the cardiovascular system and breasts.
Delatestryl (generic name: testosterone enanthate) Injectable testosterone produced by Savient. Dosage: 200 milligrams per milliliter.	Developed for men; used off-label for women. Good-quality research indicates that testosterone improves sexual functioning in some women, but optimal dosage and long-term safety remain unclear.	Testosterone can cause acne and unwanted hair. Little is known about its long-term effects on the cardiovascular system and breasts.
Depo-Testosterone (generic name: testosterone cypionate) Injectable testosterone manufactured by Star. Dosage: 200 milligrams per milliliter.	Developed for men; used off-label for women. Good-quality research indicates that testosterone improves sexual functioning in some women, but optimal dosage and long-term safety remain unclear.	Testosterone can cause acne and unwanted hair. Little is known about its long-term effects on the cardiovascular system and breasts.
Testopel (generic name: testosterone) Pellets, manufactured by Bartor at a dosage of 75 milligrams, are surgically inserted under the skin, where they deliver a steady stream of testosterone for about 4 to 6 months.	Developed for men; used off-label for women. Good-quality research indicates that testosterone improves sexual functioning in some women, but optimal dosage and long-term safety remain unclear.	Testosterone can cause acne and unwanted hair. Little is known about its long-term effects on the cardiovascular system and breasts.

PRESCRIPTION HORMONES	DOES IT WORK?	POSSIBLE SIDE EFFECTS
Formulated testosterone in petroleum (or formulated testosterone in APC) Gels and creams that are formulated by compound pharmacies to match a doctor's specifications. These are available in doses ranging from 1% to 8%. They can be applied anywhere on the skin, but tend to be used on the clitoris, genitals, abdomen, or buttocks.	Developed for men; used off-label for women. Good-quality research indicates that testosterone improves sexual functioning in some women, but optimal dosage and long-term safety remain unclear.	Same side effects as other testosterone products. Plus: Doctors are reluctant to prescribe these drugs because dosage is less exact, increasing the likelihood of overuse and side effects.

PRESCRIPTION NONHORMONES	DOES IT WORK?	POSSIBLE SIDE EFFECTS
Livial (tibolone) Synthetic steroid. Not available in U.S.	Research indicates that it helps vaginal dryness and low sexual desire, while increasing bone mass and reducing hot flashes.	Clinical research is currently under way to determine its long-term safety in terms of breast and uterine cancer.

CHAPTER 7: ACHES AND PAINS

Page Note

Page 185: Bladder Diary, National Institute of Diabetes and Digestive and Kidney Diseases.

CHAPTER 9: THINKING AND MEMORY

Page Notes

Page 229: Chart, Types of Memory, Vani Rao, M.D., A Woman's Journey (conference), Johns Hopkins Medicine.

Pages 232–33: Illustrations, Alzheimer's Disease Research (ADR), a program of the American Health Assistance Foundation. Chart, D.A. Evans, N.H. Funkenstein, M.S. Albert, et al., "Prevalence of Alzheimer's Disease Revisited," *American Journal of Public Health* (1994), 84.

CHAPTER 10: BONES

Secondary Osteoporosis

Age is not the only cause of fragile bones; a number of diseases and disorders weaken the skeleton and are considered causes of secondary osteoporosis. As many as a third of postmenopausal women suffering from primary osteoporosis also have secondary osteoporosis. Some of the more common secondary causes include:

Genetic disorders
Hemophilia
Thalassemia
Hypophosphatasia in adults
Hemochromatosis
Chondrodysplasia
Cystic fibrosis

Disorders of calcium balance
Hypercalciuria
Vitamin D deficiency
Excessive intake of vitamin A from retinol

Endocrine diseases
Cortisol excess
Gonadal insufficiency
Hyperthyroidism
Diabetes mellitus, type 1
Hyperparathyroidism
Acromegaly
Hyperprolactinemia

Gastrointestinal diseases
Malabsorption syndrome and malnutrition
Celiac disease
Chronic liver disease
Gastric operations
Inflammatory bowel disease
    (Crohn's disease and ulcerative colitis)

Disorders of collagen metabolism
Osteogenesis imperfecta
Homocystinuria due to cystathionine deficiency
Ehlers-Danlos syndrome
Marfan syndrome

Drugs
Glucocorticoids such as prednisone for more
    than three months
Long-term use of certain anticonvulsants
    such as phenytoin
Excessive thyroxine
Anticoagulants (heparin, warfarin)
Cytotoxic agents
Gonadotropin-releasing hormone antagonists
Injectable contraception
Immunosuppressives
Cyclosporine

Others
Alcoholism
Tobacco use
Athletic amenorrhea
Anorexia and bulimia
Rheumatoid arthritis
Multiple myeloma
Lymphoma and leukemia
Immobilization
Chronic renal disease
Systemic mastocytosis
Autoimmune disease
Muscular dystrophies
Organ transplantation

Sources: North American Menopause Society; American Association of Clinical Endocrinologists; Cleveland Clinic; Surgeon General's Report on Bone Health and Osteoporosis.

CHAPTER 11: EYES AND EARS

Page Notes

Page 301: Cosmetic advice, "Make Up the Difference," Laura Snavely, Bobbi Brown Cosmetics.

Page 312: Chart, "The Five-Decibel Rule," National Institute on Deafness and Other Communication Disorders.

CHAPTER 12: HEART

Medicine Chest: Cholesterol		
These medications are effective in managing cholesterol and triglyceride levels. Your doctor will explain which one you should take, and why, if diet and exercise don't bring you down to healthy levels.		
TYPE OF DRUG	**PURPOSE**	**PROS AND CONS**
Statin Brand names: Lipitor, Lescol, Mevacor, Pravachol, Crestor, Zocor	To block the enzyme required for the liver to process cholesterol, removing more LDL from the blood	Statins are the most effective drugs in lowering total cholesterol and LDL, as well as raising HDL. Side effects in 1% to 2% of patients include muscle soreness and liver injury.
Bile acid sequestrant Brand names: Questran, Colestid, WelChol	To make the liver convert more cholesterol into bile acid, which is then excreted and lowers LDL	These drugs are used for people with high LDL and normal triglycerides.

TYPE OF DRUG	PURPOSE	PROS AND CONS
Nicotinic acid Brand names: Niacor, Niaspan	To decrease production of the lipoproteins that carry triglycerides	Nicotinic acid effectively raises HDL levels. It also reduces LDL and triglycerides. Skin flushing may occur 30 minutes after taking, but side effects decrease over time. These drugs should not be used by patients with peptic ulcers or gout. Diabetics should use them with caution.
Fibrate Brand names: Lofibra, TriCor, Lopid	To stimulate the activity of an enzyme that breaks down triglycerides	The most effective drugs for lowering triglycerides. They can raise total cholesterol and LDL in some people. May cause muscle aches, liver injury, gallstones.
Cholesterol absorption inhibitor Brand name: Zetia	To inhibit absorption of dietary cholesterol in small intestine; can lower cholesterol even in people on a low-cholesterol diet	Greater reductions in total cholesterol, LDL, and triglycerides when used with a statin (combination not safe for people with liver disease or elevated liver enzymes).

Source: Adapted from "The Johns Hopkins White Papers 2005: Coronary Heart Disease."

CHAPTER 13: CANCER

Most Common Cancer Diagnoses in Women

In 2006, the American Cancer Society ranked cancer diagnoses and fatalities as follows:

TYPE	NUMBER OF NEW CASES PER YEAR	DEATHS PER YEAR
Breast	212,920	40,970
Lung	81,770	72,130
Colorectal	75,810	27,300
Uterine (endometrial)	41,200	7,350
Non-Hodgkin's lymphoma	28,190	8,840
Melanoma of the skin	27,930	2,890
Thyroid	22,590	870
Ovary	20,180	15,310
Bladder	16,730	4,070
Pancreas	16,580	16,210
Leukemia	15,070	9,810
Kidney	14,240	4,710
Cervix	9,710	3,700
Brain	8,090	5,560
Multiple myeloma	7,320	5,630
Vulvar	3,740	880
Vaginal	2,420	820

CHAPTER 14: DIET AND EXERCISE

Page Notes

Page 378: List, "Obesity-Related Diseases," The Endocrine Society.

Page 384: Graphic, "Bloated Portions," National Heart, Lung and Blood Institute.

Page 389: Chart, "A Better Way," National Heart, Lung and Blood Institute.

CHAPTER 15: LOOKING GOOD

Your Skin: Is It Aging or Something Else?

Some skin changes are just part of the aging process, but other symptoms could signal a serious illness. Here are some signs of possible problems:

Symptom	What It Might Mean
Skin lesion that appears as: • Scaly red spot or cluster of slow-growing, shiny red or pink lesions • Mole that changes shape, color, or size • New skin growth • Mole or other skin lesion that bleeds or itches • Age spot that becomes large, flat, and dark and has irregular borders • Bruise that does not heal or seems to heal and then reappears • Brown or black streak under a nail • Translucent, pearl-shaped growth	• Skin cancer
Sore that does not heal or seems to heal and then reappears	• Circulatory problem • Diabetes • Skin cancer
Skin lesion with any of the following characteristics: • Dry, scaly, rough-textured patches ranging in color from skin tone to reddish brown and in size from a pinhead to larger than a quarter • Diffuse scaling on the lower lip that cracks and dries; the lip may have a whitish discoloration • Lesion of the skin that resembles an animal horn *Note: These lesions develop on skin that has received years of unprotected sun exposure. Usually, the skin is dry, itchy, and wrinkled.*	• Actinic keratosis (AK) • Actinic cheilitis (an AK on the lip)
Itching and very dry skin that's not relieved by moisturizers	• Dermatitis • Psoriasis
Pain, usually with a headache, followed by blisters on the skin	• Shingles
Vein in the leg that bulges or is very tender	• Varicose veins

Source: American Academy of Dermatology.

Page Notes

Page 433: Graphic, "Danger Signs in Pigmented Lesions of the Skin," National Cancer Institute.

Page 434: "How to Examine Yourself for Skin Cancer," M.D. Anderson Cancer Institute.

Page 435: Chart, "What Your Nails Say About You," American Academy of Dermatology.

Appendix II: Resources

*I*n the course of our research, we discovered dozens of helpful websites and books. The list that follows represents a sampling of some we found particularly useful and accurate. When you're looking for information online, be aware of the source. Government websites, especially those sponsored by a scientific organization like the National Institutes of Health, are generally the most dependable. Sites from major professional organizations, such as the American College of Obstetricians and Gynecologists, are also reliable. In all of these, you should look for some indication of when the site was last updated. Some organizations are better about this than others. Sites run by individual practitioners may have a point of view that colors their opinions; read these with skepticism. Drug companies also set up sites to explain the diseases their medications are intended to cure. These can be very helpful on the disease part; generally, they include snazzy animations that can simplify explanations. However, you should always keep in mind that the goal is to sell something.

AN OVERVIEW

GENERAL HEALTH

Combined Health Information Database
http://chid.nih.gov/index.html
A searchable database produced by agencies of the National Institutes of Health.

Medline Plus
http://www.nlm.nih.gov/medlineplus/
From the U.S. National Library of Medicine. Great features include Health Topics (type in the name of a disease or condition and you'll get a full rundown of the latest information on the topic) and an easy-to-use medical dictionary.

Directory of Health Organizations
http://dirline.nlm.nih.gov/
A searchable database of U.S. health organizations and research resources.

Healthfinder
http://www.healthfinder.gov/
A health information website for consumers developed by the U.S. Department of Health and Human Services and other federal agencies. This is a good place to start a basic search.

Merck Manual
http://www.merck.com/mmhe/index.html
Searchable online version of the widely used medical text.

Canadian Health Network
http://www.canadian-health-network.ca/
From Canada's Public Health Agency, an all-in-one site.

American Board of Medical Specialties
http://www.abms.org
A reliable place to search for a specialist or expert who can give you a second opinion. The *Official ABMS Directory of Board Certified Medical Specialists* provides doctors' names as well as their specialty and their educational background. (Click on "who's certified.") A hardcover version of the directory is available in most public libraries. You can also get the names of specialists from your local medical society, a nearby hospital, or a medical school.

WOMEN'S HEALTH

American Medical Women's Association
http://www.amwa-doc.org/
The AMWA represents 10,000 women physicians and medical students. The Patient Information section contains clear explanations of diseases affecting women.

National Women's Health Network
http://www.womenshealthnetwork.org/about/index.php
Founded in 1975 to give women a greater voice within the health-care system, the NWHN does not accept financial support from pharmaceutical companies, tobacco companies, or medical device manufacturers. Go to the Resources section for health information useful to women of all ages.

National Women's Health Resource Center

http://www.healthywomen.org/

NWHRC, a nonprofit group, offers up-to-date women's health essentials in a well-designed format.

Society for Women's Health Research

http://www.womenshealthresearch.org/site/PageServer

Consumer Information pages cover a wide range of subjects, from oral health to addiction.

The New Harvard Guide to Women's Health, by Karen J. Carlson, M.D., Stephanie A. Eisenstat, M.D., and Terra Ziporyn, Ph.D. (Harvard University Press, 2004)

Comprehensive, easy to understand, lots of clear illustrations.

MENOPAUSE

National Women's Health Information Center

http://www.4women.gov/menopause/

A good starting point for accessing U.S. government resources on menopausal health issues.

North American Menopause Society

http://www.menopause.org/

A leading professional organization dedicated to menopausal medicine. Go to the Consumer page for the helpful Menopause Guidebook and Early Menopause Guidebook.

POSTMENOPAUSAL HORMONE THERAPY

National Institutes of Health

http://www.nhlbi.nih.gov/health/women/

Sponsored by the NIH and the Department of Health and Human Services, this site features links to important material related to the hormone controversy.

The Women's Health Initiative

http://www.nhlbi.nih.gov/whi/

Everything you need to know about this major women's health study.

Office of Research on Women's Health

http://orwh.od.nih.gov/menopause.html

A comprehensive site with information on current research.

American College of Obstetricians and Gynecologists

http://www.acog.org

The Green Journal Supplement on Hormone Therapy, October 2004, is a technical explanation of fairly current research.

The Greatest Experiement Ever Performed on Women, by Barbara Seaman (Hyperion, 2003)

and

Hot Flashes, Hormones & Your Health, by JoAnn Manson, M.D., with Shari Bassuk, Sc.D. (McGraw-Hill, 2006)

SPECIFIC HEALTH TOPICS

ALTERNATIVE MEDICINE

National Center for Complementary and Alternative Medicine
http://nccam.nih.gov/
From the NIH, basic information on the state of current research.

M.D. Anderson Cancer Center
http://www.mdanderson.org/departments/ CIMER/
A rich resource, with Spanish and Mandarin translations, from the renowned Texas cancer center.

Mayo Clinic
http://www.mayoclinic.com/health/ alternative-medicine/
An excellent introduction to the topic with useful links.

Office of Dietary Supplements
http://ods.od.nih.gov/
The latest research on dozens of herbs, vitamins, and minerals.

Alternative Medicine Foundation
http://www.amfoundation.org/
Founded in 1998 to provide reliable information about alternative medicine to the public and health professionals.

American Geriatrics Society
http://www.healthinaging.org/ agingintheknow/
Check out the Complementary and Alternative Medicine page for a useful chart listing herbal remedies and their possible interactions with various medications.

BLEEDING

TREMIN Research Program on Women's Health (formerly known as the TREMIN Trust)
http://www.pop.psu.edu/tremin/
Oldest ongoing research project on menstruation and women's health, now operating out of Pennsylvania State University. Look under Documentation for a copy of their monthly menstrual calendar cards, which can help you keep close track of your bleeding patterns.

Society for Menstrual Cycle Research
http://menstruationresearch.org/
A nonprofit interdisciplinary research organization.

NoPeriod.com
http://www.noperiod.com/FAQ.html
This site focuses on menstruation suppression and is sponsored by Dr. Leslie Miller, an associate professor of obstetrics and gynecology at the University of Washington.

CANCER

National Cancer Institute
http://www.cancer.gov
Comprehensive and current information from the National Institutes of

Health; available in English and Spanish *(http://www.cancer.gov/espanol).*

American Cancer Society
http://www.cancer.org
Information available in English and Spanish.

Women's Cancer Network
http://www.wcn.org
Developed by the Gynecologic Cancer Foundation and CancerSource. Click on "risk assessment" to see how vulnerable you are.

Susan G. Komen Breast Cancer Foundation
http://www.komen.org

National Alliance of Breast Cancer Organizations
http://www.nabco.org

National Ovarian Cancer Coalition
http://www.ovarian.org
The Cancer Information Service, at 1-800-4-CANCER, has information about treatment facilities, including cancer centers and other programs supported by the National Cancer Institute.

Mayo Clinic Guide to Women's Cancers, by Lynn C. Hartmann, M.D., and Charles L. Loprinzi, M.D. (Kensington Publishing Corporation, 2005)
This is the best women's cancer guide we found. It's easy to understand and up-to-date.

DIET AND EXERCISE

National Heart, Lung and Blood Institute Obesity Education Initiative
http://www.nhlbi.nih.gov/health/public/heart/obesity/lose_wt/index.htm
A good starting place.

National Heart, Lung and Blood Institute
http://www.nhlbisupport.com/bmi/
An easy-to-use BMI calculator.

U.S. Department of Agriculture
http://www.mypyramid.gov
How to tailor a diet suitable for your age and activity level. The site also has lots of other helpful features—and it's free!

U.S. Department of Agriculture
http://fnic.nal.usda.gov/
Look here for accurate info on food content, including calories.

American Dietetic Association
http://www.eatright.org
Nutrition information as well as a directory of registered dietitians.

American College of Sports Medicine
http://www.acsm.org
Click on "public resources."

The National Strength and Conditioning Association
http://www.nsca.com
Includes a list of certified personal trainers.

Yoga Journal
http://www.yogajournal.com
Provides information on the different types of yoga, streaming video on how to

do a variety of poses, and a national directory of yoga teachers.

Tai Chi Productions

http://www.taichiproductions.com
Website of Dr. Paul Lam, a medical doctor and Tai Chi Gold Medal winner who explains why this form of exercise is good for balance, osteoporosis, back pain, and arthritis.

American Heart Association No-Fad Diet (Clarkson Potter, 2005)
Advice on how to get motivated, plus easy recipes.

ACSM Fitness Book, American College of Sports Medicine (Human Kinetics, 2003)
A great program for getting started; written by fitness experts.

Action Plan for Menopause, by Barbara Bushman, Ph.D., and Janice Clark Young, Ed.D. (Human Kinetics, 2005)
From the American College of Sports Medicine, an easy-to-use guide specifically for midlife women.

The Pilates Body, by Brooke Siler (Broadway Books, 2000)
If you're interested in learning about Pilates, this is a good beginner's book.

Stretching, by Suzanne Martin (DK Publishing Inc., 2005)
A good basic guide with excellent how-to pictures.

EARS

National Institute on Deafness and Other Communication Disorders

http://www.nidcd.nih.gov
From the NIH, an easy-to-use entry point for information on the state of current research. Click on "health information"; we particularly liked their Wise Ears section.

The American Academy of Otolaryngology—Head and Neck Surgery (AAO-HNS)

http://www.entnet.org
Click on "health info."

EYES

Women's Eye Health Task Force

http://www.womenseyehealth.org
Top researchers from around the country provide information on how eye diseases disproportionately affect women. User-friendly and thorough.

National Eye Institute

http://www.nei.nih.gov
From the NIH, an easy-to-use entry point for information on the state of current research.

The Sjögren's Syndrome Foundation

http://www.sjogrens.org

The Macular Degeneration Partnership (part of the nonprofit Discovery Eye Foundation)

http://www.amd.org

FEET

American College of Foot and Ankle Surgeons
http://www.footphysicians.com

American Podiatric Medical Association
http://www.apma.org

American Academy of Podiatric Sports Medicine
http://www.aapsm.org

American Orthopaedic Foot and Ankle Society
http://www.aofas.org/

FERTILITY

Centers for Disease Prevention and Control
http://www.cdc.gov/ART/index.htm
Success rates of reproductive technologies.

FIBROIDS

National Institute of Child Health and Human Development
http://www.nichd.nih.gov/publications/pubs/fibroids/index.htm
Basic information also available in Spanish.

Mayo Clinic
http://www.mayoclinic.com/health/uterine-fibroids/UF99999
Good explanation of treatment decisions.

Society of Interventional Radiology
http://www.sirweb.org/patPub/uterineTreatments.shtml

A clear guide to the latest treatment techniques.

National Uterine Fibroids Foundation
http://www.nuff.org/health_riskfactors.htm
Helpful information about risk factors and treatment.

HEADACHES

American Headache Society
http://www.americanheadachesociety.org/

American Council for Headache Education
http://www.achenet.org/

National Institute of Neurological Disorders and Stroke
http://www.ninds.nih.gov/disorders/headache/headache.htm

HEART DISEASE

The American Heart Association
http://www.americanheart.org

The Heart Truth Campaign
http://www.nhlbi.nih.gov/health/hearttruth/index.htm

HeartHealthyWomen
http://www.hearthealthywomen.org/

National Center for Chronic Disease Prevention and Health Promotion
http://www.cdc.gov/dhdsp/library/fs_women_heart.htm
Fact sheet on women and heart disease.

National Women's Health Information Center
http://womenshealth.gov/faq/heartdis.htm

American Academy of Family Physicians
http://familydoctor.org/

WomenHeart: The National Coalition for Women with Heart Disease
http://www.womenheart.org/

The Women's Healthy Heart Program, by Nieca Goldberg, M.D. (Random House, 2006)
Tools to assess your risk, plus up-to-date information on hormones and heart disease.

HISTORY

Museum of Menstruation & Women's Health
http://www.mum.org/
Quirky site with lots of historical information about menopause and menstruation.

The Meanings of Menopause: Historical, Medical, and Cultural Perspectives, by Ruth Formanek (The Analytic Press, 1990)

The Wandering Womb, by Lana Thompson (Prometheus Books, 1999)

The Technology of Orgasm: "Hysteria," the Vibrator, and Women's Sexual Satisfaction, by Rachel P. Maines (Johns Hopkins Studies in the History of Technology, 2001)

HOT FLASHES

Mayo Clinic
http://www.mayoclinic.com/health/hot-flashes/HQ01409

National Center for Complementary and Alternative Medicine
http://nccam.nih.gov/health/menopauseandcam/

MEMORY AND THINKING

National Institute of Mental Health
http://www.nimh.nih.gov/

National Institute of Neurological Disorders and Stroke
http://www.ninds.nih.gov/

National Institute on Aging
http://www.nia.nih.gov/alzheimers/
Information on Alzheimer's disease.

Understanding the Mini-Mental
http://www.alzheimers.org.uk/How_is_dementia_diagnosed/Diagnosis_process/info_mmse.htm
The British Alzheimer's Society website (above) offers the easiest-to-understand explanation of the Mini-Mental (the most common test used in diagnosing dementia) that we have found. The information provided here was produced with the help and approval of Psychological Assessment Resources Inc., which holds the copyright on the test.

Overcoming Dyslexia: A New and Complete Science-Based Program for Reading Problems at Any Level, by Sally Shaywitz, M.D. (Knopf, 2003)
Some women's reading problems worsen, or are first diagnosed as dyslexia, during the menopause transition.

MOODS AND EMOTIONS

National Institute of Mental Health
http://www.nimh.nih.gov/

American Psychological Association
http://apa.org/
Click on Psychology Topics under the Public Publications link.

American Psychiatric Association
http://healthyminds.org/

Center for Mental Health Services
http://www.mentalhealth.samhsa.gov/

Depression and Bipolar Support Alliance
http://www.dbsalliance.org/

National Alliance on Mental Illness
http://www.nami.org/

National Mental Health Association
http://www.nmha.org/
Click on Mental Health Information for fact sheets and brochures on various disorders.

University of Pennsylvania Positive Psychology Center
http://www.authentichappiness.sas.upenn.edu
Features the work of Dr. Martin Seligman.

Women's Moods: What Every Woman Must Know About Hormones, the Brain and Emotional Health, by Deborah Sichel, M.D., and Jeanne Watson Driscoll, M.S., R.N., C.S. (Quill, 2000)

OSTEOARTHRITIS

National Institute of Arthritis and Musculoskeletal and Skin Diseases
http://nihseniorhealth.gov/arthritis/toc.html
Detailed information about joints and aging.

National Institute on Aging
http://www.niapublications.org/agepages/arthritis.asp
A Spanish page available.

Arthritis Foundation
http://www.arthritis.org/resources/gettingstarted/default.asp
Comprehensive resources.

U.S. Food and Drug Administration
http://www.fda.gov/fdac/features/2005/205_pain.html
Treatment options.

American College of Rheumatology
http://www.rheumatology.org/public/factsheets/herbal.asp
Facts about herbal treatments.

Cleveland Clinic

*http://www.clevelandclinic.org/health/
health-info/docs/0500/0561.asp?index=
4266*

A guide to physical and occupational therapy.

American Academy of Orthopaedic Surgeons

http://www.aaos.org/

Look for the Patient/Public Information page to get specific information on how arthritis affects different joints.

OSTEOPOROSIS

Osteoporosis and Related Bone Diseases—National Resource Center

http://www.niams.nih.gov/bone/

Information on bone development and diseases provided by the National Institute of Arthritis and Musculoskeletal and Skin Diseases, which is part of NIH.

Bone Health and Osteoporosis: A Surgeon General's Report (2004)

http://www.surgeongeneral.gov/

Click on "reports and publications" and then click on "Public Health Reports of the Surgeon General." Scroll down the list until you find the bone health report.

Strongwomen.com

http://www.strongwomen.com

Up-to-date information on osteoporosis, bone and joint issues, plus a free newsletter, exercise programs, and recipes for optimal nutrition.

Growing Stronger: Strength Training for Older Adults

*http://nutrition.tufts.edu/research/
growingstronger*

Strength-training program developed by the Centers for Disease Control and Prevention (CDC) and Tufts University experts. Plus, you can download their free book of exercises.

National Osteoporosis Foundation

http://www.nof.org/

Foundation for Osteoporosis Research and Education

http://www.fore.org/

Oregon State University Bone Density Research Lab

*http://oregonstate.edu/research/oregon/
health.htm*

Click on Osteoporosis Prevention and then scroll down to the section that describes how weighted vests can help build backbone in postmenopausal women. To order Dr. Christine Snow's research-based exercise video, call 888-431-9455.

Strong Women, Strong Bones,

by Miriam E. Nelson, Ph.D., with Sarah Wernick, Ph.D. (Perigee, 2000)

RHEUMATOID ARTHRITIS

National Institute of Arthritis and Musculoskeletal and Skin Diseases

http://www.niams.nih.gov/

Click on "health information" and then select a topic.

American College of Rheumatology
http://www.rheumatology.org/directory/geo.asp
A geographical guide to doctors specializing in rheumatology.

Strong Women and Men Beat Arthritis, by Miriam Nelson, Ph.D. (Perigee, 2003)

SEX AND RELATIONSHIPS

American Association for Marriage and Family Therapy
http://www.aamft.org/
A professional association representing more than 23,000 marriage and family therapists throughout the United States, Canada, and abroad. Resources include a searchable database of articles and books and a directory of therapists.

Coalition for Marriage, Family and Couples Education
http://www.smartmarriages.com
Look for the directory of couples workshops.

Association of Reproductive Health Professionals
http://www.arhp.org
This website contains great information for consumers. For a thorough explanation of female sexual dysfunction, read ARHP's Clinical Proceedings entitled: Women's Sexual Health at Midlife and Beyond. Find it by scrolling down to the topic list and clicking on "sex and sexuality." Look for the link on the left side of the page.

Sexuality Information and Education Council of the United States
http://www.siecus.org

American Association of Sex Educators, Counselors, and Therapists
http://www.aasect.org
A quality source listing certified sex therapists.

Columbia University's Health Education Program
http://www.goaskalice.columbia.edu

Medline Plus: Sexually Transmitted Diseases
http://www.nlm.nih.gov/medlineplus/sexuallytransmitteddiseases.html
Current information on sexually transmitted diseases, provided by the U.S. National Library of Medicine and the National Institutes of Health.

Sex Toys, Lubrication, and Moisturizers
Many different purveyors can be found online. Here's a sampling to get you started:

- **Eve's Garden**
  http://www.evesgarden.com

- **Toys in Babeland**
  http://www.babeland.com

- **Good Vibrations**
  http://www.goodvibes.com

Seven Principles for Making Marriage Work: A Practical Guide from the Country's Foremost Relationship Expert, by John Gottman, Ph.D., and Nan Silver (Three Rivers Press, 2000)
Gottman is one of the rare authors of marriage-advice books who relies on solid, evidence-based research as well as clinical experience. Other Gottman titles include *Ten Lessons to Transform Your Marriage.*

Reconcilable Differences,

by Andrew Christensen, Ph.D., and Neil S. Jacobson, Ph.D. (The Guilford Press, 2002)
Written by two of the country's top relationship researchers, the book explains why couples fight about the same things over and over, and offers effective ways to accept your differences and establish more peaceful, loving relationships.

Pleasure: A Woman's Guide to Getting the Sex You Want, Need and Deserve, by Hilda Hutcherson, M.D. (Putnam, 2006)

Sex Matters for Women: A Complete Guide to Taking Care of Your Sexual Self, by Sallie Foley, MSW; Sally A. Kope, MSW, and Dennis P. Sugrue, Ph.D. (The Guilford Press, 2002)

SKIN AND HAIR

American Academy of Dermatology
http://www.skincarephysicians.com/ agingskinnet/basicfacts.html
How skin ages and what you can do about it.

http://www.skincarephysicians.com/ agingskinnet/cosmeticpro.html
Cosmetic procedures.

http://www.aad.org/public/Publications/ pamphlets/HairLoss.htm
Explanation of hair loss.

American Academy of Family Physicians
http://familydoctor.org/210.xml
Information on excess hair (hirsutism).

American Osteopathic College of Dermatology
http://www.aocd.org/skin/dermatologic_ diseases/female_pattern_hai.html
Female-pattern hair loss.

National Institute of Arthritis and Musculoskeletal and Skin Diseases
http://www.niams.nih.gov/hi/topics/ alopecia/alopecia.htm
Good information on alopecia areata.

Mayo Clinic
http://www.mayoclinic.com/health/ smoking/AN00644
How smoking affects your skin.

http://www.mayoclinic.com/health/nails/ WO00020
Caring for your nails.

SLEEP

National Center on Sleep Disorders Research
http://www.nhlbi.nih.gov/about/ncsdr/index.htm
See the Patient and Public Information link.

National Sleep Foundation
http://www.sleepfoundation.org
A well-designed site with specific resources for women.

American Academy of Sleep Medicine
http://www.aasmnet.org/
Primarily for health professionals, but the directory is a good place to look for a sleep center or sleep doctor in your area.

National Institute of Neurological Disorders and Stroke
http://www.ninds.nih.gov/disorders/brain_basics/understanding_sleep.htm
Great explanation of the brain and sleep.

National Institute on Aging
http://nih.seniorhealth.gov/sleepandaging/toc.html
How getting older affects sleep patterns.

National Heart, Lung and Blood Institute
http://www.nhlbi.nih.gov/health/public/sleep/healthy_sleep.htm
Download "Your Guide to Healthy Sleep," a 60-page booklet.

http://www.nhlbi.nih.gov/cgi-bin/tfSleepQuiz.pl
An interactive quiz to see if you're suffering from sleep problems.

A Woman's Guide to Sleep Disorders,
by Meir H. Kryger, M.D.
(McGraw-Hill, 2004)
This sleep doctor is also the author of a major sleep medicine textbook. This guide is very easy to understand and informative, full of useful tips.

THYROID PROBLEMS

Mayo Clinic
http://www.mayoclinic.com/health/hyperthyroidism/DS00344
Hyperthyroidism.

http://www.mayoclinic.com/health/hypothyroidism/DS00353
Hypothyroidism.

http://www.mayoclinic.com/health/graves-disease/DS00181
Graves' disease.

American Thyroid Association
http://www.thyroid.org/patients/brochures/Thyroiditis.pdf
Booklet on thyroiditis.

http://www.thyroid.org/patients/brochures/Thyroid_and_Weight.pdf
Thyroid and weight.

National Women's Health Information Center
http://www.4women.gov/faq/hashimoto.htm
Hashimoto's thyroiditis.

Hormone Foundation
http://www.hormone.org/public/
thyroid.cfm
Thyroid disorders.

URINARY PROBLEMS

National Kidney and Urologic Diseases Clearinghouse
http://kidney.niddk.nih.gov/kudiseases/
pubs/utiadult/
Urinary tract infections in adults.

http://kidney.niddk.nih.gov/kudiseases/
pubs/uiwomen/index.htm
Urinary incontinence in women.

American Academy of Family Physicians
http://familydoctor.org/190.xml
Urinary tract infections in women.

American Urological Association
http://www.urologyhealth.org/
Patient information site with links to various topics.

National Center for Complementary and Alternative Medicine
http://nccam.nih.gov/health/cranberry/
All about cranberries.

Acknowledgments

*W*e are grateful to the many authorities on women's health who helped us by providing guidance in their areas of expertise or reviewing portions of the manuscript for accuracy. They include:

Alice J. Adler, Ph.D.
Senior scientist, Schepens Eye Research
    Institute, Boston
Associate professor of ophthalmology,
    Harvard Medical School
Member, Executive Committee,
    Women's Eye Health Task Force

Andrew Berchuck, M.D.
Professor of gynecologic oncology;
    director, Division of Gynecologic
    Oncology, Comprehensive Cancer
    Center, Duke University
President-elect, Society of Gynecologic
    Oncologists

John P. Bilezikian, M.D.
Director, metabolic bone diseases
    program, New York–Presbyterian
    Hospital
Chief, Division of Endocrinology;
    associate chair, Department of

Medicine; professor of medicine and
    pharmacology, College of Physicians
    and Surgeons; associate director,
    Partnership for Women's Health,
    Columbia University

Glenn D. Braunstein, M.D.
Chairman, Department of Medicine,
    Cedars-Sinai Medical Center
Professor of medicine, David Geffen
    School of Medicine at UCLA
Past president, Endocrinologic and
    Metabolic Drugs Advisory
    Committee, U.S. Food and
    Drug Administration

Jill C. Buckley, M.D.
Urologist, University of California,
    San Francisco

Zachary Chattler, D.P.M.
Podiatric surgeon, Baltimore, Maryland

Diana L. Dell, M.D.
Director, Maternal Wellness Program; assistant professor, Departments of Psychiatry and Behavioral Sciences and Obstetrics/Gynecology, Duke University

Lorraine Dennerstein, Ph.D.
Director, Office for Gender and Health, Department of Psychiatry, Faculty of Medicine, Dentistry and Health Sciences, University of Melbourne, Australia

Robert R. Freedman, Ph.D.
Professor, C.S. Mott Center for Behavioral Medicine, Wayne State University School of Medicine, Detroit, Michigan

Robert D. Frisina, Ph.D.
Professor of otolaryngology, surgery, neurobiology & anatomy, and biomedical engineering, University of Rochester Medical Center
Researcher, National Technical Institute for the Deaf at Rochester Institute of Technology

Ilene K. Gipson, Ph.D.
Senior scientist, Schepens Eye Research Institute
Professor, Department of Ophthalmology, Harvard Medical School
Chair, Executive Committee, Women's Eye Health Task Force

David J. Gordon, M.D.
Division of Heart and Vascular Diseases, National Heart, Lung and Blood Institute, National Institutes of Health, Bethesda, Maryland

Bernadine Healy, M.D.
Former director, National Institutes of Health
Columnist, *US News and World Report*

Victor W. Henderson, M.D., M.S.
Professor, Departments of Health Research & Policy (Epidemiology) and Neurology & Neurological Sciences, Stanford University

Hilda Hutcherson, M.D.
Assistant professor of obstetrics and gynecology, Columbia University
Codirector, New York Center for Women's Sexual Health

Richard Jadick, D.O.
Staff physician, Section of Urology, Medical College of Georgia

Suzanne Jan de Beur, M.D.
Director, Division of Endocrinology; associate director, General Clinical Research Center, Department of Medicine, Johns Hopkins University

Lore E. Kantrowitz, Ed.D.
Psychologist, Concord, Massachusetts

Niki E. Kantrowitz, M.D.
Director, Cardiac Catheterization Lab, Long Island College Hospital, Brooklyn, New York

Bruce Kessel, M.D.
Associate professor, Department of Obstetrics and Gynecology and Women's Health, John A. Burns School of Medicine, University of Hawaii
Former president, North American Menopause Society

Jana Klauer, M.D.
Diet and exercise expert, New York, New York

Samuel Klein, M.D.
William H. Danforth Professor of Medicine; director, Center for Human Nutrition, School of Medicine, Washington University, St. Louis

Fredi Kronenberg, Ph.D.
Professor of clinical physiology in rehabilitation medicine
Director, Richard & Hinda Rosenthal Center for Complementary & Alternative Medicine, College of Physicians and Surgeons, Columbia University

Meir Kryger, M.D.
Director, Sleep Disorders Centre, St. Boniface Hospital Research Centre, University of Manitoba Medical School, Canada

Carol Landis, D.N.Sc., R.N., F.A.A.N.
Professor of biobehavioral nursing and health systems, University of Washington

Joan M. Lappe, Ph.D., R.N., F.A.A.N.
Professor of medicine; professor of nursing; director, Clinical and Pediatric Studies, Osteoporosis Research Center, Creighton University

Lenore J. Launer, Ph.D.
Chief, Neuroepidemiology Unit, Laboratory of Epidemiology, Demography, and Biometry, National Institute on Aging, National Institutes of Health

Kathryn A. Lee, R.N., Ph.D., F.A.A.N.
Professor and Livingston Chair, Department of Family Health Care Nursing, University of California, San Francisco

Elliot Levy, M.D.
Member, The Endocrine Society
Clinical professor of medicine, Miller School of Medicine, University of Miami

Charles L. Loprinzi, M.D.
Division of Medical Oncology, Mayo Clinic, Rochester, Minnesota

Barb Malat, C.P.N.P.
Cochair, Menopause and Hormone Therapy Committee, Association of Reproductive Health Professionals, Olmsted Medical Center
Adjunct faculty member, Family Nurse Practitioner, Winona State University

Phyllis Kernoff Mansfield, Ph.D.
Professor of women's studies and health
  education, Pennsylvania State
  University
Director, TREMIN Research Program
  on Women's Health

JoAnn E. Manson, M.D.
Chief, Division of Preventive Medicine,
  Brigham and Women's Hospital
Professor of medicine and Elizabeth F.
  Brigham Professor of Women's
  Health, Harvard Medical School

Jean K. Matheson, M.D.
Sleep Disorders Center, Beth Israel
  Deaconess Medical Center
Associate professor of neurology,
  Harvard Medical School

Michael McClung, M.D., F.A.C.E.,
  F.A.C.P.
Director, Oregon Osteoporosis Center

Susan H. McDaniel, Ph.D.
Associate chair, Department of Family
  Medicine; Professor of psychiatry
  and family medicine; director,
  Family Programs and the Wynne
  Center for Family Research in
  Psychiatry, University of Rochester
  Medical Center

Laura Miller, M.D.
Associate professor of psychiatry; director,
  Women's Mental Health Program
  and clinical services, Department of
  Psychiatry, University of Illinois,

John O'Neill, M.D.
Dermatologist, Bethesda, Maryland

James W. Orr, M.D.
Oncologist, Fort Myers, Florida
Past president, Society of Gynecological
  Oncologists

Noreen Oswell, D.P.M.
Chair Podiatric Surgery, Cedars-Sinai
  Medical Center, Los Angeles

Edward Partridge, M.D.
Professor and vice chairman,
  Department of Obstetrics and
  Gynecology, Division of
  Gynecologic Oncology, University
  of Alabama at Birmingham

Rochelle L. Peck, M.D.
Ophthalmologist, on staff at
  Montefiore Hospital Center
  and in private practice in the
  New York City area

Judith Penski, D.D.S.
Washington, D.C.

Lawrence G. Raisz, M.D.
Science editor, Surgeon General's
  Report on Bone Disease and
  Osteoporosis
Director, Musculoskeletal Institute,
  University of Connecticut Health
  Center

Vani Rao, M.D.
Assistant professor, Division of
  Geriatric Psychiatry and
  Neuropsychiatry, Department
  of Psychiatry and Behavioral
  Sciences, Johns Hopkins
  Hospital

Marcie K. Richardson, M.D.
Assistant director of obstetrics and gynecology for clinical quality, Harvard Vanguard Medical Associates

Lisa McPherson Robinson
Social worker specializing in sexual problems, Bethesda, Maryland

Clifford Rosen, M.D.
Director, Maine Center for Osteoporosis Research and Education
Adjunct staff scientist, Jackson Laboratory, Bar Harbor, Maine

Zev Rosenwaks, M.D.
Director, Center for Reproductive Medicine and Infertility; professor of obstetrics and gynecology, Weill Medical College, Cornell University

Jacques Rossouw, M.D.
Women's Health Initiative project officer, National Institutes of Health

Gail Royal, M.D.
Ophthalmologist, Myrtle Beach, South Carolina

Anne B. Sagalyn, M.D.
Assistant clinical professor of psychiatry, George Washington University School of Medicine

Debra Schaumberg, Sc.D., O.D., M.P.H.
Assistant scientist, Schepens Eye Research Institute
Associate epidemiologist, Brigham and Women's Hospital
Assistant professor, Harvard Medical School

Isaac Schiff, M.D.
Joe Vincent Meigs Professor of Gynecology, Harvard Medical School
Chief, Vincent Memorial Obstetrics and Gynecology Service, Women's Care Division, Massachusetts General Hospital
Editor in chief, *Menopause*

Peter J. Schmidt, M.D.
Principal investigator, Division of Intramural Research, National Institute of Mental Health, Bethesda, Maryland

Sally E. Shaywitz, M.D.
Professor; codirector, Yale Center for the Study of Learning and Attention, Yale University School of Medicine

Jan L. Shifren, M.D.
Director, Menopause Program, Vincent Memorial Obstetrics and Gynecology Service, Massachusetts General Hospital
Assistant professor of obstetrics, gynecology and reproductive biology, Harvard Medical School

James A. Simon, M.D.
Clinical professor of obstetrics and
    gynecology, George Washington
    University School of Medicine
Former president, North American
    Menopause Society

John J. Stangel, M.D.
Specialist in reproductive endocrinology
    and infertility, Rye, New York

Marcia L. Stefanick, Ph.D.
Professor of medicine (research), Stanford
    University School of Medicine

Wulf H. Utian, M.D., Ph.D.
Founder and executive director, North
    American Menopause Society
Consultant, Cleveland Clinic

Arden Wilkins
Physical therapist, Silver Spring,
    Maryland

R. Stan Williams, M.D.
Harry Prystowsky Professor of
    Reproductive Medicine; associate
    chairman, Department of Obstetrics
    and Gynecology; chief, Division of
    Reproductive Endocrinology and
    Infertility, University of Florida

We would also like to thank Judy
Cerne, president annd CEO of McKinney
Advertising and Public Relations; Marcia
Stein, formerly at the National Sleep
Foundation; Ann McCall and Rachel Fey
at the Association of Reproductive Health
Professionals; Mary Hyde and Greg
Phillips at the American College of
Obstetricians and Gynecologists; Sharan
Jayne, Terry Long, and Diane Striars at the
National Institutes of Health; Busola
Afolabi at the American Cancer Society;
Karen J. Westergaard at the American
Macular Degeneration Foundation; John
M. Lazarou, senior media relations repre-
sentative for Johns Hopkins Medicine;
and Amy Niles at the National Women's
Health Resource Center.

We are indebted to the talented team
at Workman Publishing who made our
vision come to life: Peter Workman,
Walter Weintz, Brian Belfiglio, Doug
Wolff, Irene Demchyshyn, Janet Parker,
Janet Vicario, Ron Longe, Kate
Hanzalik, Katie Workman, Elizabeth
Shreve, Kristina Peterson, Munira Al-
Khalili, Victoria Roberts, Lynn Strong,
Randall Lotowycz, Megan Nicolay, and
last but not least, our brilliant editor,
Susan Bolotin. Suzie, we were blessed to
have you on our side from day one.

We are also grateful to our agent,
Rafe Sagalyn, who believed in us from
the beginning and was a constant source
of enthusiasm and good counsel.

Our editors at Newsweek were gener-
ous in their support of this project. We
received special encouragement from
Mark Whitaker, Newsweek's editor when
we began, and his successor, Jon
Meacham. We would also like to thank
Ann McDaniel, Danny Klaidman,
Alexis Gelber, Debra Rosenberg, Deidre
Depke, Lisa Miller, and Jennifer Barrett
Ozols. Our colleagues Wes Kosova,
David Noonan, Claudia Kalb, Anne

Underwood, and Karen Springen graciously contributed their time and expertise on many occasions. Ruth Tenenbaum provided invaluable research assistance. Sharon Begley, our former *Newsweek* colleague who is now the science columnist for *The Wall Street Journal*, was a great resource on programs for exercising the brain.

Pat would like to thank Ann McDaniel for her friendship, wisdom, and incredible generosity throughout this project; Bernadine Occhiuzzo, whose help made it possible for her to do this book; her children, Daniel, Laura, and Jack (and her special kids, Stas, Carina, and Ben) for putting up with the take-out food, extra chores, and crazy hours with humor and grace; and finally, Brian, whose love, flexibility, and support amazed even her.

Barbara would like to thank the women in her book club (the greatest focus group ever); Joan Liebmann-Smith and Robin Marantz Henig for sharing wisdom over coffee and lunch; Jennet Conant for valuable counsel at all stages of this book; Deborah Heiligman for coming up with the title; Susan Heide for being on the other end of the phone; Lore and Andrea for their love and support during a very difficult time in all our lives; Michael for the use of his room; Ben for technical support; and finally, Dan—for making sure I crossed the finish line. Yes, the book is *finally* done!

INDEX

Index

C

𝔐